LAPAROSCOPIC
SUTURING

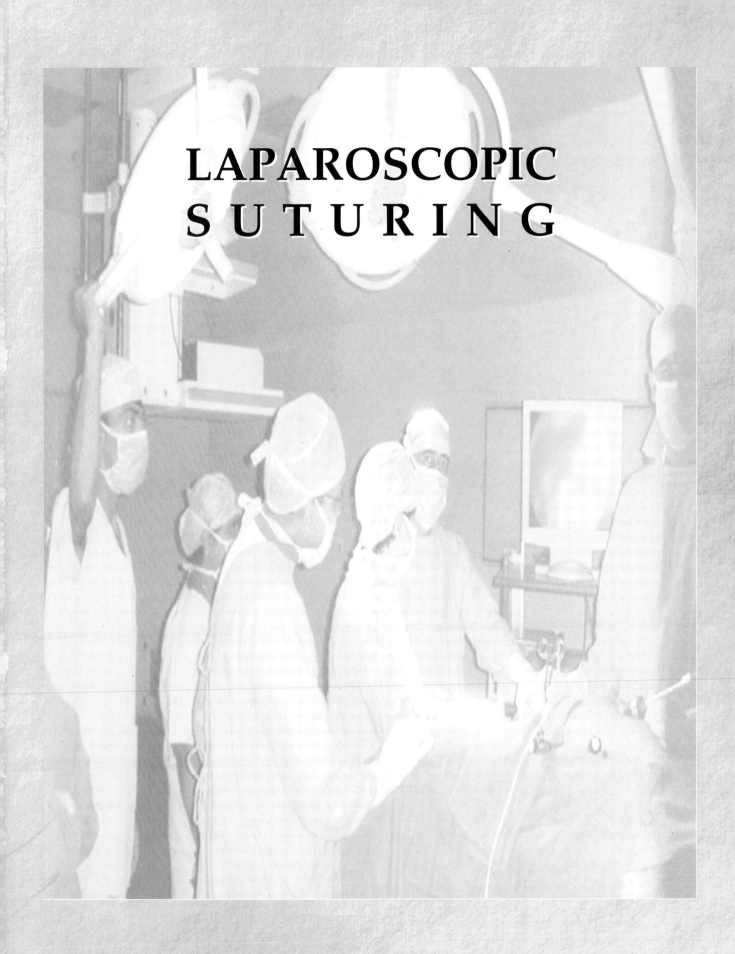

LAPAROSCOPIC SUTURING

Editor

Nutan Jain
MBBS MS (Obs and Gyne)
Endoscopic Surgeon and Infertility Specialist
Vardhman Infertility and Endoscopy Centre
Muzaffarnagar
India

Foreword by
Prof Dr Med L Liselotte Mettler

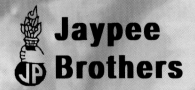

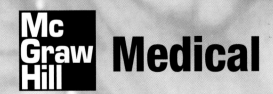

First published in India by

Jaypee Brothers Medical Publishers (P) Ltd
EMCA House, 23/23B Ansari Road, Daryaganj, New Delhi 110 002, India
Phones: +91-11-23272143, +91-11-23272703, +91-11-23282021, +91-11-23245672
Fax: +91-11-23276490, +91-11-23245683   e-mail: jaypee@jaypeebrothers.com
Visit our website: www.jaypeebrothers.com

First published in USA by The McGraw-Hill Companies, 2 Penn Plaza, New York, NY 10121-2298. Exclusively worldwide distributor except South Asia (India, Nepal, Sri Lanka, Bhutan, Pakistan, Bangladesh).

NOTICE

Medicine is an ever-changing science. As new research and clinical experience broaden our knowledge, changes in treatment and drug therapy are required. The authors and the publisher of this work have checked with sources believed to be reliable in their efforts to provide information that is complete and generally in accord with the standards accepted at the time of publication. However, in view of the possibility of human error changes in medical science, neither the editors nor the publisher nor any other party who has been involved in the preparation or publication of this work warrants that the information contained herein is in every respect accurate or complete, and they disclaim all responsibility for any errors or omissions or for the results obtained from use of the information contained in this work. Readers are encouraged to confirm the information contained herein with other sources. For example and in particular, readers are advised to check the product information sheet included in the package of each drug they plan to administer to be certain that the information contained in this work is accurate and that changes have not been made in the recommended dose or in the contraindications for administration. This recommendation is of particular importance in connection with new or infrequently used drugs.

ISBN   0-07-148579-1
ISBN 13 9780071485791

This book
is
dedicated
to
my dear parents Mrs Vimla and
Mr Ramesh Chandra Gupta
for whom I feel a deep sense of gratitude for
having guided me through my formative years

and
my children Mansi and Anubhav for their endless,
loving support all through the formation of this book.

Contributors

Arnold P Advincula MD
Assistant Professor
Director of Minimally Invasive
Surgery Program and Fellowship
Department of Obstrics and
Gynecology
University of Michigan Medical
Center
L 4000 Women's Hospital
1500 East Medical Center Drive
Ann Arbor, MI 48109

Ginger Cathey MD
Fellow Urogynecology
Department of Obstetrics
Gynecology and Women's Health
University of Louisville
Louisville, KY

Greg Cario MD
Director of the Sydney Women's
Endosurgery Centre
Sydney
Australia

Danny Chou
Sydney Women's
Endosurgery Centre
1 South St
Kogarah 2217
NSW Australia

Pradeep Chowbey MS MNAMS FIMSA
FAIS FICS
Chairman
Department of Minimal Access
Surgery
Sir Ganga Ram Hospital
New Delhi
India

Nick Elkington
Gynecological Laparoscopic
Surgeon
St George Private Hospital
Suite 14, Level 3
Kogarah NSW 2217

Mark Erian LRCP (Edin) LRCS (Edin)
LRCP & S (Glasg) D Obst RCPI FRCOG,
FRANZCOG
Senior Lecturer, Senior Consultant
Obstetrician and Gynecologist
University of Qeensland, Royal
Brisbane and Women's Hospital
Herston, Brisbane Q 4029
Queensland
Australia

Bahareh Fazilat
Minimal Invasive Surgery / GYN
Laparoscopy Fellow
The Mount Sinai Hospital
New York

Ebtihaj Hashim
Gynecological Laparoscopic
Surgeon
St George Private Hospital
Suite 14, Level 3
Kogarah NSW 2217

Nutan Jain MS
Director, Vardhman Infertility and
Endoscopy Centre, A-36
South Lines, Mahavir Chowk
Muzaffarnagar (UP), India

Keith Johnston
Research Fellow of the Sydney
Women's Endosurgery Centre
Sydney
Australia

Neeraj Kohli MD
Urogynecology and Reconstructive
Pelvic Surgery
Harvard Medical School
Cambridge MA, USA

Sankar Das Mahapatra DGO MS
Clinical Research Fellow
Vardhman Infertility and
Endoscopy Centre, A-36, South Civil
Lines, Mahavir Chowk
Muzaffarnagar (UP), India

Marshall Mark MD PhD
Director of Endoscopic Training and
Informatics
Dept of Obstetrics and Gynecology
Banner Good Samaritan Medical
Center

Glenda McLaren MBBS (Queensland),
FRCOG, FRANZCOG
Senior Lecturer
Senior Consultant Obstetrician and
Gynecologist
University of Queensland
Mater Mothers Hospital
Raymond Terrace Q 4101
Queensland, Australia

John R Miklos MD
Urogynecology and Reconstructive
Pelvic Surgery
Atlanta Urogynecology Associates
Atlanta, GA, USA

Charles Edward Miller MD FACOG
Clinical Associate Professor
Dept OB / GYN
University of Illinois / Chicago
Clinical Associate, Dept OB / GYN
University of Chicago
2101 South Arlington Heights Road
Suite195, Arlington Heights
IL 60005, USA

Robert D Moore DO
Urogynecology and Reconstructive
Pelvic Surgery
Atlanta Urogynecology Associates
Atlanta, GA, USA

Camran Nezhat MD FACOG FACS
Director, Stanford Endoscopy
Centre for Training and Training
and Technology
Clinical Professor of Surgery and
Obstetrics and Gynecology
Stanford University School of
Medicine Stanford
California

Ceana Nezhat MD
Associate Clinical Professor of
Obstetrics and Gynecology
Stanford University School of
Medicine, Stanford, California
Director, Centre for Special Pelvic
Surgery
Atlanta, Georgia

Farr Nezhat MD FACOG
Clinical Professor of Obstetrics and
Gynecology
Stanford University School of
Medicine, Stanford, California
Department of Gynecologic-
Oncology
The Mount Sinai Hospital
New York

Iris Kerin Orbuch MD
Director of Advanced Gynecologic
Laparoscopy Center
202 Spring Street
New York, USA
Assistant Clinical Professor
Lenox Hill Hospital
New York, New York
and
Mount Sinai Medical Center
New York, New York

Marie Fidela R Paraiso MD
Staff, Department of Obstetrics and
Gynecology
The Urological Institute, Women's
Health Center, and Center for
Innovative Surgery
Assoc. Fellowship Director
Urogynecology and Reconstructive
Pelvic Surgery
The Cleveland Clinic Foundation
Cleveland, OH, USA

Resad Paya Pasic MD PhD
Associate Professor
Department of Obstetrics, Gynecology
and Womans Health
University of Louisville
Louisville, KY

David B Redwine MD
Endometriosis Treatment Program
St. Charles Medical Center-Bend
2500 NE Neff Road
Bend, Oregon 97701
USA

Harry Reich MD FACOG
Advanced Laparoscopic Surgeons
Shavertown, PA

Tamer Seckin MD FACOG
Department Chief of Gynecology and
Laparoscopy
Kingsbrook Jewish Medical Center
585 Schenectady Avenue
Brooklyn
New York
Attending Physician
Lenox Hill Hospital
New York
New York

Anshumala Shukla-Kulkarni
Laparoscopy Fellow
Sydney Women's Endosurgery
Centre, 1 South street
Kogarah NSW 2217.

Johan Van der Wat MB BCh FCOG (SA)
Hon. Consultant University
Witwatersrand Department OB/GYN
Director Endometriosis Institute
South Africa
Board Member International Society
for Gynaecology Endoscopy
Private Practice
Parklane Clinic, Johannesburg
South Africa

Foreword

Microinvasive surgery (MIS) with its technical developments and advances has opened up endless possibilities. Nevertheless, we appear to be at a crossroads with regard to suturing technology. The professional goal of the incorporation of advanced laparoscopy into surgical residency programs has begun. It is, therefore, time to reflect once again on our basic tools. Intra- and extracorporeal suturing in endoscopic surgery has to be a basic requirement for everyone in our speciality.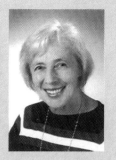

It is an honor for me to introduce this well-written book on the different aspects of suturing. I still remember the words of our teacher in laparoscopic surgery, Kurt Semm, who said, "If you don't know how to suture, you had better stop doing laparoscopy".

How can a surgeon be deemed as competent in suturing? As described in this book, he has to undergo a meticulous curriculum to build up his knowledge and his manual skills. Over the last decade many tools have been developed to provide an objective, valid and reliable assessment of surgical skills. Suturing skills are timed and evaluated according to their accuracy. Virtual reality trainers, with regular training, provide the possibility of becoming competent in suturing. Nevertheless, despite the best surgical training, not all those who endeavour to become skilled minimal invasive surgeons will be able to do so. It is, therefore, necessary to evaluate basic human performance resources as predictors of performance of laparoscopic surgery. Suturing definitely has to be included within this context.

In many of our university teaching programs scientific knowledge and analyzing skills are tested, but no one seems to be testing surgical skills. Suturing is a surgical skill. It has to be learnt, tested and can then be applied with the best possible success. To write a book on laparoscopic suturing may seem ridiculous to the uninitiated surgeon; however, all specialists recognize that laparoscopic suturing is much more difficult than laparotomic suturing. There is a genuine need for the knowledge contained within this book to be fully taught and understood. I wish this book a wide distribution and a good acceptance within our gynecological surgical speciality.

Professor Liselotte Mettler
Clinic for Obstetrics and Gynecology
Michaelisstrasse 16
D-24105 Kiel
Germany

Preface

Today, minimally invasive surgery is a highly acclaimed surgical modality amongst both patients and medical practitioners. It appears that Laparoscopy is applicable in almost every clinical situation, be it a huge myoma, multiple laparotomies, extensive endometriosis or pelvic floor repair. Laparoscopic surgery is the answer to all of the above situations. This sea change from Laparoscopy in "Challenging Situations" to laparoscopy becoming commonplace has been brought about exclusively by the increased manual dexterity in laparoscopic suturing. The approach is much bolder now, laparoscopic complications which occur in situations like bladder, bowel, ureter or vascular injury can now be managed in the same Laparoscopic procedure without conversion to laparotomy. An average endoscopist can be transformed into an advanced endoscopic surgeon by acquiring proficiency in suturing. Anybody can do an LAVH but the ones skilled in the art of endosuturing would gladly take a total lap hysterectomy and offer a Hi-McCall culdoplasty or a Burch colposuspension at the time. So, it can be aptly said "SUTURE IS FUTURE".

This book has been crafted keeping in mind the indispensable need of every endoscopist, i.e. enabling or enhancing the suturing skills of laparoscopic surgeons. A group of dedicated endoscopic surgeons have toiled together to compile this textbook cum Atlas which covers each and every aspect of suturing. All possible know-how that a surgeon needs to have before starting and then mastering endosuturing is present within a single textbook. Not only has the text been written by the world's leading experts, the surgical techniques too are shown through high quality pictures from actual surgeries. To further expedite the reader's learning and understanding, all chapters have been provided on a DVD-ROM which shows the applications of suturing through streaming videos with audio narration or subtitles.

The introduction emphasizes to the reader the need for effective suturing skills. The subsequent chapter deals with the required surgical armamentarium and operation theater facilities. In order to enable the surgeon to be more precise with what is needed for a particular surgery separate chapter has been included which elaborates upon the appropriate choice of suture materials, needles and needle holders. The need and application of pelvic trainers and virtual stimulators has been dealt with in exquisite detail. There are separate chapters to explain Extracorporeal and Intracorporeal suturing. Specific applications like sliding knots have been covered in an entirely different chapter. So the basics of Endosuturing have been discussed in great detail and presented in a manner that is easy to understand and apply.

Pioneered by Dr Charles H Koh is the concept of Ipsilateral suturing which is a major breakthrough in learning stress free, precise, targeted and prolonged suturing. An entire chapter has been dedicated to this concept and its clinical applications. This promises to take the reader through a complete journey of all the applications of laparoscopic suturing.

Hysterectomy, the most common surgical procedure can be more complete if the vault closure is done with a reinforcing Hi-McCall culdoplasty. The exact technique for this procedure has been described by the pioneer of this technique.

The section on laparoscopic management of myomas by Laparoscopy and lap assisted minilap: LAM are duly covered in two separate chapters. Most challenging situation is suturing of deep multiple myomas and the exact technique has been dealt with very well.

Laparoscopic pelvic floor repair has been getting a lot of attention and is on its way to gaining the same acceptance as a laparoscopic hysterectomy. Gradually critics will be fewer and aspirants for learning to treat this day-to-day problem will be more as the proportion of elderly women in the world's population is increasing. Greater stress has been laid on elucidating the different techniques of suturing applications for stress incontinence, cystocoele, rectocoele, entrocoele and post hysterectomy vault prolapse and nulliparous prolapse. There are several chapters describing the various ways of treating them like mesh and site specific repair. This employs the use of both intracorporeal and extracorporeal suturing.

The next section deals with accidental or intentional repair of bowel, bladder and ureter. The dilemma of many before starting rectal mobilization for advanced endometriosis or hysterectomy with multiple caesarean sections. Once the surgeon is empowered to deal with hollow viscous injury many surgical opportunities and challenges will lie ahead.

Applications in General surgery like Hernia repair, Gallbladder and Appendectomy are all dealt with exclusively by experts in their field. It promises to be an equally beneficial atlas for the gynecologist and the general surgeon alike. All surgical procedures have been showcased through pictures and videos.

Lastly the latest and most advanced application of suturing, i.e. laparoscopic microsurgery has been extremely well elaborated and will instantly prompt the reader to venture into this new modality.

Advances in Robotic suturing promise to make 'endoscopic suturing wizards' without the pre-requisite for acquiring manual dexterity. The latest applications of robotic suturing have been amply highlighted by the pioneers in this field.

This atlas, with its unique theme and purpose, i.e. propagation of suturing applications, promises to be a most useful creation on laparoscopic suturing. The richness of text, references, and high quality color photographs, further supported by surgical videos are the highlights of this atlas and textbook on suturing.

Nutan Jain
Phones: +91-131-2600049, +91-131-2407437, +91-131-2600052
Fax: +91-131-2409737
e-mail:jainutan@hotmail.com
Visit our website: www.vardhmanhospital.com

Acknowledgements

It has been such a pleasure planning, working, executing and finally bringing out this "State of the Art Atlas and Textbook of Laparoscopic Suturing". Right from inception to the final completion, it has been a great learning experience. Though science knows no boundaries, interacting and working with so many renowned endoscopic surgeons from around the globe has been an memorable experience. It gave enormous insight into human behavior, differences in ethnic, linguistic and cultural practices, but the one thing that remained common was their commitment to Endoscopic Surgery. The keen desire to promote and propagate safe practices of Endoscopic Surgery was the common platform they shared, which brought them together. It was my endeavor to bring forth a book containing the best possible expertise from around the world on suturing.

I express my heartfelt gratitude to all contributing authors, pioneers in their specific fields who despite their busy schedules put in their best efforts to compile chapters of immense scientific value. Their valuable suggestions, constructive criticism and words of encouragement during the compilation of the book went a long way in keeping me motivated towards this task. Their valuable contributions collectively have taken the shape of a fine textbook and atlas which will enlighten budding and established gynecologists and general surgeons practicing endoscopy on laparoscopic suturing. I take this opportunity to express my sincere gratitude to all my teachers, who taught me, nurtured my skills and enabled me to work for the cause of Endoscopic Surgery.

I profusely thank the Publishers M/s Jaypee Brothers Medical Publishers (P) Ltd. and especially Shri Jitendar P Vij (Chairman and Managing Director), Mr Nitin Goyal , Mr Tarun Duneja (General Manager Publishing), and their efficient team. They put in tremendous efforts to bring out this book timely and to give it excellent print and picture quality. It was a pleasant experience working with them.

My sincere thanks to dear friends like Mrs and Dr Kame, Mrs and Dr Gada, Mrs and Dr Dilip Pal, Mrs and Dr Narayana Hegde, Mrs and Dr Sunil Ahuja, Mrs and Dr Satish Bhutani, and Mrs. Shashi Dawar, Dr Suchi Kushwaha, Dr Vinod Kushwaha and Dr Mayank Jain. It is their continued support, which has been instrumental in bringing out this book.

I would like to acknowledge the efforts of Dr Sankar Das Mahapatra and Dr Mamta who have been very keen on this project and helped me a lot in the compilation of this book. I sincerely thank my own hospital staff especially Mr. Ashish, Vishram and Basu who have worked day and night for the compilation of this book. They deserve full credit for their excellent work and dedication.

I greatly appreciate the wholehearted support of all my family members. My parents have been a great source of inspiration for me. My husband Dr Mukesh and children, Mansi and Anubhav have in their capacity been extremely caring and helpful and never complaining about the lesser time spent with them. Their unwavering support helped me tide over the difficult phases during the compilation of this book.

In the end, I would like to thank all my patients who have posed faith in me and the newer modality of Endoscopic Surgery. If I can assure safe propagation of more advanced endoscopic surgery by means of this atlas, which, promises to sharpen the existing skills of endoscopists in suturing, it will be the ultimate fulfillment of a cherished dream.

Contents

DVD Contents

DVD - 1

DVD - 2

Introduction

NUTAN JAIN

Chapter One

"Today's Empowerment in suturing skills paves the way for tomorrow's success." This meaningful adage by Dr Charles H Koh will be the starting point of this comprehensive atlas cum textbook of laparoscopic suturing. It will go a long way to prove that laparoscopic surgeons empowered by suturing skills can take up more demanding surgeries which carry the risk of visceral damage. Once a surgeon is endowed with suturing skills more advanced procedures like deep infiltrating endometriosis and pelvic floor repair can be undertaken.

Minimal access surgery poses a challenge to the surgeon right from the word go. It is in no way similar to the traditional laparotomic approach the students master at medical schools. The beginner first passes the hurdles of newer entry techniques, creating pneumoperitoneum and knic-knacks of electrosurgery (Figs 1.1A to F). It takes time to get used to the lack of depth perception as the procedure is viewed on a two-dimensional video screen, there is lack of direct tactile feel of the tissue. Those who are able to adjust to this newer way of working with long handled instruments looking at a video screen away from the surgical field, Survive.

The survivors then carry out simpler procedures, which may initially not require suturing, as it may sound quite intimidating in the beginning to introduce curved or straight needles in the abdominal cavity. But the followers of this unique modality of surgery, i.e. minimal access soon realize that without recourse to extracorporeal or intracorporeal suturing they are left with very few surgical procedures in their armamentarium. Certain procedures such as pelvic floor reconstruction and myomectomy, or the repair of lacerations of the bowel or bladder are still best accomplished by a suture based approach. Prescient pioneers such as Courtney Clarke[1] of Canada and Kurt Semm[2] of Germany demonstrated that, with creativity, practice and patience, most, if not all the techniques developed for "open" surgery could be applied to endoscopically directed procedures. Clarke, in 1972, first described his set of instruments and a technique that could be used to suture-ligate tissue and transfer standard knots created extracorporeally into the peritoneal cavity via endoscopic ports or cannulas. Semm demonstrated that prettied knots and loops could be introduced, placed around defined pedicles for secure and hemostatic ligation.[2] Although these techniques received scant attention when first introduced, in the late 1980s and early 1990s endoscopic suturing and knot tying was rediscovered by surgeons such as Reich[3–5] and Corfman. Other innovators have added to the currently available list of needle drivers, suture positioners, knot manipulators and techniques that collectively allow for the application of suturing techniques to virtually any procedure. While many of these techniques have been published[6–9] there exist a variety of effective non-published variations.

After an early phase of mastering simpler procedures and having gained sufficient proficiency in basic laparoscopic skills, it is quite natural for the endoscopist to progress to more advanced procedures which demand suturing back, the intended or accidental incisions made in the body tissue.

In laparoscopic surgery innovators tried hard to bring in industry based innovations to replace the traditional laparotomic suturing. Earlier innovations like clips, staples, Endo GII fires, fibrin glue, tackers etc. were all directed towards a simpler shortcut to suturing. But in any modality of surgery and especially more so in gynecology, certain procedures like myomectomy, pelvic floor repair and tubal recanalization cannot be carried out utilizing the above. Also the invariable risk of injury to bladder, bowel and ureter must be tackled only by suturing. So this poses a challenge to progressive endoscopists and they have to embrace the fascinating world of laparoscopic suturing. The art and science of laparoscopic suturing is neither too complex to understand, nor too difficult to master.

Most critical to the successful use of the suturing techniques in laparoscopy is appropriate training at a dedicated training facility. It implies a long learning curve, more so, because initially the techniques are required less frequently.

So earlier attempts at applying these techniques in the operating room will be inappropriate, inefficient and at worst, unsafe. When the trainee tries doing all this instantly in the patient, it could wreak havoc and dampen his morale for another couple of months. So it is highly recommended that the prospective laparoscopist who contemplates suturing, master his skills on a pelvic trainer.[10] The most rudimentary trainer could be made using a

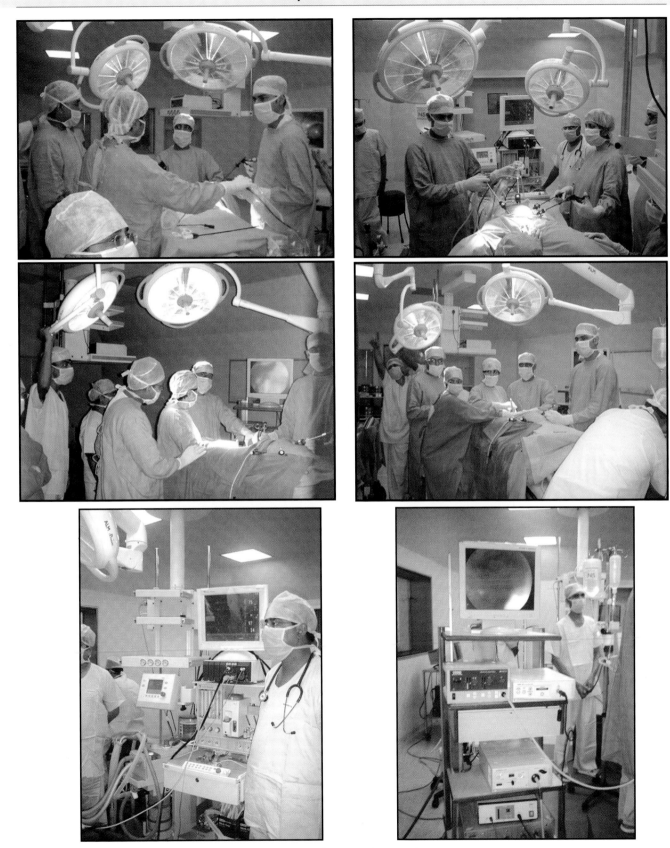

Figs 1.1A to F: Endoscopic operation room

cardboard box with a video camera attached to a color television. This gives the trainee ample opportunity to master the suturing skills within a home setting. Another trainer could be made utilizing a simple inexpensive small, sting camera worth 10 dollars, which transfers the images to the TV monitor. This obviates the need of telescope, light cable and a light source making it versatile to be used anywhere (Figs 1.2). Capturing images by computer soft-wave and videos during surgery and reviewing them later in the evening also adds a great deal to discover the shortcomings and improvising steps of improving them (Fig. 1.3). Another versatile tissue for practicing suturing after one has acquired reasonable skills in introducing needles into the peritoneal cavity and learnt to grab the needle in the correct fashion is to practice the intracorporeal or extracorporeal knots on the round ligament. In the female pelvis it is the best form of surgical tissue where one or two knots can be practiced as it is anterior, no danger of any important viscera close to it, does not bleed on passage of needle and lastly after the knot is done at the end of the procedure, the knot can be undone. Many times in simpler infertility evaluations when one gets time this could be easily accomplished. I have learnt all newer knots and tried new needle holders on the round ligament itself. It is far safer to do a couple of knots on the round ligament rather than to jump on to a myomectomy and be unable to complete it. Therefore, a realistic progression from pelvic trainers and virtual simulators to relaxed suturing on the round ligament and then finally to an intended or accidental surgical tissue approximation by suturing should be attempted. At least, I learnt and mastered suturing this way.

Gynecological endoscopists are required to put their suturing skills to test while carrying out a myomectomy. Earlier limitations of myoma no more than 5 cm made way for extracorporeal knot tying. But now, as endoscopic myomectomy knows no boundaries, the only limitation[11] is the surgeons suturing capability. A 10 cm deep myoma would require extensive suturing of the myoma bed preferably in two or three layers. Here's where the real need for suturing in a more advanced manner arises.

LAVH was the beginning towards offering the benefits of minimally invasive surgery and was quickly embraced by gynecologists all over. But soon

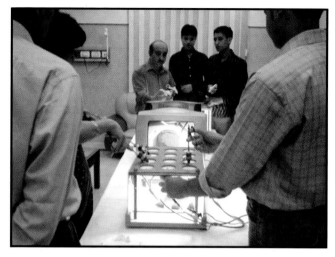

Fig. 1.2: Instructing laparoscopic suturing on a simple pelvic trainer utilizing an inexpensive sting camera, obviating the need of telescope, fiber optic light cable and laparoscopic camera (assistant pointing at the 2.5 cm small sting camera)

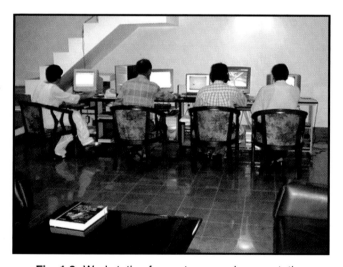

Fig. 1.3: Workstation for postsurgery documentation

the limitations of hybrid surgery, having three distinct steps of laparoscopic, vaginal and then final laparoscopic route made it rather cumbersome. Total laparoscopic hysterectomy wherein all steps of hysterectomy are done by the laparoscopic route, started gaining more popularity. It also became more versatile as pelvic reconstruction could be done at the same time and bigger uteri could be dealt with by laparoscopy. But transition from LAVH to TLH is possible only if one has adequate suturing skills. So once again there is need to learn intra- or extracorporeal suturing to effectively tackle the uterine arteries and laparoscopic closure of vaginal vault with vault suspension.[12]

Laparoscopic microsurgery is another exciting field, which puts the IVF specialist at bay and can empower the endoscopist to accomplish the same microsurgical feats as the open microsurgeon. Without recourse to operating microscope, laparoscopic microsurgery easily carries out tubo-tubal reanastomosis, tubo-cornual implantation, eversion of fimbria at neosalpingostomy and many other procedures. With the use of specially designed, dedicated instruments[13,14] outstanding surgeries can be carried out. However, the bottom line remains acquiring proficiency in suturing.

Deft intraoperative recognition and management of bladder, bowel and ureteric injuries is imperative for safe outcome of the procedure, avoidance of prolonged morbidity or even mortality and future litigations. A deft endoscopist is not adjudged by surgical dexterity alone but rather by promptness to recognize intraoperative visceral injury and steadily asking for reparative procedure either himself or a colleague like an urologist or colorectal surgeon. In the face of a surgical disaster to gather one's wits and carry out necessary repair with the help of a specialist goes a long way in avoidance of medicolegal complications. Needless to say, this is a situation where the guts and skills of a laparoscopist are put to test. The more proficient one is in suturing the more easily the complication is tidied over. So, if, the surgical team is efficient to do the required bowel and bladder repair the surgical morbidity does not alter much. The experienced surgeon you summon then, remains on observer and sort of just approves of your surgical procedure, rather than doing it himself. This is more of a medicolegal drill which is good to be followed. The literature is full of several case reports of bladder, bowel, ureteric injury repair.[15–19] They should only act as a stimulus to learn suturing and be able to tide a similar situation comfortably rather than scare an endoscopist.

As the world's female population is living longer so are the problems of pelvic floor defects surfacing in larger proportions. Increasing awareness that these defects like stress urinary incontinence, pelvic organ prolapse viz. cyctocole, rectocele, posthysterectomy vault prolapse can be repaired laparoscopically, a gynae endoscopist is repeatedly approached by patients concerning them. The most efficient way of treating them is, a thorough knowledge of surgical anatomy of the pelvic floor and then higher level of suturing abilities. There is no shortcut except to be a master of laparoscopic suturing to be able to give equal or better results than vaginal or abdominal route.[20–23]

For the general surgeons, laparoscopic cholesystectomy becomes a surgery, which they can easily embrace. This is simply due to the fact that it can be performed without a single tie or suture. However, if one wishes to locate anything other than cholecystectomy, it is then imperative that the methods of securing knots, placing sutures and approximating tissues be learnt. Laparoscopic hernia repair, other bowel and bladder surgeries all require suturing skills.[24–26]

This introduction to the historical development of suturing skills and their applications in the modern day endoscopic practice should be a starting point for understanding, learning and then mastering the skills of laparoscopic suturing. The only ingredients to success appear to be a passion for endoscopic surgery, ability to dedicate sufficient time for practicing on pelvic trainers and a sustained morale to overcome initial failures. A drive for learning supported by perseverance and diligence will definitely transform an average endoscopist to an endosuturing wizard.

REFERENCES

1. Clarke HC, Laparoscopy-new instruments for suturing and ligation. Fertil Steril 1972;23:274-77.
2. Semm K. Tissue puncher and loop-ligation-new ideas for surgical therapeutic pelviscopy (Laparoscopy) endoscopic intra-abdominal surgery. Endoscopy 1978;10:119-24.
3. Reich H, McGlynn F. Laparoscopic repair of bladder injury. Obstet Gynecol 1990;76:909-10.
4. Marrero MA, Corfman RS. Laparoscopic use of sutures. Clin Obstet Gynecol 1991;34:387-94.
5. Reich H. Clarke HC, Sekel L. A simple method for ligating with straight and curved needles in operative laparosopy. Obstet Gynecol 1992;79:143-47.
6. Hasson HM. Suture loop techniques to facilitate microsurgical and laparoscopic procedures. J Repro Med 1987;32:765-67.
7. Natanson LK, Easter DW, Cuschieri A. Ligation of the structures of the cystic pedicle during laparoscopic cholecystectomy. Am J Surg 1991;161:350-54.

8. McComb PF. A new suturing instrument that allows the use microsuture at Laparoscopy. Fertile Steril 1992;57:396-38.

9. Weston PV. A new clinch knot. Obstet Gynecol 1991; 78:144-47.

10. Clarke HC. An improved ligator in operative Laparoscopy. Obstet Gyncol 1994;83:299-300.

11. Miller C, Johnston M, Rundell M. Laparoscopic myomectomy in the infertile woman. J Am Assoc Gynecol Laparosc 1996;3 (4):525-32.

12. Koh CH. A new technique and system for simplifying total laparoscopic hysterectomy. J Am Assoc Gynecol Laparosc 199;5(2):187-92.

13. Koh CH. Koh Ultramicro laparoscopic Suturing System-Endo World, while paper: Karl Storz Endoscopy-America, Inc 1995.

14. Koh CH. Laparoscopic microsurgical tubal anastomosis result of 40 consecutive cases (oral presentation) ASRM 52nd Annual Meeting; 2-6 November 1996:Boston:ASRM.

15. Nezhat C, Childers J, Nezhat F et al. Major retroperitoneal vascular injury during laparoscopic surgery. Hum Reprod 1997;12:480.

16. Nezhat C, Nezhat F, Ambroze W, Pennington E. Laparoscopic reapir of small bowel, colon and rectal endometriosis. A report of twenty six cases. Surg Endosc 1993;7:88.

17. Nezhat C, Nezhat F, Pennington E. Laparoscopic treatment of lower colorectal and infiltrative rectovaginal septum endometriosis by the technique of video laparoscoppy. Br J Obstet Gynaecol 1992;99:664.

18. Nezhat F, Nezhat C, Levy JS. Report of laparoscopic injuries and complications over a 10-year period. Presented at the 41st annual clinical meeting of the American College of Obstetricians and Gynecologists, Washington DC, 1993.

19. Nezhat F, Nezhat CH, Admon D, et al. Complications and results of 361 hysterectomies performed at Laparoscopy. J Am Coll Surg 1995;180:307.

20. Miklos JR, Kohli N. "Paravaginal Plus" Burch procedure: a laparoscopic approach. J Pelvic Surg 1998;297-302.

21. Liu CY. Laparoscopic treatment of genuine urinary stress incontinence. Clin Obstet Gynecol 1994;8:789-98.

22. Ross JW. Laparoscopic Burch repair compared to laparotomy Burch for cure of urinary stress incontinence. Int Urogynecol 1995;6:323-28.

23. Lam AM, Jenkins GJ, Hyslop RS. Laparoscopic Burch results. Med J Aust 1995;162:18:22.

24. Ryberg AA, Uluap KM Cornet D, Fitzibbons Jr. RJ. Laparoscopic inguinal herniorrhaphy-transabdominal preperitoneal repair. In Brune (Ed): Laparoendoscopic Surgery Oxford: Blackwell Science 1996;263-69.

25. Matsuda M, Nishiyama M, Hanai T, Saeki S, Watanabe T. Laparoscopic Omental patch repair for perforated peptic ulcer. Ann Surg 1995;221:236-40.

26. Wexner SD, Verzaro R. Agachan: Laparoscopic colorectal carcinoma: Is it safe? Presented at the Annual Meeting of the Society of Gastrointestinal Endoscopic Surgeons. Philadelphia: Pennsylvania, 1996;13-16.

The Dedicated Endoscopic Operating Room of Today

JOHAN VAN DER WAT

Chapter Two

HISTORY

The modern operating room had its origin at the turn of the previous century when three main events occurred. These were:

1. The advent of safe inhalation anesthetics.
2. The realization that aseptic technique could improve surgical outcomes.
3. The invention of specialized equipment primarily driven by electricity like electrocautery and X-rays.

As surgical specialities diversified, so did the specific requirements related to the operating room. This eventually resulted in specialized operating rooms being developed for specific surgical specialities. For example, "laminar flow theaters" were developed with the sole purpose to diminish postoperative infections in orthopedic patients. With the advent of open cardiac surgery large operating rooms for the surgical team and technicians managing the specialized equipment like heart/lung machines became the norm for that speciality.

In the 1960s with the introduction of diagnostic laparoscopy[1] into gynecological practice, general gynecological theaters provided sufficient equipment and space to perform laparoscopies. The father of the author Dr JJ Van der Wat visited Dr Palmer in 1965 and introduced laparoscopy to South Africa. I can still remember many pioneer Laparoscopists carrying their perspex boxes with their own personal equipment to the operating room where they performed laparoscopies. Then laparoscopy was still in its infancy and considered a fad which still had to be evaluated. With the introduction of gynecological endoscopic surgery by Kurt Semm and his team from Kiel it became obvious that the specific needs of the endoscopic surgeon had to be addressed.[2] Semm's historic pictures of an endoscopic surgeon surrounded by a large array of machines peering down a laparoscope with his arms suspended on frames reminds us of the origin of the dedicated endoscopic theater. This was prior to the introduction of "video laparoscopy".

By the 1970s it became obvious that laparoscopy was here to stay and the operating room had to adjust accordingly. Laparoscopic sterilization soon became the norm and with a paper published by Victor Gomel[3] showing that salpingostomies could be performed successfully endoscopically, an astronomic rise in the procedure list followed?

With the introduction of video technology the dynamics of endoscopy changed radically because magnification, better visualization and illumination made rapid advances in surgical technique possible. In 1989, Harry Reich was the first to perform a laparoscopic hysterectomy. This set the trend for things to follow. Oncology surgery, resection of endometriosis, myomectomy, colposuspensions and other procedures soon followed. Today procedures like the endoscopic management of ectopic pregnancy, adnexal surgery and surgery for endometriosis have been established as true "endoscopic" procedures.

One of the main objectives of minimally invasive surgery was to allow the patient a quicker recovery and a shorter hospital stay. Not only did the demands in the operating rooms change but patient care also underwent dramatic changes with daycare being the norm. The Park Lane Clinic Endoscopic Unit evolved on par with the evolution of endoscopic surgery and from 1990 a dedicated endoscopic unit was developed which progressed as technology became available. This unit has been host to many distinguished surgeons and has been active in teaching since its origin. Distinguished surgeons like Harry Reich, Victor Gomel, Jim Daniell, Dan Martin, Brian Cohen, Nick Kadar, Marco Pelosi, Michelle Nisolle and others have visited this unit to teach and to perform surgery.

REQUIREMENTS AND SPECIFICATIONS

Before sitting down to plan a dedicated endoscopic operation room an array of factors will have to be taken into consideration. These include:

1. Capital expenditure budget.
2. Size of population to be served and whether the optimal use of operating room time can be achieved.
3. The capabilities and expertise of the surgeons involved.
4. Availability of intensive care and other specialized facilities, which may be required for postoperative patient care.
5. Education and teaching possibilities.

The philosophy should be to have a self-contained unit with a full complement of equipment and instruments. All sterilization and storage facilities should be contained within the endoscopic operating room complex. The golden principle is that all instruments and equipment are kept cleaned, maintained and set out within the unit and *never* leave it. A dedicated staff, in our case 2 technicians and 3 operation room sisters take responsibility for the operation and function of our unit.

The basic specifications of a dedicated endoscopic surgery unit should include the following:

a. An independent flow of patients to the operating room, separated from that of patient flow to the main operating room complex. This is essential as daycare and short-term hospital stay will be required in the majority of endoscopic cases.

b. Operating rooms with scrub facilities.

c. A recovery area.

d. Storage facility for endoscopic equipment and instruments both reusable and disposable.

e. Storage for emergency equipment like laparotomy sets.

f. Storage for sutures, drapes and anesthetic equipment.

g. Cleaning and sterilization (autoclave) facilities

h. Waste corridor and dirty linen exits.

i. Change rooms and ablution facilities.

j. Rest and catering facilities.

Attached to the operating room complex and with direct access should be the instrument and equipment storage facility with shelves, lockers and trays. Private lockup cabinets should be provided for the personal equipment of surgeons. Stock cupboards for disposable equipment and suture materials should also be provided. In the equipment facility a section must be set aside for laparotomy and emergency surgery equipment to be readily available for the quick conversion from laparoscopy to laparotomy should the need arise. Incorporated in the storage facility should be a setup area where trays can be set as needed for operations. A nice touch is a small fridge where refreshments can be kept.

Attached to this equipment and setup room should be a cleaning area with an autoclave and sterilization facilities. This area should also contain a heated cupboard for the heating of intravenous, hysteroscopy, and irrigation fluids.

The Park Lane endoscopic unit is primarily reserved for gynecologists of which there are forty working in our establishment. Operating room time in our complex is thus utilized to its full potential. It is cared for by a dedicated staff whose sole responsibility is the care and maintenance of the equipment.

Anesthetic personnel who assist the anesthetist rotate through this unit for training. In our unit the surgeons provide their own anesthetists. In many instances the anesthetist has formed a long-standing relationship with the endoscopic surgeon and together with the trained operation room nurse form a dedicated team. I have included the basic floor plan of our endoscopic surgical unit, which does not necessarily reflect that of other units but in our experience functions well for optimum utilization of time and space.

GENERAL OPERATING ROOM EQUIPMENT

1. Standard anesthetic equipment with ventilators and trolleys for anesthetic drugs. Ancillary equipment like Bair Huggers and blood warmers should be available especially when long surgical cases are planned.

2. Electronically or hydraulically controlled operating tables, which should be adjustable to the requirement of the surgeon. The operating table must be equipped with hydraulic assisted lithotomy poles and foot boots. This significantly enhances our ability to position patients for optimal comfort and access during surgery. This also allows for the leg and foot position to be changed during the operation without compromising sterility. This device secures a comfortable leg and foot position for long procedures even in obese patients. We use "Ultrafins" from the OR group.

3. Central operating room light with 2 to 3 ancillary satellite lights to light up specific areas, i.e. abdomen, perineum and cranial end of the operation table.

4. X-ray light box.

5. Dictation area.

ENDOSCOPIC INSTRUMENTS AND EQUIPMENT

Instruments

Instruments carried in a dedicated endoscopic surgery unit should be focused at two levels:

Gynae Endoscopy Surgery Suite

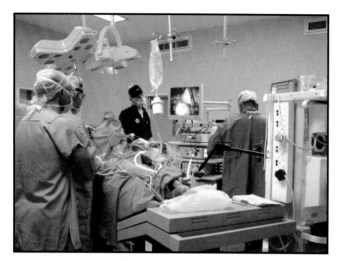

Fig. 2.1

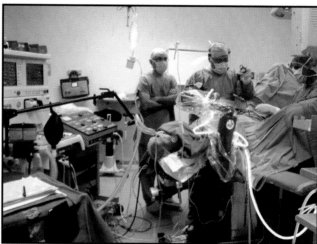

Fig. 2.2

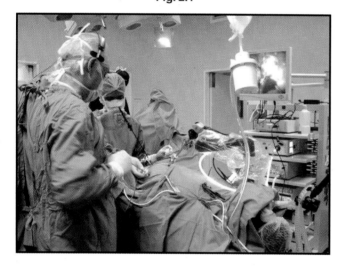

Fig. 2.3

Fig. 2.4

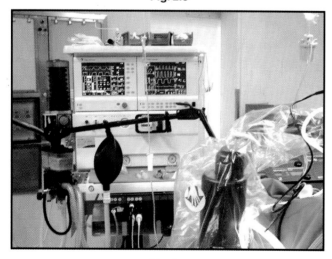

Fig. 2.5

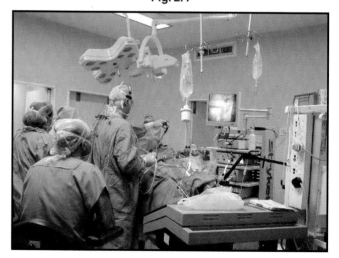

Fig. 2.6

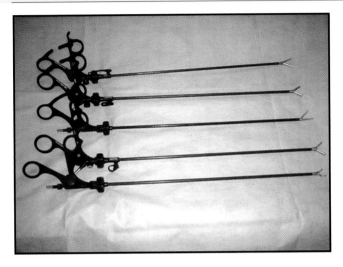

Fig. 2.7: Laparoscopic tissue graspers

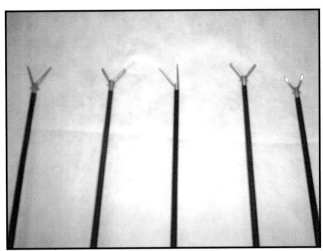

Fig. 2.8: Tip of the laparoscopic graspers

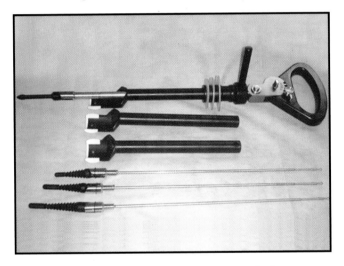

Fig. 2.9: Clermont Ferrand uterine manipulator

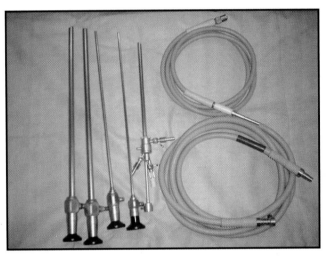

Fig. 2.10: Telescopes and fiber optic cables

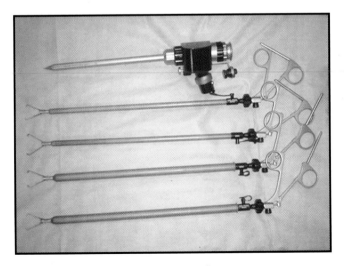

Fig. 2.11: Sawahles morcellator graspers

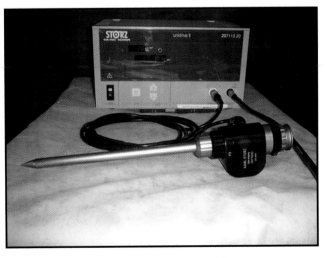

Fig. 2.12: Sawahles morcellator with generator

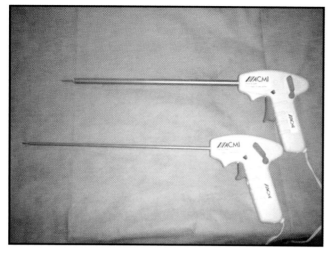

Fig. 2.13: 5 mm and 10 mm tripolar forceps

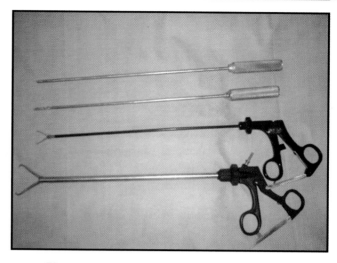

Fig. 2.14: 10 mm and 5 mm Tenaculum forceps and myoma screw

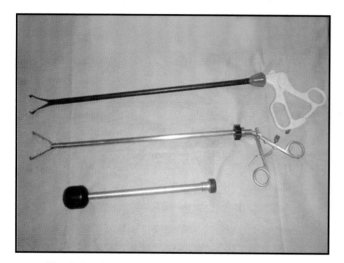

Fig. 2.15: CCL extractor and 10 mm claw forceps

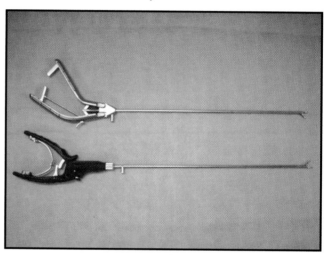

Fig. 2.16: Richard Wolf and Koh needle holders

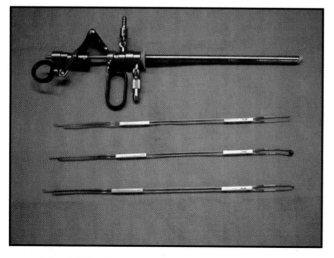

Fig. 2.17A: Resectoscope with working element

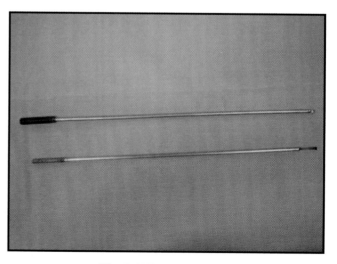

Fig. 2.17B: Knot pushers

General Instruments

This equipment is that needed to perform endoscopic surgery and hysteroscopic surgery up to level III and include laparoscopes and hysteroscopes both of large to small diameter. All the instruments like scissors, forceps, graspers and needle holders should be available in 5 mm and in some instances 10 mm sizes.

A range of insulated instruments for electrosurgery should be kept and readily available. Instruments should be easily disassembled and cleaned. Instrument tips and scissors should be mounted on replaceable shafts that can be exchanged when broken or blunt. All instruments should ideally be able to rotate and should be mounted on ergonomically designed handles. Trocars, cannulas, and uterine manipulators should be available. A complimentary set of disposable instruments and trocars should also be available. When purchasing instruments one should look for quality from a reputable firm. This is extremely important as good service and the availability of replacement instruments and parts makes for a well-run operating room and limited down time.

Specialized Instruments

Over and above the general endoscopic instruments, specialized instruments which are surgeon specific, should be catered for. These instruments are used by surgeons for specific operations and specialized techniques, which require a more sophisticated array of instruments. These include uterine manipulators, special scissors, retractors, graspers and needle holders, which are preferred by the specific surgeon. Personal lockers should be provided for individual surgeons for these instruments.

Equipment

In a dedicated endoscopic surgery suite a full compliment of equipment should be available. This includes:

Camera/light Systems

With the development in the mid 1980s of video cameras that could be coupled to laparoscopes, the surgeon was finally freed from direct visualization thought the laparoscope. Today a 3-chip high definition camera/Xenon light combination is used.

It is important that this light source is designed around the unique optical needs of the camera system. Ideally, functions like data capturing, zoom and picture quality should be controlled from the camera head. A filter to eliminate fibreoptic images from the screen is a great advantage when flexable or semi rigid endoscopes are used. Todays systems must have digital capabilities and digital output.

High Volume CO_2 Gas Insufflator

This should be capable of delivering a high volume of CO_2 in heated form to the patient. Adequate display of intra-abdominal pressure, gas flow and volume must be provided. A safety release valve must be included in the system to guard against over inflation (high pressure). A moisturizing system can be added, as it will prevent dehydration of the peritoneum with subsequent postoperative shoulder pain. Heating the CO_2 is useful to prevent mist formation and hypothermia.

Electrosurgical Equipment

This should include mono and bipolar generators with all attachments and instruments. Safety feedback circuits are mandatory to prevent intraoperative thermal injury to the patient. Argon beam capabilities could be included or coupled to existing electrocautery generators. We find this a particularly useful addition to our electrosurgical armamentarium as it provides excellent hemostatic capabilities. New plasma coagulators have become available for the treatment of superficial endometriosis (Helica Plus). They work in a similar fashion as the argon beam coagulator. New developments in bipolar technology have now produced a new generation of bipolar generators that can safely coagulate large pedicles (LigaSure, Tyco Healthcare).

Morcellators

Motorized morcellators have now become the norm and are an essential piece of equipment in the endoscopic operation room when subtotal hysterectomies, myomectomies and other procedures requiring morcellation are performed. Morcellators have been developed in reusable (Karl Storz) and disposable forms (GyneCare- Johnston & Johnston). Recently a morcellator for hysteroscopic surgery has been described.

Harmonic Scalpel: Ultracision (Ethicon Endo-Surgery)

With this instrument electrical energy is converted into mechanical motion causing vibrations at 55,500 cycles per second, which denatures protein in the tissue. It achieves precise hemostasis, cutting and dissection at low temperatures. It has found acceptance with many surgeons due to its effectiveness and ease of handling and has thus become their instrument of choice. The fully equipped endoscopic suite should have a harmonic scalpel available. It may be considered an alternative to electrosurgery but our opinion is that it is complimentary to electrosurgery and is a welcome addition to the operation room.

Suction Irrigation Equipment

This equipment is vital for performing endoscopic surgery. High-pressure fluid irrigation is essential for hydrodissection and cleaning the operating field of blood and debris. In addition good suction will allow a "smoke free" and clear operating field. We use the StrykeFlow system from Stryker and find it a great addition to our equipment. It is easy to operate and although disposable it is cost effective in our hands.

Laser Equipment

Lasers became popular during the 80s and are now established as niche products which are limited to the historically "laser active" units. Because of the high cost of the specialized equipment required for laser surgery, electrosurgery and harmonic scalpel are replacing lasers.

Endometrial Ablation Equipment

New developments in this field have provided the endoscopic surgeon with a wide choice of machines most relying on the balloon and "heated water" principle. It is not necessary to view this equipment as capital equipment as the relevant company will gladly supply the heat generators free of charge if the rather expensive disposable balloon system is frequently utilized. Microwave and Radiofrequency endometrial ablation apparatus are also available and used with good success.

Gasless Laparoscopy

This is a specialized field that requires special equipment and training. Various products have been developed to suspend the abdominal wall but to date the Laprolift system from Karl Storz has found acceptance. There are cost benefits by using gasless laparoscopy as expensive insufflators are not necessary and conventional surgical instruments can be used. It could be considered a method of choice where budget constraints exist. As yet it has not seriously challenged the traditional CO_2 pneumoperitoneum model.

Hysteroscopic Fluid Pumps and Fluid Monitors

A wide range of hysteroscopic fluid pumps and fluid monitors exist. This apparatus gives welcome and necessary information and assistance during prolonged hysteroscopic procedures like submucous myoma resection. As a rule, however, diagnostic and short surgical procedures can be adequately performed using pressurized fluid delivery systems and careful fluid loss calculations.

Robots and Robotic Surgery

Robots and robotic surgery have become a reality with many companies investing large amounts of research and development capital into this specialized field with the view to making endoscopic surgery move reproducible, cost effective and safe. The Parklane Clinic endoscopy unit introduced 'AESOP', (Automated Endoscopic System for optimal positioning) the robotic arm from Computer Motion in 1997. The AESOP robotic arm controls the camera and laparoscope by voice command to the position required by the surgeon. In our specific circumstances it has been a wonderful "assistant" under the most trying circumstances. We have found that the ability to control ones own "focal length" and visual field by voice command has greatly enhanced our surgical comfort zone. By having both hands free to operate one can experience the great advantage of true ambidexterity which can be critical for complex gynecologic cases.[10] We use the AESOP system mainly for adnexal and endometriosis surgery like endometrioma resection and rectovaginal septum surgery.

Recently the Da Vinci Robot System (Intuitive Surgical, Mountain View, CA) has been tested in gynecologic endoscopic surgery.[11] This is a tele-robotic system designed to overcome the surgical limitations of conventional laparoscopy by providing surgeons with improved dexterity and precision coupled with three-dimensional imaging that allows for the completion of complex minimally invasive procedures like microsuturing.

The Da Vinci System consists of three components comprising a stereoscopic viewer with hand and foot controls, a vision system, which provides 3-D imaging through a 12 mm endoscope and a patient side cart with 3 or 4 robotic arms. One arm holds the telescope while the other arms hold the laparoscopic surgical instruments. Although only tested on a myomectomy and anastomosis model, evolving robotic technology may further improve patient outcomes while presenting new options for the management of gynecological surgical problems.

INTEGRATED OPERATING ROOM SYSTEMS

As the armamentarium of instruments and equipment has grown, the surgeon has been faced with the task of dealing with multiple devices. Leading endoscopic equipment and instrument manufactures like Karl Storz (OR 1), Stryker (i-Suite), Wolf (CORE) and Olympus have developed integrated operating room systems, which give the surgeon the ability to control the equipment verbally, by "touch" technology or radio remote. This gives control over the entire operating room including equipment, lighting, patient records, images and documents. These systems make for the total remodeling of the existing operation room. All equipment and lighting is ergonomically mounted from ceiling booms and equipment settings can be pre-customized to be readied for different surgeons and procedures as required.

No system will be complete without digital imaging and data capture, which will allow images captured during operation to be accessed, edited, printed and saved on disc or video. Furthermore the images can be used to create and print documents relevant to these operations and then downloaded into the hospital system and onto the surgeons PC or laptop. The data captured can also be transmitted to distant locations via high-band telephone lines or even to the internet. This enables the surgeon to transmit and become interactive within the hospital or even around the world. This facility will also allow teleconferencing, telementoring, distant tutoring and in some instances telesurgery.

The OR milleu is constantly changing and it is important to purchase into an open ended arrangement which will enable the hospitals to design their own operation rooms to precisely meet their current needs as well as being able to upgrade to meet future needs and accommodate new technology.

EDUCATION AND TRAINING

Ideally attached to the unit should be a training and teaching facility. Training boxes (pelvitrainer) should be made available for formal teaching as well as casual training and skills honing that can be performed at the surgeon's leisure. Other audiovisual equipment should also be available for lecturing. We find such a facility useful as specialists in training rotate though our facility and qualified specialists who would like to enhance their endoscopic skills are always present and welcome in our unit.

HUMAN RESOURCE

This is the most vital asset for a dedicated endoscopic unit to be effective and to function optimally. To my mind we have developed a module, which functions well. For our two-operation room complex we have three operation room nurses that take full responsibility for the smooth running and operation of the unit.

Except for staff in training these nurses are the only ones responsible for taking cases and handling our instruments. They work flexible hours and must be available when needed. We also have two endoscopic technicians that must be present during all surgery. They are responsible for the maintenance of instruments and equipment. They are the key to running a successful unit as they limit down time by keeping equipment and instruments functional and in good working order. These technicians are also responsible for data capturing and IT networking. It is vitally important that a good understanding and working relationship develops and exists between the persons working together in the dedicated unit.

A team that functions efficiently in unison is definitely more desirable then a fancy new piece of equipment. Good maintenance and efficient work makes for a happy surgeon and a satisfied patient.

REFERENCES

1. Steptoe PC. Laparoscopy in Gynaecology Edinburgh, ES Livingstone, 1967;1.
2. Semm K. Endocoagulator: new possibilities for tubal surgery via Pelviscopy. Excepta Medica 1974;370:242.
3. Gomel V. Salpingostomy by laparoscopy. J Reprod Med 1977;18:265.
4. Murphy AA. Operative laparoscopy. Fertil and Steril 1987;47:18,
5. Reich H, De Caprio J. Laparoscopic hysterectomy. J Gynecol Surg 1989; 5:213-16.
6. Tulandi T. Surgical Management of ectopic pregnancy. Alin Obstet. Gynecol 1999;42:31-38.
7. Levine RL. Economic impact of pelviscopic surgery. J Reprod Med 1985;30:655.
8. Bessell JR, Karatassas A, Patterson JR, et al. Hypothermia induced by laparoscopic insufflation. Surg Endosc 1995;9:791-96.
9. Emanuel M, Wamsteker K. The Intrauterine Morcellator: A new hysteroscopic operating technique to remove intrauterine polyps and myomas. J Minimal Invas Gynecol 2005;12:62.
10. Mettler L, IB Rahim M, Jonat W. One year experience working with the aid of a robotic assistant (AESOP) in gynaecological endoscopic surgery. Human Reproduction 1998;13:2748-50.
11. Advencula A, Song A, Burke W, Reynolds K. Preliminary experience with robot—assisted laparoscopic myomectomy. J Amer Assn Gynecol Laparos 2004;11:511.

Laparoscopic Needle Holders and Knot Pushers

MARIE FIDELA R PARAISO

Chapter Three

INTRODUCTION

Laparoscopic suturing is often the skill acquired when a surgeon makes the leap from endoscopic surgeon to advanced endoscopic surgeon. It is often the learning curve associated with laparoscopic suturing that makes a surgeon an expert laparoscopist or convinces a non-laparoscopic surgeon to avoid advanced endoscopic procedures. Sometimes lack of good instrumentation dissuades a surgeon from laparoscopic suturing and knot-tying. The objective of this chapter is to introduce various needle holders and knot-pushers to the reader. Because there are no randomized trials comparing various needle holders and knot pushers, the expert endoscopic surgeons in the departments of Obstetrics and Gynecology, Urology, General Surgery, Bariatric Surgery, and Colorectal Surgery at the Cleveland Clinic Foundation were polled for their preferences.

NEEDLE HOLDERS AND SUTURING DEVICES

For standard suturing technique, needle holder preference is determined by comfort of the surgeon. A surgeon should trial various types of needles holders prior to purchasing them because the weight and type of handles vary. The weight of needle holder may facilitate intracorporeal knot-tying. The Snowden-Pencer needle holder (Snowden-Pencer, City, State) is particularly lightweight and is preferred by some surgeons who perform intracorporeal knot-tying the majority of the time (Fig. 3.1). However, this needle holder cannot handle a lot of torque and should be avoided in such situations. The flamingo-tipped and parrot-tipped needle holders (Karl Storz Endoscopy, Culver City, California) are advantageous for intracorporeal knot-tying because they facilitate wrapping the suture around the needle holder tip (Figs 3.2 and 3.3). Conventional and 90° self-righting German needle holders (Ethicon Endo-Surgery, Inc., Cincinnati, Ohio) have ratchet spring handles, which allow opening and closing the needle with ease (Figs 3.2 and 3.3). These handles are reliable because they do not spring or stick and are very ergonomic for repeated movements. The Talon curved needle drivers with spring handles (Cook OB/GYN, Spencer, Indiana) self-right the needle at an angle, either 45 or 90 degrees to the needle driver shaft, depending on the style chosen. The self-righting needle holders do not allow the freedom of needle angulation that is so important when suturing in tight spots or at difficult angles. Since the abdominal ports are fixed, motion of the driver handles is limited unless the port is placed suprapubically. The El-Med needle driver (El-Med, City State) is ideal for placement through a suprapubic port to serve as assistant driver with freedom of movement in 360 degrees. Most ratcheted needle holders can be used in the same fashion. A surgeon who is early on in the learning curve may want to use a self-writing driver; however, grasping suture with these drives is difficult and complicates suture and needle removal when performing extracorporeal knot-tying. The Storz Scarfi needle holder and notched assistant needle holder (Karl Storz Endoscopy, Culver City, California) are most like conventional needle holders used during laparotomy (Figs 3.2 and 3.3). However, the handles are difficult to maintain and may pop open after extended use, especially if CT-1 needles are the mainstay. The needle holder tips may become magnetized, which hampers needle grasping as well. The clasp handles of the three centrally located needle holders in Figure 3.2 have clasp-like handles that may not grasp very well with extended use.

Disposable suturing devices have been introduced that include the Endo-stitch (US Surgical Corp., Norwalk, Connecticut) and the Capio CL (Microvasive Boston Scientific, Inc., Natick, Massachusetts-CL stands for Cooper's ligament—Fig. 3.6). The needle is toggled back and forth with the Endo-stitch device. The Capio needle and suture are threaded through the tissue or fixation point and retrieved in the same motion. These devices may be more time efficient early on but with increased experience, the surgeon becomes more adept at standard suturing techniques and can defray the cost of these suturing devices.

KNOT PUSHERS

Extracorporeal knot-tying is preferred because of technical facility and the ability to hold more tension on the suture. The choice of an open-ended or close-ended knot pusher for extracorporeal knot-tying depends on surgeon preference. Use of a close-ended knot pusher allows the surgeon to avoid slippage of the knot pusher off of the suture. If a knot is not completely pushed down with an open-ended knot pusher, a close-ended knot pusher may be used to facilitate completion of the knot. Examples of knot pushers (Marlow, Cooper Surgical, Sheldon, Conneticut) are shown in Figures 3.4 and 3.5.

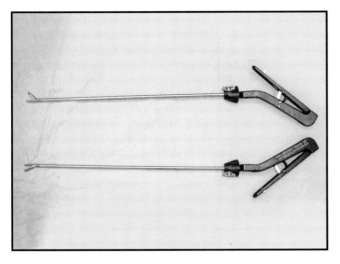

Fig. 3.1: Snowden-Pencer needle holder

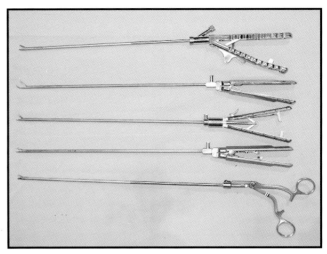

Fig. 3.2: Various types of needle holders

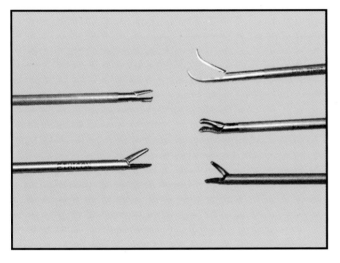

Fig. 3.3: Close-up of needle holders

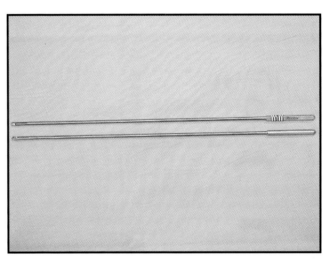

Fig. 3.4: Knot pushers

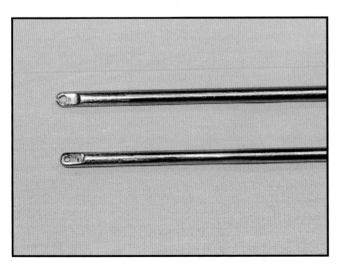

Fig. 3.5: Knot pushers (close-up)

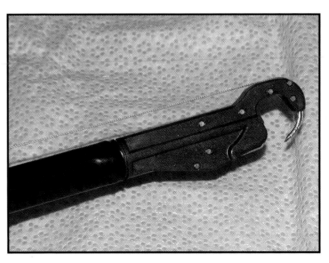

Fig. 3.6: Disposable suturing device

If a close-ended knot pusher is not available, the ends of the suture can be threaded through both eyes of a laparoscopic babcock clamp and be pushed down. The other alternative is to use laparoties (Ethicon Endo-surgery, Cincinnati, Ohio), which are absorbable clips used to fasten knots. Various clinch knots (Roeder, Westin, Fisherman's knot, etc.) may be used when performing extracorporeal knot-tying. These techniques are discussed in another chapter.

The choice of suture and needles for laparoscopic procedures is dependent on the surgeon's preference and the specific procedure. For standard total laparoscopic hysterectomy, No. 0 absorbable sutures on a CT-1 needle are appropriate for closure. Lubricating the suture with vaseline gauze makes the suture easier to handle and facilitates extracorporeal knot-tying. It is more difficult to tie sutures with high tensile strength such as polydioxanone suture (PDS, Ethicon Inc., Somerville, NJ). For myomectomy incision closure, No. 3-0 polyglycoic acid suture (Vicryl, Ethicon Inc., Somerville, NJ) should be utilized to close the endometrial layer in a continuous fashion. No. 0 or 2-0 absorbable suture should be used for the myometrial layers and No. 3-0 absorbable suture is suitable for closure of the serosa. The same techniques applied to open surgery for myomectomy closure should apply so that dead space is closed; hemostasis achieved; and adhesion formation is decreased. Closure of the peritoneum is performed with No. 2-0 or 3-0 polyglyocolyic acid suture.

With respect to laparoscopic colosuspension (Burch or Marshall Marchetti Krantz) No. 0 nonabsorbable sutures is ideal, either braided polyester with two arms on an SH or CT-2 needle (Ethibond, Ethicon Inc. Somerville, NJ) or No. 0 expanded PTFE on a CT-2 needle (Gore-tex, WL Gore, Flagstaff, AZ). The latter is not available as double armed suture. The paravaginal defect repair should be performed with No. 2-0 or No. 0 nonabsorbable sutures with a single armed CT-2 needle or UR-6 if preferred with the same type of suture as those utilized for colposuspension. For laparoscopic sacral colpopexy or uterosacral ligament vaginal vault suspension No. 0 nonabsorbable suture on a CT-1 or CT-2 needle is ideal for suture into the vagina and into the anterior longitudinal ligament of the sacrum. Ethibond should be greased with vaseline gauze. Gore-tex suture slides through tissue easily. Prolene suture sometime shears as does PDS if tied extracorporeally.

Laparoscopic tubal reanastomosis is best performed with No. 6-0 or 7-0, suture (Vicryl ethicon Inc., Somerville, NJ).

CONCLUSION

The choice of needle holders and knot pushers is based on preference and surgeon comfort. Having good equipment presents a time and cost savings when performing laparoscopic suturing and knot-tying.

Use of Pelvic Trainers and Simulators to Teach Endoscopic Suturing

MARSHALL MARK

Chapter Four

INTRODUCTION AND HISTORY

Laparoscopy has long been the primary tool of gynecologists for performing sterilization procedures, but until the late 1980s few surgeons of any other specialty utilized the technique. Then in 1987 the floodgates were opened when the first laparoscopic cholecystectomy was performed, and suddenly many other specialties seemed to suddenly recognize the potential of utilizing the laparoscopic approach for various types of procedures. This was a unique phenomenon in surgery, because within a span of only a few years the technique immediately become immensely popular and was being demanded by the public, while very few surgeons at any level of training or experience had the skills for performing advanced procedures via operative laparoscopy. Because of the abrupt and overwhelming demand for training from both general surgeons as well as gynecologists, many animal labs were opened and often surgeons learned their skills practicing on pigs or sheep in these labs. Several of the instrument companies (e.g. Autosuture, Ethicon) did provide basic box-like pelvic trainers for surgeons to practice suturing, but these were as a rule rarely used by the surgeons. In fact, the first wave of laparoscopic surgeons was not especially skillful at laparoscopic suturing; preferring instead other modalities such as endoloops, stapling and electrosurgery, and thus avoiding the necessity to have to learn to suture. During this time suturing was performed as more of a novelty, and was simply not included as a significant component of training courses during this first wave of the growth of operative laparoscopy.

Then, in the nineties surgeons became more aggressive on the types of procedures they were attempting, and the ability to suture laparoscopically became more crucial for these more advanced procedures. General surgeons began to do colon and gastric work, and gynecologists began to perform more pelvic support work; first retropubic urethropexies and later full pelvic support procedures. These accomplished surgeons were very skillful in suturing in open cases, but unfortunately these open suturing skills did not readily translate to laparoscopic skills. Consequently many surgeons became quickly frustrated and still continued to avoid procedures that required suturing. Other techniques such as screws and staples were devised, often in attempts to avoid

suturing for the surgeons without those skills; but eventually this wave of surgeons finally recognized the necessity for an advanced laparoscopic surgeon to be skilled in intra-abdominal laparoscopic suturing. This opened the door for even more complex procedures to be performed via the laparoscopic approach.

Up until this time the pelvic trainers had remained very basic, and many surgeons usually still learned their suturing skills during their surgical procedures on their own patients. Pelvic trainers started to become more sophisticated, but many practicing surgeons had already become accomplished in suturing by the volume of cases they were doing. However, as endoscopic tasks and procedures being performed became more and more complex and time intensive, practicing surgeons were even more reluctant to allow residents and apprentice surgeons to learn on their patients. Then because of the public's increasing awareness of the dramatic number of errors in medicine and surgery, and the growing demand by patients for a reduction of errors and increased patient safety; the stage was set for the evolution of more advanced pelvic trainers for training. Residents and novice laparoscopists began to utilize to pelvic trainers to learn and practice suturing techniques, and several commercial models began to appear to meet those needs.

In becoming more advanced, some trainers were improved versions of earlier ones; still box like compartments containing various exercises inside to practice upon, usually without defined objectives or specific end points. However, some companies began to develop software which employed computer sensing of the movements of the instruments, measuring the efficiency of the techniques of the operator. Others measured time and errors and derived a score based upon the McGill classification of surgery. Many of these still used the traditional box like structure but with computer technology integrated inside for the exercises.

At this time computerized trainers were being developed which used virtual reality for training, but the first of these were very simplistic and poorly accepted by surgeons. The image generating software lacked sufficient sophistication and the images were still unrealistic, and the lack of touch or feeling (force input) of the instruments made the exercises appear even more unreal to the surgeons. However, now the surgeon could practice; repeating the clinical scenario over and over without danger or damage to a live patient, and could practice (and fail safely) as often as it took to develop the necessary suturing skills. Gradually the imaging became more realistic, and programming was developed that could integrate haptics (the sense of feel or force feedback) into the models. Today simulators of both types are finally becoming accepted for developing task skills for use in the operating room.

CURRENT TYPES OF SURGICAL SIMULATION TRAINERS

There are two main types of surgical trainers available today. One is the advanced version of the old pelvic box trainer, and although it has become much more sophisticated today with several advantages over the computerized ones, basically it is still a box-like structure using actual surgical instruments. These may vary from simple home-made devices to those more elaborate and expensive. These newer training devices utilize virtual reality (VR), with computer generated images and computerized intra-abdominal instruments that you manipulate, much like the computerized play stations games of today (Figs 4.1 to 4.3). And there are also combinations, or hybrids, of the two. Each type has its advantages and disadvantages, and both can assist in effectively learning operative skills in laparoscopic suturing.

COMPARISON OF BOX TRAINER AND VIRTUAL REALITY TRAINER

The box or pelvic trainer is significantly cheaper than the VR trainers, and there are even reports on how to make one very cheaply from everyday household items. Others are much more elaborate; utilizing a full laparoscopic set up with a genuine laparoscope, camera, light source and container shaped like an abdomen and pelvis for working. One advantage with this type of trainer is that one can use authentic laparoscopic instruments, and usually the surgeon can practice with the actual instruments to which he/she is accustomed. These instruments obviously have exactly the same feel and shape as the ones they use in live surgery, and thus feel very familiar and comfortable to the surgeons. And probably most

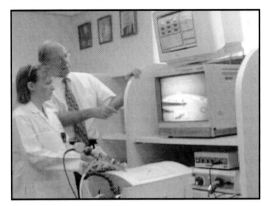

Fig. 4.1: This is an instructor teaching a student on the LTS 2000 ISM-60 by RealSim Systems, one of the pelvic box models that has computerized measurements of skill levels integrated into the exercises. This is one example of immediate feedback, but is a less efficient method in training because it requires the full time commitment of the instructor in a one on one setting. (Used by permission by RealSim Systems)

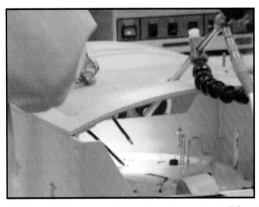

Fig. 4.2: This type of pelvic trainer, the LTS 2000 ISM-60, utilizes actual objects for the exercises for training, thereby providing real force feedback in training with no need for haptics development. (Used by permission by RealSim Systems)

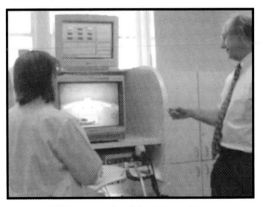

Fig. 4.3: This type of pelvic trainer does use computerization and objective measurements of skill levels in training, unlike the original pelvic box trainers (see top computer screen in picture). (Used by permission by RealSim Systems)

importantly, they have true force feedback as they are physical objects, and this feedback appears to be an important component to many surgeons and makes the exercises feel much more realistic. As many surgeons prefer an actual touch and feel for a more realistic sensation of the exercise materials, presently most still prefer the box trainers for training.

Learning suturing on pelvic box trainers also requires actual sutures and needles, another cost which has to be incurred. However, at the same time this also offers the flexibility to use different types of sutures and needles, and offers the surgeon the ability of using the same suturing materials that they are familiar with or commonly use in their own procedures. It also allows for learning the characteristics of various types of knots as well as different suture materials. This allows them to develop their suturing skills using the exact suture and techniques that they use in the ORs, a distinct advantage in the learning process. However, the cost and nuisance factor of providing conventional instruments and suture materials can be a disadvantage of pelvic trainers.

Simulation trainers, or those using computer generated images or virtual reality, are understandably more expensive than pelvic trainers because of the extent of the technology and computerization involved. They are usually self-contained, i.e. one does not have to supply instruments or suture materials as its images are programmed into the VR exercises. However, because of the complexity of coding and imaging of these exercises there is usually only one type of instruments and suture available, so that the surgeon does not have options or the flexibility of learning or practicing on different instruments, sutures and needles.

FEEL OR HAPTICS

One disadvantage with the earliest VR simulators is that the instruments had no feel; that is, there was no sense of resistance when one touched something in the virtual field, or when one picked up a needle or tied a suture. Initially when endoscopy began to become popular and surgeons were first learning, they had to forgo the ability to reach in and touch an organ or structure with their hand. This transition was difficult for many surgeons, as open surgery relies heavily on this sense of touch both for identifi-

cation of structures as well as for the surgical procedure itself. Consistency of organs, firmness of tissues and planes, the sense of feel of tissue being retracted or transected, tension applied to knots that were laid down; these are all examples of how surgeons use their hands and their sense of touch and resistance (force feedback) in open surgery.

In laparoscopy surgeons were then left with only the sense of feel through a long thin instrument, and to compound their transition further they were reduced to only a two dimensional view of the operative field. They learned to compensate in many ways for not having the ability to touch the tissue with their hand, but they did retain some sense of touch with the laparoscopic instruments. When the first VR simulators came out without any sense of touch at all, it was another difficult transition for them. The early VR simulators had no sense of touch at all for the surgeons, and this was generally unacceptable as it was too unrealistic for genuinely practicing suturing and other procedures. This sense of touch is called haptics, and has been a recognized science for a long time in areas other than medicine. Haptics are beginning to be developed and integrated into the newer medical simulators, but still are not quite as sophisticated and realistic as surgeons would prefer. And, the difficulty of the programming continues to make this an expensive component of the VR simulators. Nevertheless, haptics programming is advancing rapidly and becoming more and more realistic, and soon will probably closely mimic those experienced in live surgeries.

VALIDATION STUDIES

One of the reasons for the slow acceptance of simulators is the lack of documented validity for them. When simulators are utilized, until now there has been little data that the skills gained on simulators transfer efficiently to the operating room. Just because you are good on a particular exercise on a simulator does not necessarily mean you are good at suturing, the association has to be proven. There are many attempted validation studies where a novice turns out to be equally adapt at an exercise as an expert surgeon, but obviously is not near as skillful in the operating room.

When one develops his/her skills in doing the actual live surgery itself, then the skill acquired is obviously the one that is required for the procedure, and this is the apprentice method of learning that has traditionally been used in medicine. Ironically, although used for many centuries, the apprentice method of teaching has never formally studied or documented to be an effective or efficient method of training surgeons! However, it was the only available method of teaching and learning over 4000 years ago, and over time has become deeply ingrained in surgical teaching with very few changes (or validations). Any replacement teaching methodology has to be proven to be at least if not more effective than the current apprentice method. And so the validity confirmation of teaching with simulators or pelvic trainers has been adamantly required for acceptance for this type of training and learning, certainly to a higher level than the apprentice method ever was.

This confirmation is obtained through validation studies, and includes different types of validation. Face validity, or the task on the simulator *looks* like the task being trained for; content validity, or you are training and measuring is the exact surgical skill you really want to teach; and construct validity, that it accurately differentiates various levels of skills of different levels of surgeons (novice vs. intermediate vs. expert). There is also the issue of reliability; will training on that exercise on the simulator repeatedly produce the same results in different surgeon populations? So, the road to acceptance has been slow for surgical simulators, but these validation studies have now been documented for most simulators as they come to the market.

However, the ultimate holy grail today for acceptance in medicine has to be an improvement in clinical outcomes, and finally there are studies appearing that are showing that training on simulators result in more efficient surgeries (on live patients) and a reduction of errors when the surgeons take those skills learned on a simulator to the operating room. Even though resistance of many surgeons in the surgical fields is still substantial, the data today shows that learning surgical skills on simulators is more effective, more efficient, and in the long run safer for the patient, even to the point that many credentialing organizations are starting to require that simulation be a required component of surgical training.

EVALUATION METRICS

One difficulty with pelvic box trainers is that in general metrics are more difficult to integrate into them than with VR trainers. The importance of objectively quantifying the surgeons' progress and proficiency, or the accumulated skill level, is becoming increasingly emphasized today, and this is one advantage of simulation trainers. Several pelvic or box trainers today do have metrics and measurable parameters integrated into their systems, and there are also other advantages of the pelvic box trainers. One example is the ability to test the integrity of the suture knot; today's simulated trainers do not have that ability, while there are box trainers that can test the integrity of the knot after the surgeon completes it. Another example is that simulated trainers do not have the capability of being able to practice extracorporeal knots, while either intra- or extracorporeal knots can be learned and practiced on a pelvic box trainer.

One of the major advantages of simulation trainers is that they have objective and standardized metrics built into them, so that a surgeon's progress and skill can be objectively and accurately assessed. This becomes important in training students, such as surgical residents, to monitor their progress and ensure that they are learning required suturing skills. Moreover, it appears that it will also become of even more importance in the future, as most authorities believe that eventually surgeons will be required to demonstrate a minimal skill level or proficiency for accreditation and credentialing purposes. This is a major advantage of computerized trainers; that by being computerized the trainers have the ability to measure and assess skill and proficiency levels programmed into the machine.

Another distinct and increasingly important advantage of simulation training is that simulators can often provide immediate feedback to the student. It is well documented that the best and most efficient way of learning procedures is by receiving immediate feedback and instructions. This was never a problem in the traditional learning experiences of most surgeons, in that the professor would be operating with the student, and providing constant feedback as the student would be suturing and tying their knots (And often probably was much more unsympathetic feedback than the student preferred). When students are practicing on pelvic trainers, a proctor is not always able to be present, so that this learning advantage is frequently missed. Practice is not as beneficial in this setting, in fact may even be detrimental if incorrect techniques are practiced and ingrained, so this must be a consideration if using pelvic box trainers for training in suturing that do not have immediate feedback. Virtual reality simulators can provide this ongoing and immediate feedback via computer programming, so this is a distinct advantage of the VR simulators (Fig. 4.4).

LEARNING ON A SIMULATOR

There are both advantages and disadvantages of the two simulators as discussed above, and one should choose the one that best fits with one's needs in regards to training objectives, budgets, etc. Most simulators available today also come with training exercises programs and devices, whether virtual or real, and these should be incorporated into an overall training program. One should plan the training sessions, and set goals and objectives for the sessions. It should be remembered that a surgical procedure can be broken down into many complex tasks, and that each task in turn consists of several individual skills required to accomplish that particular task. Thus, novices should concentrate on first learning individual skills; things like becoming familiar with use of the instruments and a sense of where they are inside the abdomen. They should work on skills such as depth perception, touching structures with an instrument (Fig. 4.5), opening and closing instruments, and then move on to grasping and transferring objects between instruments, and then eventually grasping the needle itself. While many beginners want to go straight to suturing, there will be little progress made in learning how to suture until these basic single skills are mastered, and mastered well.

The surgeon with intermediate skills might move on to putting these skills together in learning to suture, and in order start practicing how to properly grasp the needle in the correct orientation for suturing (Figs 4.6 to 4.8), how to stabilize tissue with the second instrument for entering it with the needle, and how to pronate the hand holding the needle holder until the tip of a curved needle is perfectly perpendicular to the tissue before entering the tissue. This is a very important step, and one that novices commonly forget to include as they are concentrating

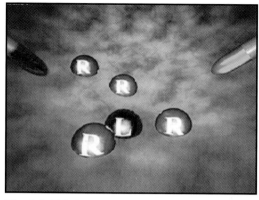

Fig. 4.4: This is an example of using simulation or virtual reality to teach laparoscopic pointing and touching skills, the first basic skills for a novice to master before attempting to suture. This software is LapSim developed by Surgical Science, and uses the AccuTouch laparoscopic surgical workstation (hardware interface device) developed by Immersion Medical. (Used by permission from Immersion Medical)

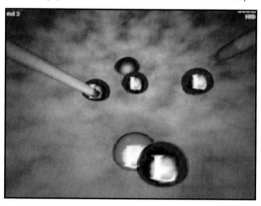

Fig. 4.5: Next the exercises move on to games with the point and touch learning, requiring that both hands are being used, using the LapSim software on the Accutouch. (Used by permission from Immersion Medical)

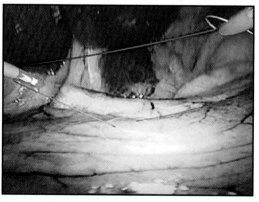

Fig. 4.6: Then the exercise advances to a virtual reality suturing exercise on a simulated organ, here placing a suture in the bowel. Note the circle on the bowel inside which the suture has to be placed (Used by permission from Immersion Medical)

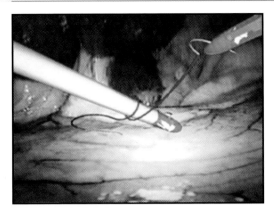

Fig. 4.7: Here the loops are thrown for intracorporeal knot tying in virtual reality (Used by permission from Immersion Medical)

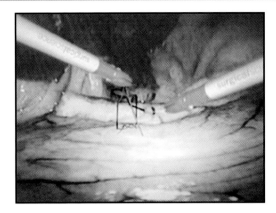

Fig. 4.8: And here the knot is completed and being cinched down, all in virtual reality. (Used by permission from Immersion Medical)

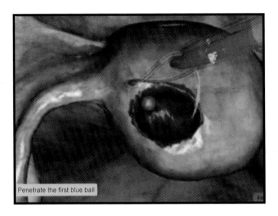

Fig. 4.9: Here is a simulated repair of a uterine defect after myomectomy, again in virtual reality and using the LapSim and AccuTouch. The blue dot in the defect represents the correct area where the needle should enter the tissue to begin suturing to close the defect (Used by permission from Immersion Medical)

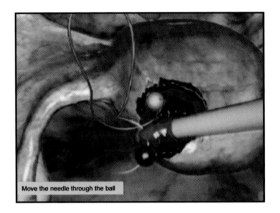

Fig. 4.10: Here is the second pass of the suture in repair of the myomectomy defect. The blue dot is where the second pass of the suture should be placed. Note the blue dot for the first pass has turned green, signifying that the first suture pass was placed correctly. This is an example of immediate feedback using computerization and virtual reality. This allows students to practice on their own without an actual instructor having to be present, but still with maximal learning potential from immediate feedback in using correct techniques. (Used by permission from Immersion Medical)

so intently on bringing the needle tip to the tissue. Then they should practice passing the needle through the tissue in a circular motion with supination of the hand and wrist, minimizing the size of the needle tract as the needle passes through he tissue (Figs 4.9 to 4.11). The second phase of passing the needle through tissue is how to grasp the tip of the needle as it emerges from the tissue with the second needle holder. The first needle holder should hold the needle and tissue steady, with the needle tip visible as it emerges from the tissue. The needle tip should be grasped by a second needle holder, and then the

pass of the needle completed through the tissue with pronation of the second hand and wrist, but keeping the needle in the proper orientation for passing the needle back to the first needle holder. This step is crucial in that it avoids the more time consuming step of reorienting the needle into the primary holder each time for the next tissue pass.

The more advanced surgeon would practice on intracorporeal instrument knot tying of the suture, while the less advanced would most like be practicing their extracorporeal knot tying (Figs 4.12 to 4.14). Here the student should learn the basic steps of

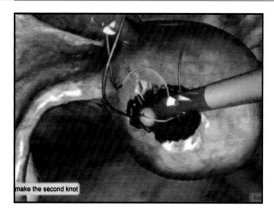

Fig. 4.11: And now that the suture has been placed correctly in the myometrium (the two green dots merge into one), the knot is tied intracorporeally in virtual reality. (Used by permission from Immersion Medical)

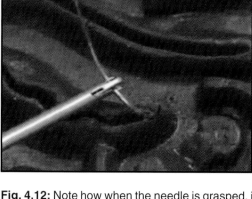

Fig. 4.12: Note how when the needle is grasped, it is righted in the needle holder as a result of the design of the jaws, and avoids the often cumbersome step of proper orientation of the needle for suturing when initially grasping it. These types of needle holders are often good to begin to learn suturing, otherwise the novice spends too much time and becomes frustrated with this first and often difficult step in suturing

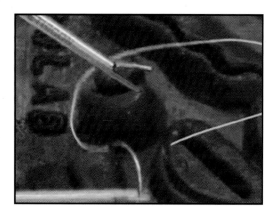

Fig. 4.13: Here the surgeon is starting to tie an intra-corporeal knot. This image demonstrates three very basic but critical steps for easy intracorporeal knot tying: (1) The suture has been cut appropriately and pulled through the tissue, so that the tail of the suture to be grasped once the loops are thrown is short. It is carefully placed directly beneath the second needle holder, BEFORE the loops are thrown, so that all the surgeon has to do is go directly down and grasp it with the second needle holder after the loops are thrown, (2) The needle is grasped at right angles and at the tip by the first needle holder, levering it as a side arm and making it easier to throw the loops around the second needle holder, (3) The jaws of the second needle holder are held open while throwing the loops, this helps to keep the loops on the needle holder once they are thrown

intracorporeal knot tying. First to place the tail of the suture directly beneath the second needle holder around which the loops will be thrown, and this

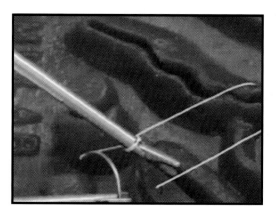

Fig. 4.14: Once the loops are thrown, then the second needle holder is simply advanced down to the pre-placed tail for grasping and completing the knot

should be done first so that once the loops of suture are on it no additional movements other than picking up the suture tail are required. Second is to use the needle itself as an accessory extension of the first needle holder in throwing the loops, and finally to open the second needle holder if the loops are tending to slide off. It should be reminded that only the box trainers provide the ability to practice the extracorporeal knot tying, while both the box and VR trainers provide the ability to train on intracorporeal knot tying.

When practicing on a trainer of either type, one should attempt to stand in a manner that is comfortable and is their usual stance and position in the operating room. If one is using a box trainer, then one should make ever effort to use the same or similar instruments and suture and needle that one usually uses in their own surgeries. The more closely one can approximate the practice experience to their own operating room setting, the more likely the skills learned will transfer into the operating room on live patients. Trocar placement is extremely important, on the simulator just as it is on a live placement. The trainee must learn the technique of triangulation with the instruments by proper placement of the trocars and avoiding putting the operating trocars too close together, although often on the VR trainers the trocar sites are already established on the exercise.

It is well accepted that receiving immediate feedback is the most effective method of learning, and attempts should be made to either have a proctor work with the trainee or to have some other method of instant feedback (many of the VR trainers have feedback built into the system). This is especially true in the beginning, when one is first learning the proper steps and techniques. To practice at length using poor and incorrect technique is not only ineffective, but may lead to the ingraining of improper techniques that at best have to be unlearned, and at worse may be dangerous to their patient in the operating room. Thus, all attempts should be made to obtain some type of immediate proctoring or feedback, at the very least when beginning to learn suturing.

Training sessions should be repeated; studies show that skills are best retained with repetition of practice sessions. Certainly advancing skills may be incorporated into the continuing training sessions; and if one is not active in surgery or has been through a period of absence from the operating room, maintenance of skills is easily accomplished by regular sessions on a training simulator.

It is well recognized that the teaching of endoscopic surgical skills and tasks such as suturing are only one component of the training of an endoscopic surgeon, and skill development should be integrated into a structured curriculum with other critical components. Any competent surgeon has to have a very complete and extensive knowledge of anatomy, the best surgical skills in the world are useless if one has no idea what structure to cut and what structures to suture. Likewise, skill and experience in intra-operative decision making is another critical skill of a good surgeon, one that can make or break even a surgeon with good knowledge of anatomy and good technical skills. Thus, the teaching of skills and suturing should always be incorporated into a broader curriculum with other components as well.

FUTURE OF SIMULATION TRAINING

Simulators in surgical training are becoming accepted world-wide, and most if not all major academic centers have build or are building simulation training resources on their campuses. There is no question that they are starting to address growing needs in endoscopic training such as less experience in the OR, due to less training time for student surgeons is available and the growing reluctance of patients to be "practiced upon". Suturing remains one of the more complex tasks in endoscopic surgery, requiring extensive practice to master. Simulators provide the ability to gain this experience and practice without endangering actual live patients during their own surgeries. As simulators gain more and more acceptance, it does not take a crystal ball to see that simulators will eventually be used to measure proficiencies, and after that will inevitably be used for accreditation and credentialing processes. The role of simulation training in surgery, from robotics to training to accreditation, will continue to grow as simulators are integrated more and more into the learning process in minimally invasive surgery.

CONCLUSION

Simulation in endoscopic training has gone through several phases of evolution, and currently there are box like pelvic trainers, virtual reality trainers, and hybrids of the two available for teaching and learning suturing. Each has advantages and disadvantages, and these factors have to be kept in mind when one is considering selecting a simulator and learning by simulation. When one selects a simulator on which to learn, then the advantages of using some type of immediate feedback must also be kept in mind, either through computer generated feedback or by using a proctor. And, learning and practice sessions must be repetitive, skills are not adequately learned and retained with only a single learning session on a simulator.

Equally, one has to remember that teaching or learning suturing is only a single skill set among many skill sets and complex tasks required to perform an endoscopic surgical procedure, and that simulators only assist with the acquisition of these skills. As such, simulation training should be only a component of a training program; the development of a sound data-base (e.g. basic knowledge of anatomy and pathology) and training in surgical decision making processes are other crucial components of training that are equally important in training endoscopic surgeons. Nevertheless, today surgical simulators bring many advantages to the teaching and learning of these skills, and as they continue to improve and become recognized as more efficient and effective methods of teaching, the inefficient and outdated teaching model of "see one, do one, teach one" is destined to soon become a relic of the past. It has served us well for many centuries, but the future of surgical simulation training beckons us and it is time to move on.

BIBLIOGRAPHY

1. Fenner DE. Training of a gynecologic surgeon [see comment]. Obstetrics and Gynecology 2005;105(1):193-96.
2. Frede T, Stock C, Renner C, Budair Z, Abdel-Salam Y, Rassweiler J. Geometry of laparoscopic suturing and knotting techniques. Journal of Endourology 1999;13(3):191-98.
3. Gallagher AG, Ritter EM, Champion H, Higgins G, Fried MP, Moses G, Smith CD, Satava RM. Virtual reality simulation for the operating room: proficiency-based training as a paradigm shift in surgical skills training.
4. Gallagher AG, Ritter EM, Satava RM. Fundamental principles of validation, and reliability: rigorous science for the assessment of surgical education and training [see comment]. Surgical Endoscopy 2003;17(10):1525-29.
5. Grantcharov TP, Kristiansen VB, Bendix J, Bardram L, Rosenberg J, Funch-Jensen P. Randomized clinical trial of virtual reality simulation for laparoscopic skills training. British Journal of Surgery 2004 ;91(2):146-50.
6. Harold KL, Matthews BD, Backus CL, Pratt BL, Heniford BT. Prospective randomized evaluation of surgical resident proficiency with laparoscopic suturing after course instruction. Surgical Endoscopy 2002;16(12):1729-31.
7. Larsson A. Intracorporeal suturing and knot tying in surgical simulation. Studies in Health Technology and Informatics 2001;81:266-71.UI: 11317754
8. O'Toole RV, Playter RR, Krummel TM, Blank WC. Cornelius NH. Roberts WR. Bell WJ. Raibert M. Measuring and developing suturing technique with a virtual reality surgical simulator.[see comment]. Journal of the American College of Surgeons 1999;189(1):114-27.
9. Rogers RM Jr, Julian TM. Training the gynecologic surgeon [see comment]. Obstetrics and Gynecology 2005;105(1): 197-200.
10. Satava RM. Now is not soon enough [comment]. Surgical Endoscopy 2003;17(8):1326-27.
11. Satava RM. Disruptive visions: surgical education. Surgical Endoscopy 2004;18(5):779-81.
12. Wanzel KR, Hamstra SJ, Caminiti MF, Anastakis DJ, Grober ED. Reznick RK. Visual-spatial ability correlates with efficiency of hand motion and successful surgical performance. Surgery 2003;134(5):750-57.

Laparoscopic Extracorporeal Suturing

GINGER CATHEY

RESAD PAYA PASIC

Chapter Five

INTRODUCTION

Laparoscopic surgeons often avoid suturing laparoscopically. They complain that laparoscopic suturing is cumbersome and too difficult to learn. But as laparoscopic gynecological surgery becomes an increasingly accepted method for treatment, the need for laparoscopic suturing skills also increases. Just as one must be able to suture proficiently to perform open gynecological surgeries, one must also be able to suture effectively when undertaking laparoscopic cases such as hysterectomy, prolapse repair, advanced endometriosis and other advanced endoscopic procedures.

Typically, an endoscopic surgeon must master the skill of extracorporeal laparoscopic suturing prior to tackling intracorporeal suturing. The following equipment is needed for laparoscopic extracorporeal suturing:

1. Two laparoscopic needle holders
2. Laparoscopic knot pusher (closed or open)
3. Laparoscopic scissors
4. Suture (typically 36 in/70 cm suture is needed to easily perform extracorporeal knot tying).

To become skilled at laparoscopic suturing, the surgeon must possess hand to eye coordination, steady hands and patience. Both depth perception and direct tactile sensation are absent when one sutures laparoscopically. The surgeon must be comfortable in using both his right and left hands, as two-handed manipulation is a must.

EQUIPMENT

A zero-degree laparoscope is used to permit direct visualization. The assistant must hold the camera and laparoscope in a steady fashion always keeping the operator in the center of the field of view.

Proper placement of trocars is imperative for optimal extracorporeal suturing. Most right-handed surgeons begin by learning to suture from the patient's left. As skills progress, advanced endoscopic surgeons will suture with ease from either side of the patient. With the laparoscope typically in the umbilical region, ancillary ports are placed lateral to the inferior epigastric vessels. Lower ports are 1 to 2 cm medial to the anterior superior iliac spine though some surgeons may prefer a single suprapubic port.

Laparoscopic suturing in the pelvis is made easier by placing the upper trocar(s) high, approximately parallel to the umbilicus, in the same lateral line as the lower quadrant port(s) (Fig. 5.1). For intensive suturing, a 10-12 mm trocar is needed to accommodate a CT-1 needle. A 7/8 mm trocar can be used for an SH needle or smaller. This larger trocar should be placed in the upper, lateral port position. Alternatively, a 5 mm trocar can be used using a "back-loading" technique.

There are a multitude of laparoscopic needle holders commercially available. The two basic designs are:
1. Self-righting needle holders with a fixed locking jaw mechanism
2. Standard, articulating jaw needle holders that mimic open needle drivers. Self-righting needle holders, such as the Cook needle holder, allow the needle to be grasped in an upright position, perpendicular to the needle driver with little effort. One of the limiting factors of self-righting needle holders is that you cannot grasp the suture with needle holder. Doing so may cause damage to the suture. Most advanced endoscopic surgeons, however, prefer the standard articulating jaw design that allows them to angle the needle perfectly for a given stitch and to manipulate the suture. Needle holders come in standard and long lengths. Long length needle holders allow the surgeon access to deep pelvic structures. This is particularly useful when suturing ports are placed high (Fig. 5.2).

Knot pushers also exist in two basic designs—open and closed knot pushers (Fig. 5.3). The tip of a closed knot pusher requires the surgeon to thread the suture through the knot pusher prior to tying his knot. This may be more of a challenge for those of us whose vision is not as keen as it used to be. The advantage of this type of knot pusher is that the suture material will stay in place while tying. Open knot pusher may inadvertently slide off of the suture while tying.

Chose of suture material is operator dependent. Pop-off sutures should be avoided. The suture, however, must be 36 inch/70 cm to be tied extracorporeally with ease.

INTRODUCTION OF SUTURE

The suture is grasped with the needle holder approximately 2 cm from the needle and introduced

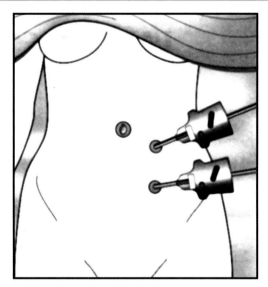

Fig. 5.1: Port placement for suturing

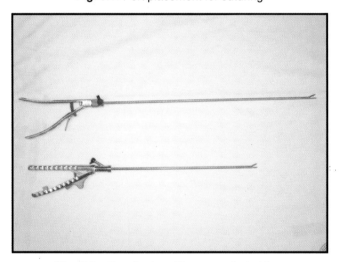

Fig. 5.2: Standard and long needle holders

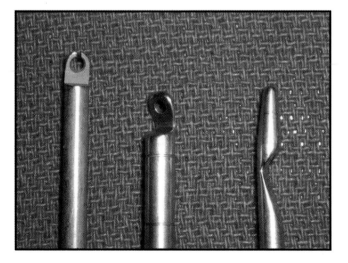

Fig. 5.3: Tips of knot pushers open and closed end

through the upper, larger (10 mm) trocar into the peritoneal cavity. This should be performed under direct visualization. It is important to always keep the exposed needle visible.

If only a small amount of laparoscopic suturing is anticipated, such as in simply closing the vaginal cuff after a laparoscopic hysterectomy, the suture may be "back-loaded" through a 5 mm trocar.

In "back-loading" the suture, the upper 5 mm trocar is removed from the abdominal wall (Fig. 5.4). The assistant or surgeon must plug the open site to prevent excessive loss of pneumoperitoneum. The laparoscopic needle holder is then introduced through this trocar (Fig. 5.5). The needle holder grasps the end of the suture material pulling the end of the suture back through the trocar. The needle holder is placed again through the trocar, now with the suture also traveling through the trocar, and grasps the suture 3-4 cm from the needle (Fig. 5.6).

The needle holder, holding the suture, is then placed through the upper port site. Under direct laparoscopic visualization the surgeon will watch as his needle holder enters the peritoneal cavity though the previously made incision. As the needle holder is pushed deeper into the pelvis, the needle will slide through the incision following the needle holder. The 5 mm trocar sleeve can then be pushed over the needle driver, thus replacing the trocar to its original location (Fig. 5.7).

PLACEMENT OF LIGATURES

Now that the suture is in the peritoneal cavity, the surgeon can proceed with suturing. To grasp the needle properly, the suture should be held 2 cm from the needle hub with a needle holder in the lower port site. The needle is allowed to dangle or is positioned such that the needle tip is facing the patient's left side. If difficulty is encountered in pointing the needle tip to the patient's left, the needle may be stabilized against a pelvic structure and then slowly turned to the patient's left.

Through the upper trocar, a needle holder is used to grasp the needle two-thirds away from the needle tip. The needle should be grasped at a 90° angle with the tips of the needle holder's jaws. The needle can be "righted" in the needle holder by grasping the suture 2 cm above the needle hub and gently tugging the suture (Fig. 5.8). This technique is employed to perfect the angle of the needle in the needle holder

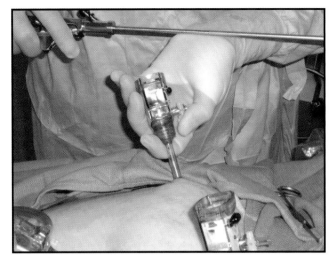

Fig. 5.4: Pulling the trocar out in preparation of suturing

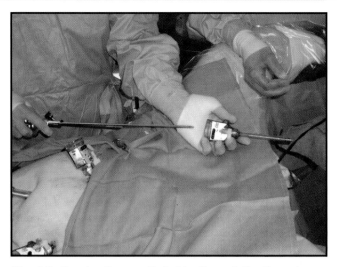

Fig. 5.5: Passing the needle holder through the 5 mm trocar

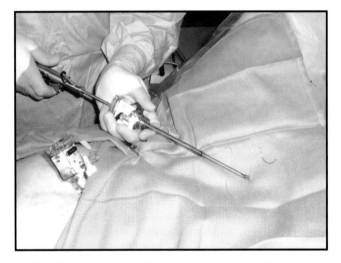

Fig. 5.6: Back loading the suture into the needle holder

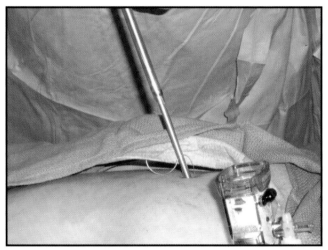

Fig. 5.7: Inserting curved needle inside the abdomen by Clarke-Reich technique

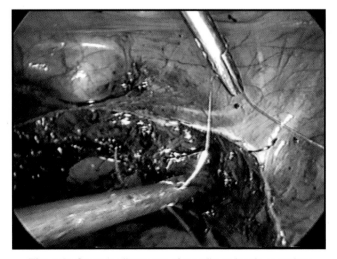

Fig. 5.8: Correct alignment of needle to begin suturing

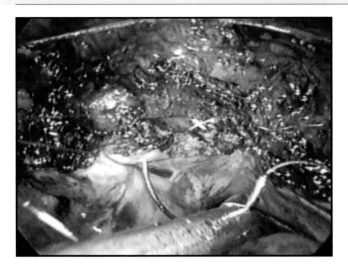

Fig. 5.9A: Passing suture through posterior vaginal wall

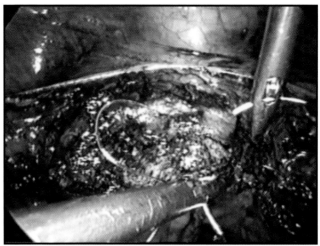

Fig. 5.9B: Passing curved needle suture through anterior vaginal margin. The tip of the exiting needle grasped by second needle holder

prior to suturing. The camera should zoom in closely to promote easier needle positioning.

When the needle is properly positioned, suturing is performed by a gentle initial push through the tissue followed by rotation of the wrist (Fig. 5.9A). Having your assistant stabilize the tissue to be sutured with a laparoscopic tissue grasper is sometimes helpful. You should be prepared with a needle holder through your lower trocar to grasp the needle tip and continue rotation of the needle through the tissue if needed (Fig. 5.9B).

Straight needles may also be used for laparoscopic suturing. These needle are easily placed through a 5 mm cannula and are easily manipulated with laparoscopic instruments. However, since it is difficult to suture pedicles with a straight needle, they are rarely used by advanced gynecological endoscopic surgeons.

EXTRACORPOREAL KNOT TYING

If a larger trocar was used for suturing (10/11 mm trocar for CT-1 needle, 7/8 mm trocar for SH needle), the needle can be removed from the abdomen through the same trocar prior to tying your knot. Again, the suture should be grasped 2 cm above the needle hub. The needle is then removed under direct laparoscopic visualization through the 10/11 mm trocar. Watching all needles exit the abdomen is recommended. The trocar valve should be depressed to allow removal of the needle. If one is not careful the needle can become caught on the trocar sleeve and dislodged from the suture.

With the needle outside the body, it is cut from the suture. Both ends of the suture are now exposed exiting the trocar. If a closed knot pusher is chosen, one free-end of suture is threaded through the knot pusher and secured with a hemostat (Fig. 5.10). A simple knot is then tied distal to the knot pusher and pushed down until the tissue is ligated. Both ends of the suture are held in the non-dominant hand while the laparoscopic knot pusher, held in dominant hand, pushes the knot through the trocar (Fig. 5.11). Again this is performed under direct laparoscopic visualization (Fig. 5.12). The second throw of the sutures is placed in the same direction as the first, creating a "granny-knot." This is done so that the second knot will slide into place. When a sufficient number of knots have been placed the suture is cut laparoscopically.

With an open knot pusher the suture does not have to be threaded through the knot pusher. A knot is first tied. The open end of the knot pusher is then placed above the tie and used to push it into place. The open knot pusher sometimes becomes dislodged while pushing the knot into place. If this occurs, the suture should be grasped inside the peritoneal cavity until the knot can be seen laparoscopically. The knot pusher can then be replaced above the knot under direct vision. If the knot cannot be located, the entire suture should be pulled inside the abdomen and untangled. The free suture ends can then be taken out through the trocar and a new knot placed.

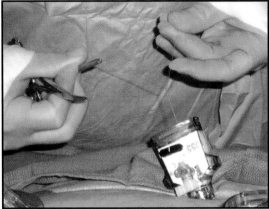

Fig. 5.10: Making extracorporeal knot

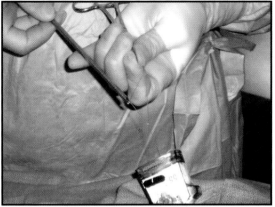

Fig. 5.11: Applying knot pusher to pass the extracorporeal knot. The free end is held taut by an artery forceps giving it upward traction

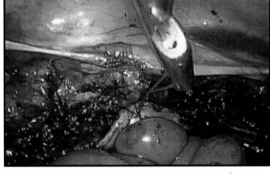

Fig. 5.12: Extracorporeal knot placed at the vault for closure

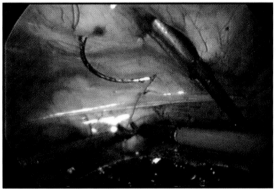

Fig. 5.13: Cutting away the extra suture by scissors

If the suture was "back-loaded" through the 5 mm trocar into the abdomen, the needle must be cut in the abdomen after the stitch has been placed. The needle is placed into the anterior abdominal wall and the suture is cut at least 2 cm above the needle (Fig. 5.13). The suture tail is than grasped and pulled out of the abdomen for knot-tying. With knot-tying completed, the suture is cut with the laparoscopic scissors. The needle is than removed by grasping the suture tail and pulling it from the anterior abdominal wall. The 5 mm trocar is first slid out of the abdomen with the needle holder and exposed needle following. It is important to not pull the needle into the 5 mm trocar as this will likely result in the needle being dislodged from the suture. The trocar has to be pulled out first and than the needle holder with the needle (Fig. 5.14). Careful observation of the needle is recommended as it exits the peritoneal cavity.

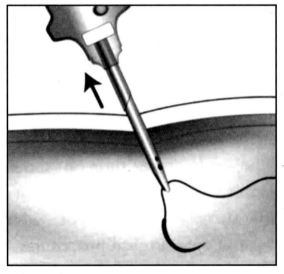

Fig. 5.14: Taking the needle out of the peritoneal cavity by holding the suture 2 cm away from the hub of the needle and withdrawing the trocar from the abdominal wall

Intracorporeal Suturing

NUTAN JAIN

SANKAR DAS MAHAPATRA

Chapter Six

INTRODUCTION

Laparoscopic suturing is an endoscopic skill necessary for the successful performance of a variety of advanced and complex laparoscopic procedures. Although some attempt to dismiss endosuturing as unnecessary but most experienced endoscopic surgeons recognize that neither energy sources, clips nor stapling devices can replace the need for suturing. As with conventional open surgery, laparoscopic suturing techniques permit restoration of normal anatomical relationships, organ reconstruction, approximation of tissue planes and establishment of hemostasis. Of the suturing and knot-tying methods adopted for laparoscopic surgery the intracorporeal method remains the most difficult to master. Intracorporeal suturing is defined as the placement of suture and subsequent tying of a secure suture knot within the peritoneal cavity.

Once limited only to short straight or ski needles, endosuturing can now be performed with a variety of curved needles and different suture materials. The ability to utilize curved needle suturing provides the surgeon with greater operative flexibility. Curve needle suturing has totally changed the dimension of laparoscopic surgery. That is how nowadays laparoscopists are doing complex surgeries like uterine prolapse repair, burch colposuspension, tubo-tubal anastomosis etc. New curved needle holders have been designed to firmly hold the needle with minimal instability at the tip. This permits SH, CT3 needle to be driven through the tissue of various thickness and consistency. Suturing dominated traditional open surgery for centuries. Laparoscopic suturing techniques were introduced and utilized by Kurt Semm[1] in gynecology in mid 1970s The first significant step in the evolution of laparoscopic instruments was mating of the microsurgical handle to the laparoscopic instrument, permitting free movement and full rotation. Also important was the introduction of two handed suturing technique and the design of instruments as a matched pair with each performing its specific role of needle driving or assisting grasper. To become skilled in laparoscopic suturing endoscopic surgeons must learn to adept to the laparoscopic operating environment, i.e. acquire the skill of proper depth perception, hand eye coordination, direct tactile sensation, steady practice and above all patience.

EQUIPMENT

The following equipment are necessary for intra-corporeal suturing:
1. Two laparoscopic needle holders or one laparoscopic needle holder and a grasper.
2. Suture materials.
3. Laparoscopic scissors.

A zero degree telescope is used to permit direct visualization. The assistant holds the camera in a steady fashion always keeping the target area in the center of the field of view. Proper placement of trocars is required for optimal intracorporeal suturing. As skills progress advanced endoscopic surgeon will suture with ease from either side of the patient and with either hand, right or left. Telescope with camera is placed in the umbilical region. Ancillary ports are placed lateral to the inferior epigastric arteries. Lower ports are placed 2-3 cm medial to the anterior superior iliac spine though some surgeon may prefer a suprapubic port midway between pubic hairline and umbilicus and the other in the lower quadrant on the side from where he is operating. Laparoscopic suturing in the pelvis is made easier by placing the upper trocar high approximately at the level of umbilicus for continuous and prolonged suturing. A 10 mm trocar is needed to accommodate a CT-1 needle. A 5 mm trocar can be used for SH needle or smaller needles. The larger trocar to be placed in the upper lateral position. Alternatively 5 mm apple valveless trocar can be used with 'back loading' technique.

NEEDLE HOLDERS

a. Self-righting needle holder with a fixed locking jaw mechanism
b. Standard articulating jaw needle holders that mimic open needle drivers.

Self-righting needle holders such as cook needle holders, Endopath (Johnson & Johnson) needle holder allows the needle to be grasped in an upright position, perpendicular to the needle driver with little effort. One of the limiting factors of the self-righting needle holders is that one cannot grasp the suture with needle holder, as it can damage suture materials during the time of holding. Most advanced endoscopic surgeons, however, prefer the standard articulating jaw needle holder (Karl Storz, Wolf) that allows them to angle the needle preferably for a given stitch and to manipulate the suture . Needle holders are of two sizes long and standard. Long needle holders will allow the surgeon access to deep structures in the pelvis.

PREREQUISITE FOR INTRACORPOREAL SUTURING

Be in top physical and mental condition. Slow movements are important for the beginners until proper skill develops. Motor skills determines the performance of a successful surgical procedures. Familiarity with open microsurgery facilitates the transition from open traditional surgery to laparoscopic surgery. Video magnification and camera factors will provide video picture that is adequate for most suturing procedures. Tissue needs to be handled as gently as possible. For a practicing gynecologist a dedicated endotraining will be the first step of learning. Ultimate success will come from motivation, will power, discipline, persistence and consistency. So one must get trained in proper way to perform intracorporeal suturing.

BASIC TECHNIQUE

1 The natural position for surgeon.
   — The laparoscope located between the right or left instrument
2 The offset position
   — The instruments are located to one side of the laparoscope (left or right)

Ideally needle holder to be parallel to the suture line. The assisting grasper to be at least 60-90 degree and set 6-7 inches apart to avoid a "Chopstick effect". A distance of 75-100 mm between endoscopic instrument tip and target tissue is optimal ergonomic condition for suturing.[2]

Optimal condition for proper suturing are needle holding angle greater than 90 degree and angle of needle insertion into the target tissues of 80 degree to 100 degrees. The needle to be gripped at the junction of anterior two-third and posterior one-third from tip of the needle The needle can be introduced inside the peritoneal cavity by the following methods:
1. Through 5 mm port.
2. Through 10 mm port with a 5 mm reducer.

Among these methods when small surgical area suturing is required introduce the needle through 5 mm port (Reich method). When prolonged suturing is required and frequent introduction of needle is necessary then 10 mm port is used with a 5 mm reducer.

ADJUSTING THE NEEDLE

Beginners will attempt to reposition the needle by holding it back and forth between assisting grasper and needle holder, hoping to adjust it in the process. This technique is sometimes frustrating for the beginners.[3]

Better method is to rest the tip of the needle on solid tissue, e.g. uterus and release grip followed by moving the needle holder till correct alignment is reached. When correct alignment is achieved then suturing can be started. Needle can be adjusted by manipulating suture by left needle holder. Needle can also be corrected by placing needle over a tissue and putting the needle holder with jaw open position over the needle and pressing it by upper jaw of the needle holder. This instantly snaps needle in a correct position and then the jaws can be closed and the needle is aligned correctly.

The plane of the needle should be perpendicular to the shaft of the instrument and the needle should be perpendicular to the suture line. During the time of needle insertion satisfactory counter pressure is provided and the needle is slowly driven into the tissue, making sure that the direction of penetration is properly maintained. During the time of entrance bite and exit bite the selection of site is very important. The amount of bite needs to be precisely calculated for each structure keeping in mind the function of the organ and reconstruction goal. Too small bite may tear the margin on the other hand too large bite may cause tissue necrosis or a bulky suture line.

TECHNIQUE OF INTRACORPOREAL SUTURING

Laparoscopic intracorporeal suturing is a difficult and complex task involving several integrated skillful movements, i.e. needle handling, suturing and knotting. But it is an acquired skill. One can master intracorporeal suturing by regular practice and following the principles of suturing technique. The intracorporeal suturing is accomplished by continuous, interrupted or a combination of both types of suturing. Factors to be kept in mind before choosing suture material and type of needle to be used are length of incision, body tissue to be sutured, function of tissue. Length of suture to be taken depends upon length of incision. The common mistake in suturing is to work with too long or too short a piece of suture. For a single stitch thread should be approximately 14 cm long. A good rule of thumb for a running suture is to allow 14 cm for the first stitch and about 2-3 cm for each additional stitch. A suture incision ratio of 9:1 is best for longer suture lines and 10:1 is better for short suture lines.[2]

Interrupted suturing may be applied to approximate tissue that may be under tension or where visibility is needed for placement of further sutures. This is usually the type of suturing one attempts in the beginning of his or her suturing endeavors. Suture should be placed evenly bringing the tissue together without excessive tension. More often used in closure of vault of vagina after TLH (Total Laparoscopic Hysterectomy) repair of myoma bed, some times approximation of ovarian tissue.

Continuous suturing is quicker but more difficult to perform correctly. The continuous suturing technique begins and ends in an anchoring knot. The initial knot of the running suture can be formed by a standard square knot. For running portion of the suture one may use simple over and over running suture without locking. It is important that the assistant picks up the slack and keeps uniform tension during suturing. During training one should practice suturing in both directions. A golden rule is to identify anatomy before the start of suturing.

TECHNIQUE OF INTRACORPOREAL KNOTS-TYING

Intracorporeal knot-tying requires substantial practice for mastery and is a challenge for the novice. Advanced laparoscopic surgeries are hampered by the inability to perform intracorporeal knotting. The advantages of intracorporeal suturing are, lesser tissue trauma as compared to extracorporeal knot-tying.

Ideal knot is the traditional square knot. Basic knot is essential for open as well as laparoscopic surgery. First single half knot is followed by another half knot in opposite direction. It is prone to slippage when tissues are under tension. At least one needle driver is needed for passing the needle in the tissues,

the other instrument is the assisting instrument and can be another needle holder or simply a grasper. It is needed for stabilizing the tissues, needle or suture during suturing.

EXACT TECHNIQUE

Usually two needle holders are used. The needle is introduced in the abdomen by Clarke-Reich technique.[4-5] Small suture length is pulled inside the abdomen. The needle is aligned and held in the right needle holder. The left grasper or needle holder assists in optimizing needle entry into targeted tissue. The needle exits the tissue and is held at the tip by left needle holder. Then again it is pulled out of the tissue by the right needle holder. A "C" loop is formed by the right needle holder after pulling the suture and leaving a 3-4 cm suture at the tail end. So the suture now has two arms, the tail end and the standing part. The standing part makes a C loop and the left needle holder enters it from below and takes two throws. After the throws are completed the left needle holder picks up the tail end (Figs 6.1 to 6.12). Now at this point the throws are spilled from the tip of the left needle holder. It could be good to keep the left needle holder static and move the right needle holder only so that the throws spill easily from the tip and do not get strangulated, which may damage the suture. After the throws are spilled the needle holders are pulled apart in opposing direction to tie the first half of the knot. Then the second half of the square knot is applied by taking a single throw by the left needle holder and picking up the tail end. When this is done in opposite direction to the first knot, it forms a complete secure square knot. The suture is cut away and the needle is removed from the abdomen by grasping it with the end of the suture and the apple trocar is removed bringing the curved needle out of the abdomen along with it.

TIPS

- Know the anatomy well.
- Always keep the needle under view .
- The suture must be short in case of beginners
- If C loops can made to stand-up in front of the camera, the wrapping and knotting can be done conveniently and rapidly .
- Following wrapping the tail must be grasped as near the tip as possible.

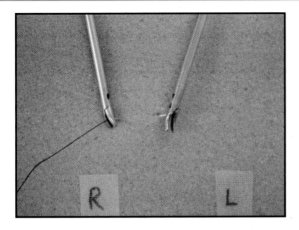

Fig. 6.1: Passing the curve needle by holding in the right needle holder. Needle is regrasped by the left needle holder as it exits from the tissue

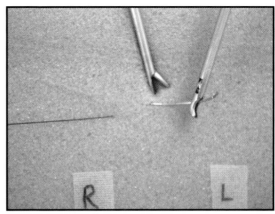

Fig. 6.2: Needle egress from the tissue is facilitated by counter pressure by the right needle holder

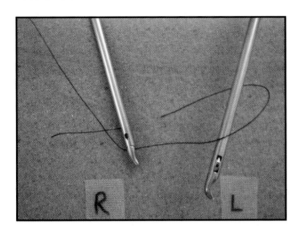

Fig. 6.3: With the right needle holder making a "C" loop the left needle holder enters from below and makes the throws

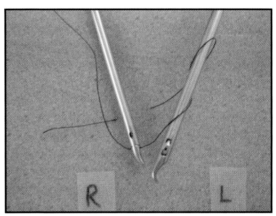

Fig. 6.4: The first throw by the left needle holder is completed

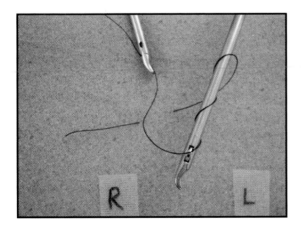

Fig. 6.5: Two throws are completed over the left needle holder, ready for tying the first half-knot

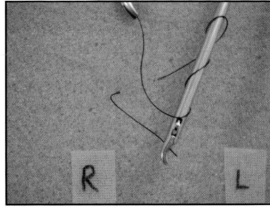

Fig. 6.6: Holding the tail end of the suture by the left needle holder after two throws have been taken

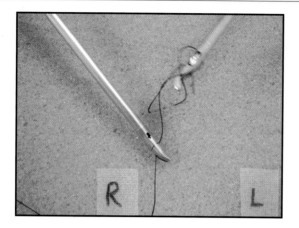

Fig. 6.7: keeping the left needle holder static, right needle holder spills the throws over the tip of the left needle holder

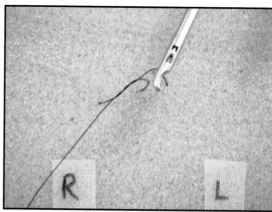

Fig. 6.8: The throws forming the first half-knot spilled over the left needle holder, ready for tying the knot

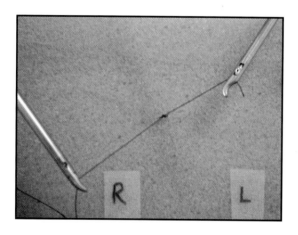

Fig. 6.9: The two needle holders holding the tail and standing part of suture pull in opposite direction to secure the knot

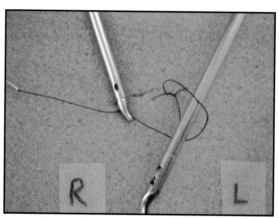

Fig. 6.10: "C" loop is formed and left needle holder passes below the "C" loop ready for second half knot

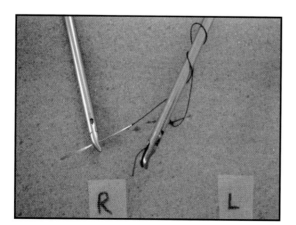

Fig. 6.11: Second half of the knot is formed by picking the tail end of suture and spilling the throws over the left needle holder

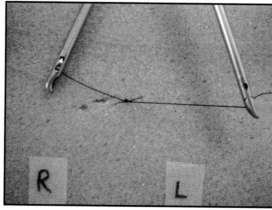

Fig. 6.12: Second half knot-tying is completed by pulling the both needle holder opposite to the direction of first half knot

- Don't pull the tail end first .
- For secure knotting the wrapping and pulling of the second component of the knot must be in reverse direction of the first.
- Close camera work aids in depth perception.

Everybody learns by mistakes, laparoscopic intracorporeal suturing is learnt by practice and has a learning curve. Experience is the name every one gives to their mistakes.

Suggested point where beginners can stuck up and remedy.

LOOSENING OF KNOT

The first half knot loosens during the time second knot is being tied, this phenomenon is known as loosening. Tightening the first half knot while second half knot is being configured in the following way. First wrap the second half knot over the instrument and pick the tail of the suture do not spill the wrap over the tip at this stage. Then continue to tighten with the wraps over the assisting instruments without spilling over the wrap of second half knot. When the first half knot will begin to tighten then spill the wrap of the second half knot over the tip of the assisting instruments followed by tightening of second half knot.

Some times short suture length will cause problems during continuous suturing or during multiple interrupted suturing. During this trouble shooting period one can hold the needle near the tip and form C-loop utilizing the length of the needle and follow the steps of knot-tying.

Some times needle deflection will occur during the time of driving the needle through the target tissue. At that point drive the needle slowly so that if deflection occurs the direction of penetration can be corrected.

COMPLICATIONS OF LAPAROSCOPIC SUTURING

The needle may traumatize the vessels or adjacent structure. So, precaution is to be taken during introduction and taking out the needle from the peritoneal cavity. Handle the needle only by the attached suture except when driving through the tissue.

Some times needle may be lost in the peritoneal cavity so always keep the needle under vision to avoid this complication. Needle to be parked in a safe position which is easily seen at all times during the surgery, like the pouch of Douglas. Some times radiological localization or visualization under C-arm may be helpful in such extreme situations.

CONCLUSION

Laparoscopic surgery is evolving and its applications are growing to include most gynecological operations. Today endoscopic surgeon is driven by the desire to perform a given procedure under laparoscopic guidance with the same expertise or even better than laparotomy. This passion can only be overcome with good performance of Intracorporeal suturing. Intracorporeal suturing application empowers the surgeon to accomplish a wide array of complex surgical procedures which could otherwise by unimaginable. With this background and more research done on improving existing surgical equipment, many less experienced endoscopists could learn and master laparoscopic intracorporeal suturing.

REFERENCES

1. Semm K. Tissue puncher and loop-ligation – new ideas for surgical therapeutic pelviscopy (Laparoscopy) endoscopic intra-abdominal surgery. Endoscopy 1978;10:119-24.
2. Desai PJ, Moran ME, Calvano CJ, Parekh AR. Running suturing: The ideal length facilities this task. J Endoural 2000;14:191-94.
3. Nathanson LK, Nathanson PDK, Cuschieri A. Safety of vessel ligation in laparoscopic surgery. Endoscopy 1991;23:206-09.
4. Clarke HC. Laparoscopy—new instrument for suturing and ligation. Fertil Steril 1972;23:274-77.
5. Reich H, McGlynn F. Laparoscopic repair of bladder injury. Obstet Gynecol 1990;76:909-10.

Sliding Knots

DANNY CHOU, NICK ELKINGTON
ANSHUMALA SHUKLA-KULKARNI
EBTIHAJ HASHIM

Chapter Seven

INTRODUCTION

All laparoscopic surgeons should be familiar with laparoscopic suturing and with both intracorporeal and extracorporeal knot tying. These techniques are useful for ligating blood vessels, approximating tissue planes or creating anastomoses. The ability to suture laparoscopically opens the door to performing more complex surgical procedures. This means that many operations that have traditionally been performed at laparotomy may now be accomplished laparoscopically.

Extracorporeal knot-tying is unique to endoscopic surgery. It can be learned easily and tends to be technically easier and quicker than intracorporeal knot-tying. Extracorporeal knots can be made either by tying individual square knots, that are pushed down repeatedly with a knot pusher, or by tying a sliding knot that is slipped or pushed down with the single pass of a knot pusher. Although there are a number of different sliding knots, it is not necessary to master them all, but it pays to become familiar with one or two and then to become adept at tying them.

This chapter aims to give a practical guide on how to perform three types of extracorporeal sliding knot: the sliding square knot, the modified Roeder knot and the Weston knot. The advantages and disadvantages of each knot are discussed and when they are most appropriately used.

THE SLIDING SQUARE KNOT

This is a relatively simple technique consisting of a series of alternating square knots, with each knot being pushed down with the repeated passage of a knot pusher.

After suturing or ligating a pedicle, the suture ends are brought out through the same port. Initially, a single throw (double throws tend not to run well) is made and a knot pusher engages one arm of the suture. The knot is "pushed down" with the knot pusher whilst the suture arm, which is not engaged with the knot pusher, is tensioned (but with less tension on the other arm) allowing the knot to slide down (Fig. 7.1A).

The knot pusher should be pushed beyond the knot (rather than onto the knot) with a technique called "pass pointing" (Fig. 7.1B). This avoids an

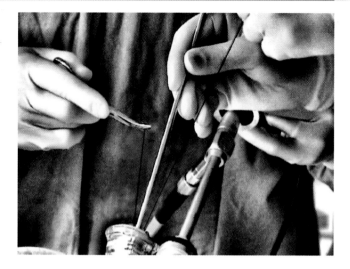

Fig. 7.1A: A sliding square knot

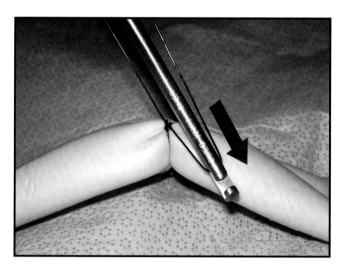

Fig. 7.1B: 'Pass pointing' during a sliding square knot

inadvertent "stabbing" injury to the pedicle and produces the ideal line of opposing tension for maximum knot security. The line of tension should be through the knot close to the pedicle to minimize pulling on the tissue. A series of alternating surgical square knots are repeated, the number of repetitions depending on the suture material and the strength of the knot required.

The sliding square knot works well with both monofilament and braided sutures. However, knot tension, particularly with the first throw is better maintained with braided sutures. Sutures need to be at least ninety centimeters long to provide enough length to make a tie outside the port.

There can be some technical problems associated with this technique. Maintaining adequate tension on the first knot can be difficult at times, particularly with monofilament sutures. In this situation a repeat throw in the same direction allows the second knot to tighten the first knot. Throws should alternate thereafter to minimize knot loosening. Entanglement of two arms of the suture can occur and this can be disentangled by rotating the knot pusher with its engaged arm, around the other arm. To minimize this, one should avoid changing sides of the ends of the suture.

Maintaining engagement of the knot pusher to one arm of the suture until it is tensioned can also be challenging. Re-engagement can be difficult, particularly if disengagement occurs with the knot inside the trocar. If this occurs the suture can be brought into laparoscopic view by using another instrument through another port and the suture re-engaged. A more efficient way of performing a sliding square knot is with the use of a knot pusher with a closed opening through which suture can be threaded (Fig. 7.2).

In this technique, after the two ends of the sutures are brought out through the port, one end is threaded through the opening and held loosely with an artery clip by the assistant. The surgeon holds the other arm of the suture with a non-dominant hand and the knot pusher with the dominant hand (Fig. 7.1A). Knots are tied with single hand technique and pushed down with the knot pushed immediately afterward while maintaining more tension on the arm held by the surgeon. At the point of 'pass pointing' the assistant provides just enough resistance to the push of the knot pusher to achieve good tension. This technique eliminates the repeated need to engage the knot pusher to the suture arm and the potential trouble of disengagement so is quicker.

Another common difficulty arises on knowing which, arm to maintain tension and how much. This comes with practice and generally with too much tension not only will the knot not run down but one also risks excessive pulling and tearing of the pedicle.

Maintaining the pneumoperitoneum can be a problem as gas can leak out through the port around the suture (during knot tying) and suture and knot pusher (during knot pushing). This can be particularly troublesome during the learning phase but can be minimized as one becomes more proficient. This can

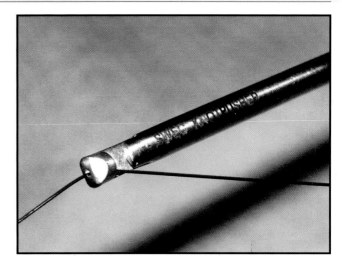

Fig. 7.2: The SWEC-Carlton knot pusher

be overcome by having the assistant's a finger placed over the top of the trocar to stop gas escaping during the extracorporeal throws. Some trocars are better at maintaining a seal than others. If there is significant loss of gas, one needs to stop the leak and re-establish an adequate pneumoperitoneum. Raising the rate of insufflation, and checking other potential sources of gas leakage (e.g. smoke evacuator) may be helpful.

This type of sliding knot, with practice, can be extremely efficient and quick. This laparoscopic square-sliding knot has comparable strength to conventional surgical knots (Dorsey, 1995). It can be used for a variety of tasks including ligation of major vessels including uterine artery and infundibulo-pelvic pedicles. It can also be used in reconstructive surgery, such as colposuspension suspensory sutures, paravaginal repair and McCall culdoplasty sutures.

THE MODIFIED ROEDER KNOT

A number of modifications to the original Roeder have been published in attempt to strengthen this slipknot. We favor the 4S-modified Roeder knot (Sharp, 1996), which has comparable strength to the conventional open square knots. The modification consists of four (4), instead of three wraps around the suture loop and securing the loop in place with a Square knot (two nonidentical half hitches) instead of a single half-hitch to the original knot. This knot is tied by initially making a single throw (Fig. 7.3A). One end is then wound around the two strands of the suture four times in a clockwise direction (Fig. 7.3B). The end that has been wrapped around

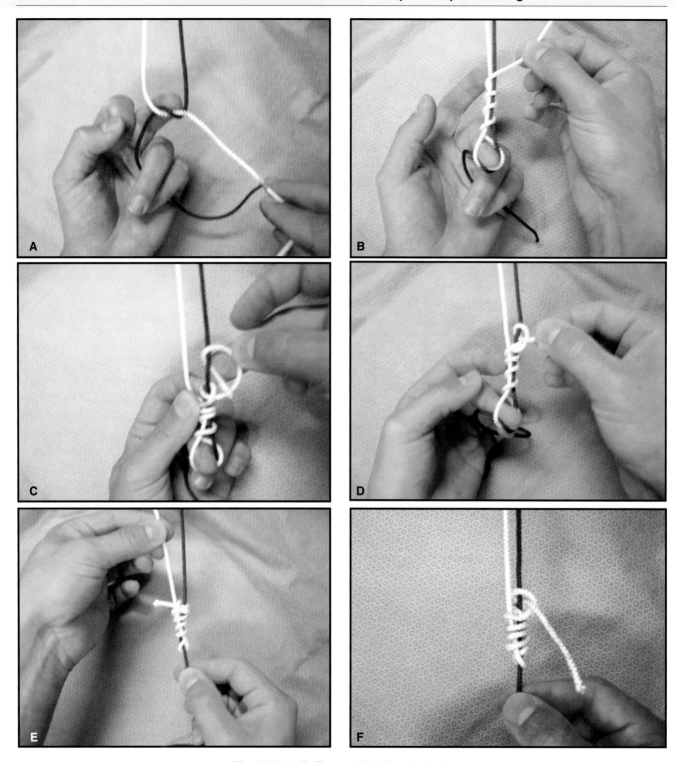

Figs 7.3A to F: The modified Roeder knot

is used to make two nonidentical half hitches to lock the suture (Figs 7.3C and D). The knot is then gathered together, by pulling the non-wound loop (Fig. 7.3E). The needle is then cut off and the short tied end trimmed (Fig. 7.3F). The long end that was not involved in the tying is then threaded through the eye of a knot-pusher and the knot is slid down onto the pedicle.

We feel the best knot pusher for pushing this type of robust, strong slipknot is one with a closed opening like the Carlton-SWEC knot pusher. This provides good uniform pressure around the knot allowing good axial counter tension right through the knot. Other grooved knot pushers tend to cause problems with knot disengagement. In the absence of a knot pusher, a grasper can be used to grasp the knot tight and push it down. However, this risks squashing the knot and the knot may not run nor tighten as well.

It is important to note that the knot is actually pushed by the knot pusher down onto the pedicle while the traction on the remaining end of the suture is only to provide counter traction. This allows the knot to slide down and reduces the loop around the pedicle as the knot is pushed down on it. At the final stage of tightening, one should have the tip of the knot pusher, with the knot, abutting against the tissue while applying traction on the remaining end. This minimizes any undesirable pull on the pedicle. There may be some loose loops that need to be "snuggled" down to ensure maximum knot security.

The modified Roeder knot is most suited when using monofilament sutures, such as PDS, Nylon or Monocryl sutures. With braided sutures, such as Vicryl, the knot is not likely to slide as well and risks the knot locking prematurely. Furthermore as the slipknot involves having the suture going through the tissue as the knot is being pushed towards the pedicle, there is a greater "sawing" effect on the tissue. The knot can occasionally lock "prematurely" before achieving desired tightening, even with the use of monofilaments. Some monofilament sutures like Monocryl, tend to be softer and easier to form a tight knot and may have a better tendency to lock, while Nylon, tends to be stiffer and has more "memory" and is less likely to create a tight knot. A common cause of "premature" locking occurs when the 4 loops override one another resulting in locking. Thus, maintaining a nice spiral configuration during knot tying can be helpful. A very tightly wound knot can be difficult to slide so it is best to keep it slightly loose and tighten it with the knot pusher. If "premature" locking occurs it is very important to realize the pushing should be the net force and resist excessive pull. In most cases the knot can be slid down with additional force, however, if the "prematurely" locked knot cannot be "unlocked", the knot may need

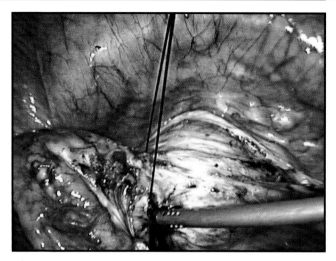

Fig. 7.4: Right uterine pedicle

to be cut and repeated or alternatively, tied intracorporeally.

The modified Roeder knot is a very strong sliding knot that is easily mastered with a little bit of practice. An advantage of this knot is that it only involves one passage of the knot pusher thus minimizing problems with potential loss of pneumoperitoneum. As the knot can be pushed down onto a pedicle, a modified Roeder knot is suitable for tying vascular pedicles. For this reason, this is our knot of choice for securing uterine artery pedicle (Fig. 7.4) and large infundibulopelvic ligaments.

The modified Roeder knot is also a strong helpful knot for reconstituting the uterus after myomectomy. It can also be used for the suspensory suture in colposuspension, however as it is a robust and strong knot, it is difficult to loosen if one has to modify the tension.

THE WESTON KNOT

The Weston knot is another very efficient slip knot (Weston, 1992). This knot is a simpler knot and thus can be performed quickly because it can be slipped down without a knot pusher. However, the knot is weaker and needs to be reinforced with intracorporeal throws. Thus, it makes it a good starting knot but one does need to be proficient at intracorporeal throws.

The Weston knot is tied by performing a single hitch (Fig. 7.5A). One end is then wound under the two strands of the suture in a clockwise direction (Fig. 7.5B). This is passed over the top of only one strand and threaded between the two strands and brought to top around the other strand (Fig. 7.5C).

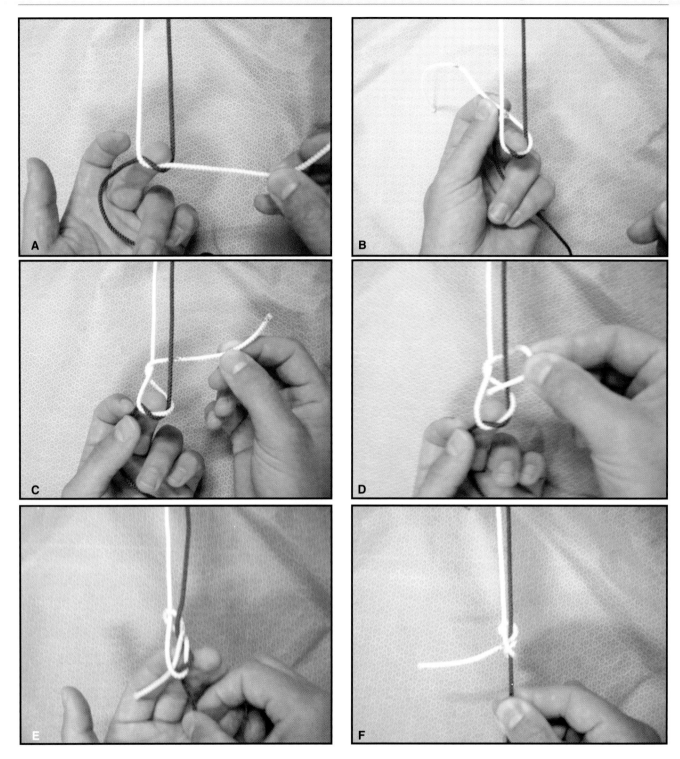

Figs 7.5A to F: The Weston knot

The end is placed through the loop form by the initial single hitch (Figs 7.5D and E). The final knot has a resemblance of a figure of eight wrapped around a suture (Figs 7.5F and 7.6A). The end of the knot should be long enough to allow easy intracorporeal knot tying.

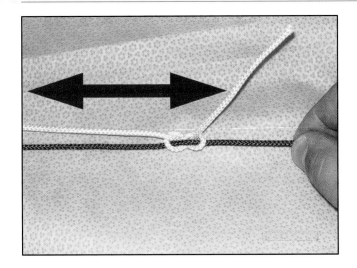
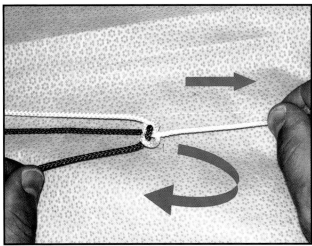

Figs 7. 6A and B: The sliding Weston knot (A) and knot locking (B)

The knot can often be slipped down through a port, with a tugging motion on the straight arm without the need of a knot pusher, depending on the suture material used and the tissue being tied. The knot can certainly be pushed down, as with modified Roeder knot but much of the attraction of this simple knot is that it can be tied quickly and slipped down quickly.

After slipping the knot down onto the pedicle, it is advisable to "lock" the knot before tying one or two intracorporeal reinforcing knots. The "locking" minimizes the knot loosening during intracorporeal knot tying. The slip knots has a common factor in the knot geometry that allows them to slip. That is, it involved one arm of the suture being maintained straight (straight arm) while the other is involved in wrapping around forming knots (wrapping arm) that will self-lock when the straight arm is pull to its limit. This can be appreciated on Figures 7.3F and 7.5F. The "locking" of Weston knot or any other slipknots is achieved by bending the straight arm. This can be easily performed by pushing the straight arm held above the knot, towards the knot itself while counter-tension is applied by pulling on the short end of wrapping arm, thus jackknifing the straight arm (Figs 7.6A and B).

This locking technique can be particularly helpful with suspensory sutures in colposuspension where slippage of the knot would result in loss of tension and this could compromise clinical outcome. Similarly this knot can almost always be "unlocked" by reversing the locking effect to loosen excessive tension.

The disadvantage of the Weston knot is its weaker strength and the need for an intracorporeal locking throw. When it is used without the knot pusher, the upward traction pulls on the pedicle as it is being tightened. This makes it unsuitable when tying delicate structures such as vascular pedicles or bowel. However, it is a quick suture that is suitable for suturing firm tissue whilst allowing the correction of excessive tension. Weston knots can also be used with some braided sutures. We favor Weston knots in procedures such as laparoscopic colposuspension (Fig. 7.7), laparoscopic pelvic floor repair, and closure of vaginal vault in total laparoscopic hysterectomy.

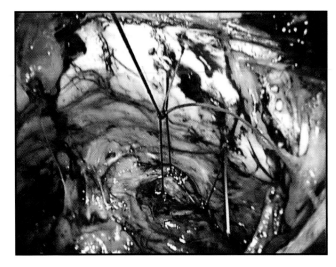

Fig. 7.7: Weston knot for laparoscopic colposuspension

KNOT PUSHERS

Knot pushers are a very important knot-tying instrument but are often unappreciated. There are several designs available (Fig. 7.8). The ideal knot pusher should be reusable, easily sterilized, 4 mm diameter and about 45 cm long. It should not have any sharp edges or points that could cut into the suture or tissue. It should also be suitable for monofilament and braided sutures of most suture diameters.

At Sydney Women's Endosurgery Centre (SWEC), Dr Mark Carlton has taken all these criteria into consideration and after several prototypes has designed and developed a very practical knot pusher that can be used for a wide range of laparoscopic knot-tying (Fig. 7.9).

The unique design allows the suture to be threaded through the "eye" at the tip of the knot pusher and be easily retrieved. It allows the knots or the suture arm to remain engaged with the knot pusher at all time throughout the knot tying.

Ethicon has developed the endoknot pack which includes a monofilament suture pre-threaded through a plastic knot pusher (Fig. 7.10). The knot pusher has a conical end, which is used to slide the knot on to the tissue. This is effective in tying all the sliding knots without using an additional knot pusher. The suture length included in it is about 107 cm, which allows one to tie multiple knots with one pack. We use it most often to tie the infundibulopelvic ligaments bilaterally with a modified Roeder knot in total laparoscopic hysterectomy.

CONCLUSIONS

Mastering laparoscopic suturing and sliding knots equips the surgeon for a wider range of advanced laparoscopic surgical procedures. Although there are many types of sliding knot, we have simply described three commonly used knots. We have found these applicable to all our surgical requirements although some are preferable in certain situations. With an understanding of the advantages and disadvantages of each type of knot, one can choose, one's preferred sliding knot for the required task. This will save time, minimize technical problems and help improve surgical outcome. Although most advanced laparoscopic procedure can be carried out with extracorporeal knot tying, intracorporeal knot tying is still recommended

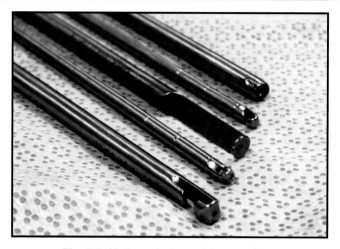

Fig. 7.8: Various designs of knot pushers

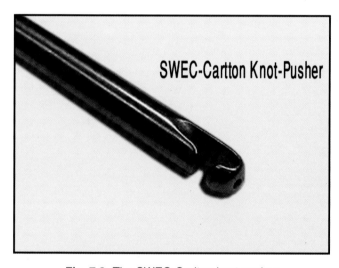

Fig. 7.9: The SWEC-Carlton knot pusher

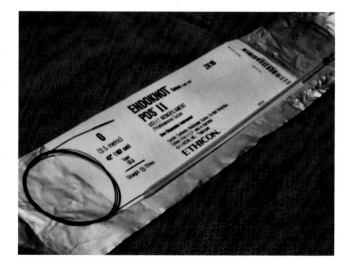

Fig. 7.10: The Ethicon Endoknot with plastic knot pusher

for closure of delicate tissues such as the bowel, bladder and for fine anastomoses of fallopian tubes and ureters.

The strength of different sliding knots can vary widely. The sliding square knot has been shown to be the strongest. The Roeder knot is not as strong as compared to conventional open square knots but a number of modifications have been reported with some being comparable to conventional square knots (Dorsey JH 1995). Weaker but simpler sliding knots, such as the Weston knot, can be used where approximation of tissues is required without tension.

From our experience of running laparoscopic courses, the best way to learn laparoscopic knot tying is by repetitive practice and surgical application, once one has familiarized from the diagrams, pictures and videos. Many challenging factors such as thin, short suture ends, slippery wet gloves, dim operating theatres and leaking ports add to the challenges. However, these can be easily overcome with persistence and practice.

REFERENCES

1. Dorsey JH, Sharp HT, Chovan JD, Holtz PM. Laparoscopic knot strength: a comparison with conventional knots. Obstet Gynecol 1995; 86(4 Pt 1):536-40.
2. Sharp HT, Dorsey JH, Chovan JD, Holtz PM. The effect of knot geometry on the strength of laparoscopic slip knots. Obstet Gynecol 1996;88(3):408-11.
3. Weston PV. A new clinch knot. Obstet Gynecol 1992; 79(1):156.

The Concept of Ipsilateral Suturing and Clinical Applications

NUTAN JAIN

Chapter Eight

Historically laparoscopic suturing was introduced with Kurt Semm[1] describing the use of Endo Loops. However this had limited applications being useful only for mobile pedicles. Since then laparoscopy and laparoscopic suturing have come a long way. All the contraindications of laparoscopy in the earlier years are now gradually becoming the day-to-day applications of laparoscopy. This wide shift in contraindications becoming standard applications of laparoscopy today has only been possible due to the excellence achieved in suturing skills. The pioneers were of course[2,3] Reich and Clarke who started the concepts of introduction of curved needles and use of knot pushers for positioning the extracorporeal knots. But it appears that prolonged applications of suturing requiring a lot of sutures as in pelvic floor repair, suturing of myomectomy bed and tubal microsurgery cannot be executed by extracorporeal suturing alone. Thus, the need for skillful intra corporeal suturing arises.

The conventional method of laparoscopic suturing[4,5] was the one in which two lower lateral ports, placed on either side of the abdomen (Figs 8.1 A and B) lateral to rectus abdominis muscle 1-2 cm above the anterior superior iliac spines were utilized. This technique remained highly popular for a very long time. This was and still is a fixed notion among many surgeons that the two needle holders should approach the intended suture line at right angles. This has been proved beyond doubt that is not true and a much better and comfortable suturing way is to approach the needle and needle holders from the same side. The drawbacks of ipsilateral suturing were obvious, the surgeon standing on the left or right of the patient was approaching the tissue to be sutured, by bringing one of his hands from a distant port placed in the lower abdomen on the contralateral side. This posed various problems.

1. Approaching the suture site by an altogether less ergonomic, unusual way where in hands cross over each other. Do we eat with the fork and knife approaching from points at 180 degrees to each other? We normally work with two hands going parallel to each other. The same is true for open surgery. Both hands of the surgeon work together in close coordination approaching the tissue in the same direction and axis. So when we do laparoscopy, as it is there is difficulty in holding needles, sutures and needle holders and this is further complicated by abnormal hand movement thereby posing a lot of difficulty in

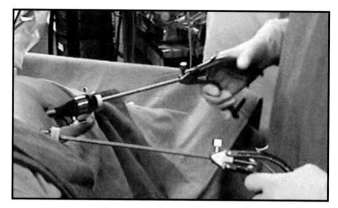

Fig. 8.1A: Ipsilateral suturing

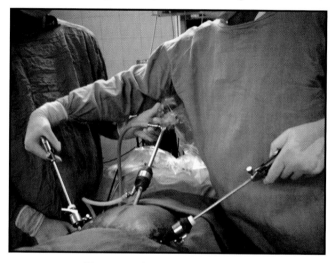

Fig. 8.1B: Contralateral suturing

learning, trying to adapt to an abnormal hand movement sequence which the surgeon has never done in his formative years.

2. Loss of precision: When the surgeon is approaching the suture site with one hand working at least 30 cm away from his own body the precision has to be low, more so when handling a delicate tissue requiring exact coaptation.

3. Surgeon's fatigue after one to two hours of prolonged suturing with hands in the crossed over position and the amount of stress posed on the surgeon's shoulder due to this position. There have been several reports of increased risk of cervical and shoulder spondylitis in laparoscopic surgeons which could easily be aggravated by assuming stressful working and suturing styles.

So to be more precise, ergonomic, less stressful and more adapted to physiological methods is the concept of ipsilateral suturing. In this way of suturing the surgeon makes the lower ports as usual, but also makes a paraumbilical port on the same side as he stands. So the Endoscopic surgeon is working in extreme comfort, using both hands in the most familiar way as he has been doing all his life in all his day-to-day activities. The concept of ipsilateral suturing pioneered by Dr Charles H Koh[6–12] is a boon to laparoscopy. It becomes an instant starting point for learning "stress free" suturing. It is additionally beneficial for short statured or female surgeons for whom approaching the contralateral port is even more difficult. The ipsilateral port is not only beneficial for suturing, it is a *total surgical style* where the hands work in their normal resting position enabling the surgeon to deliver his best skills and precision. Ipsilateral port placement actually makes the laparoscopic working style akin to the more conventional open surgical style, making it easier to learn and quicker to master.

EXACT TECHNIQUE

With this introduction of ipsilateral port placement we shall now go on to its exact technique and clinical applications.

Exact port placement for ipsilateral suturing remains like shown in Figure 8.2. Most of the surgeons operate while standing on the left side of the patient, so the ipsilateral ports are placed on the left side. There are two lateral ports as usual and additionally there is a paraumbilical port on the side the surgeon stands. If it is microsurgery the paraumbilical port is 3 mm. While usually it is 5 mm. In case of prolonged suturing applications as required in pelvic floor reconstruction then it is 10 mm so that the curved needle can be introduced directly without the need of removing the trocar every time. The distinct steps of curved needle introduction and suturing in ipsilateral style are:

1. Remove the lower left 5 mm trocar and back load the needle on a 5 mm valve less apple trocar held in a needle holder. A suture grasper can also be used but usual preference is using two needle holders for suturing (Figs 8.3A to G).
2. The suture is held in the left lower needle holder about 2 cm from the hub of the needle, and it is introduced in the peritoneal cavity like this. After the needle passage the valveless, trocar is positioned appropriately by gently securing it inside the abdominal cavity.
3. At this point introduce only small length of the suture inside the abdomen, and not the full length of the suture, as showing too much suture (Fig. 8.4A) in the laparoscopic field confuses the

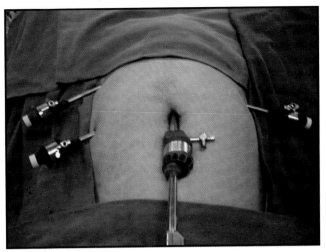

Fig. 8.2: Port placement for ipsilateral suturing

surgeon during needle passage and knot tying. The ratio of suture to incision is usually 9:1.

4. The curved needle is hung vertically by the left needle holder (Fig. 8.4B) at right angles to patient's body, with the concavity of the needle facing towards the pelvis. This is a very easy position for grasping the needle by the right needle (Fig. 8.4C) holder at junction of anterior two-thirds and posterior one-third. After a secure grip this needle is then turned in a horizontal manner so that the concavity of the needle is facing towards the anterior abdominal wall or the "Smiley Needle" (Koh).
5. Then the left handed instrument, either the needle holder or grasper, applies a little tug (Fig. 8.4D) on the suture which automatically allows needle to come in "good smiley position".
6. This is the final position of the needle ready for suturing, "smiley needle, or the half moon effect" with the convexity of the needle facing down (Fig. 8.4E)
7. The suturing is done in the vertical zone. Means, that the needle passes the tissue bites from below upwards always. The needle holder is in horizontal alignment and the needle is in the vertical zone passing through tissues from below upwards.
8. For ipsilateral suturing the surgical incision needs to be transverse to effectively carry out continuous curved needle suturing. Suturing becomes a pleasure and does not give any stress to the surgeon or assistant.
9. Needle passes through the lower flap of the surgical incision with help of delicate wrist movement. Needle is taken out of the upper flap,

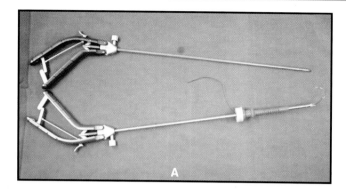

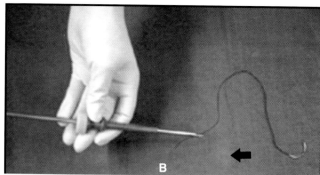

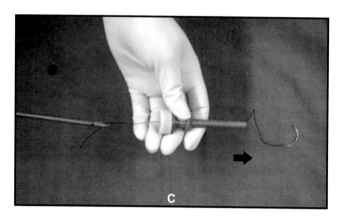

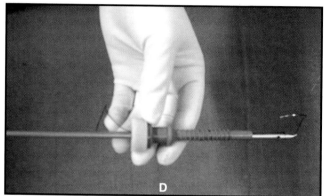

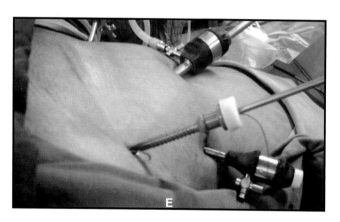

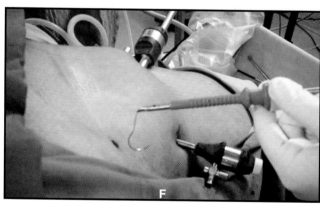

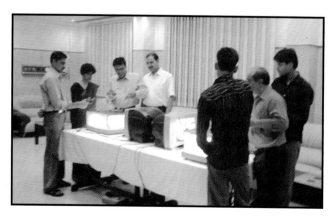

Figs 8.3A to G: Loading the needle for intracorporeal suturing: (A) Right and left handed Koh needle holder, (B) Holding free end of the suture and pulling it in the trocar, (C) Bringing the suture out through the valveless apple trocar, (D) Holding the thread 2 cm from the hub of the needle, (E) Insertion of the needle in the peritoneal cavity, (F) Removing the needle from abdominal cavity, (G) Practising ipsilateral suturing on pelvic trainers

Aligning the Needle Inside the Abdominal Cavity

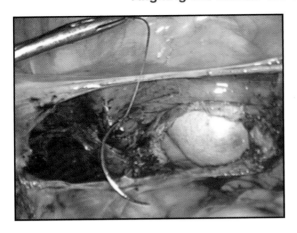

Fig. 8.4A: Introducing the curve needle by holding it 2 cm away from the hub by left needle holder

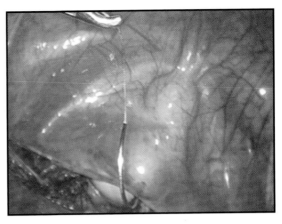

Fig. 8.4B: Hanging the needle vertically by left needle holder with the concavity of the needle facing towards the pelvis

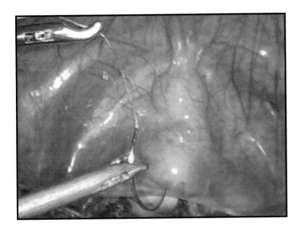

Fig. 8.4C: Grasping the needle at junction of anterior 2/3 and posterior 1/3 by right needle holder

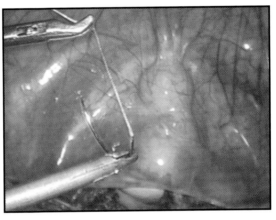

Fig. 8.4D: By a little tug on the thread from left needle holder aligns the needle in smiley position

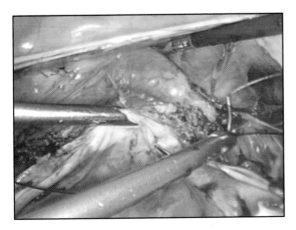

Fig. 8.4E: Needle in smiley position correctly aligned for suturing

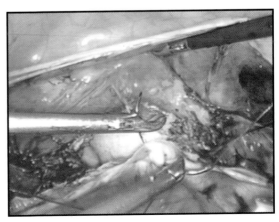

Fig. 8.4F: Regrasping the needle by left needle holder as it comes out of the tissue

while the needle holder in the left hand pushes the tissue back and this facilitates the egress of the needle through the upper flap.

10. As the needle emerges from the upper flap it is instantly held in correct "Smiley" alignment by the left needle holder (Fig. 8.4F) without allowing it to drop. This saves lot of time and frustration which could be spent on correct aligning in "Smiley position".

11. The first knot is tied as square surgeons knot. The right needle holder makes a loop or C and the left needle holders enters it from below and takes two throws and then grasps the free tail end of the suture. It is tied securely and then another throw reinforces it by pulling in opposite direction (Fig. 8.5A).

12. From here on curved continuous needle progresses in an identical manner, regrasping the needle as it emerges from the upper flap without allowing it to drop. This saves tremendous suturing effort and surgical time.

13. The continuous suture is closed by utilizing the curve of the needle (Fig. 8.6K). The needle is held in the right needle holder in a smiley position and the left needle holder enters from below takes two throws and grasp the free end and ties a secure surgeon knot. This is re-enforced by another throw.

14. The needle held by the suture is removed out of the peritoneal cavity by removing the short apple, valveless trocar (Fig. 8.5B). The movements of needle introduction and removal from the peritoneal cavity are done under direct visual control, otherwise the needle may get lost or could drag on soft tissue, causing trauma.

With this introduction of ipsilateral port placement and suturing we shall now go over to the discussion of clinico-surgical applications in various gynecological surgeries.

MYOMECTOMY

In laparoscopy if we are able to deliver the same suturing pattern as in open laparotomy then all criticism of laparoscopic myomectomy regarding fear of scar, dehiscence during pregnancy or labor become non-existent.[13-16] Traditionally in open surgery myoma bed has been sutured in two or three layers obliterating the myoma bed from deeper planes to the more superficial ones. Suturing in two or three layer gives more anatomical closure and added

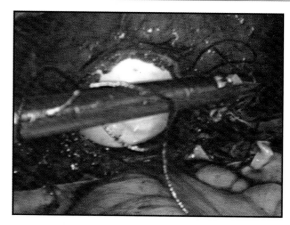

Fig. 8.5A: Making two throws by the left needle holder and picking the tail end of the suture

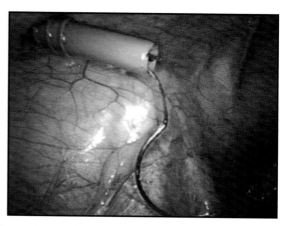

Fig. 8.5B: Removing the needle from abdominal cavity by removing the valveless apple trocar along with the needle

strength to the myoma bed which can endure the stress of pregnancy and labor.[17] There is lesser risk of hematoma or a fistula formation.[18-20] The exact technique entails the employment of ipsilateral ports for suturing on the same side as the surgeon stands, i.e. his right or left. The myoma incision is given transversely over the most bulging part of the myoma. Prior injection of pitressine reduces the bleeding from incision site. Vicryl 1-0 on a taper cut, needle is the preferred suture material. A suture about 45 cm in length is loaded on a needle holder and introduced in the peritoneal cavity by the Clarke Reich technique of removing the smaller valveless apple trocars (Figs 8.6A to F). The angle knot is taken by passing the suture on the upper and lower edges of the myoma bed. Intracorporeal knot is tied making a secure, surgeon's knot. From this point on continuous suturing is done passing the needle from the lower flap to the upper edge without locking (Figs 8.6G to L). The assistant plays an important role in

Laparoscopic Myomectomy

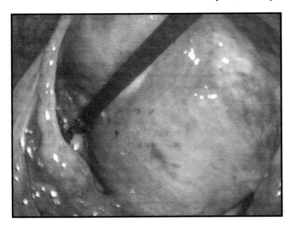

Fig. 8.6A: Initial appearance of myoma

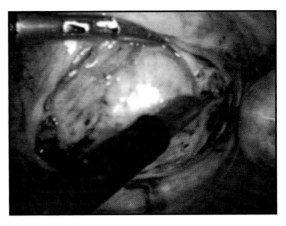

Fig. 8.6B: Transverse incision over the myoma by monopolor hook

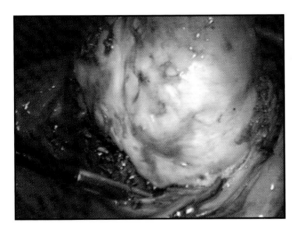

Fig. 8.6C: Enucleation of the myoma

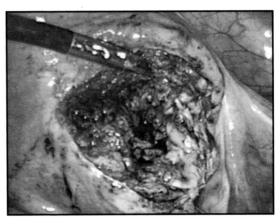

Fig. 8.6D: Cavity after removal of myoma

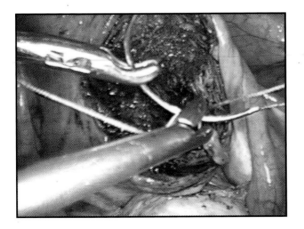

Fig. 8.6E: Smiley position of the needle

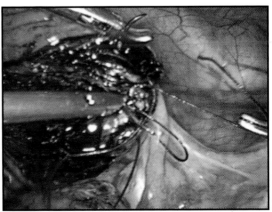

Fig. 8.6F: Passing the needle

Laparoscopic Myomectomy

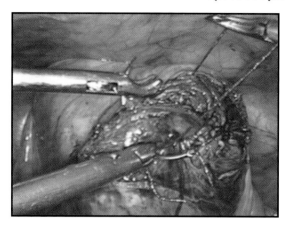

Fig. 8.6G: First layer in progress

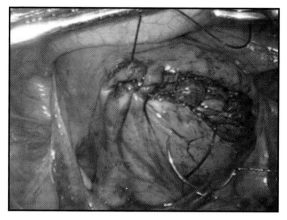

Fig. 8.6H: First layer is completed

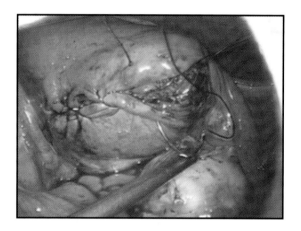

Fig. 8.6I: Second layer in progress

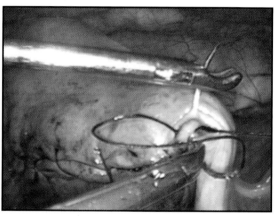

Fig. 8.6J: Second layer almost completed

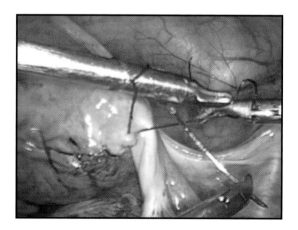

Fig. 8.6K: Tying the knot utilizing the curve
of the needle

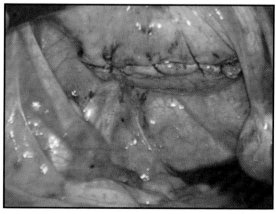

Fig. 8.6L: Final picture of myomectomy

pulling the slack of the suture and keeping adequate tension on the suture when the surgeon passes the successive sutures. Needle holders in both hands give a much better grip and needle alignment becomes easier. The needle is re-grasped as it comes out of the upper flap and is realigned immediately without letting it fall. This adds a lot of speed and convenience to continuous curved needle suturing. It is extremely important to keep aligning the needle as soon as it exits from the upper flap of the myoma bed. The bites in the tissue are taken according to the thickness of the myometrial bed and keeping in mind that it gives good anatomical closure without being too bulky or too thin, both of which will result in either inadequate or bad tortous suture line. Sutures should be placed evenly, bringing the tissue together without excessive tension or malalignment of layers. The first layer is thus completed by passing running non-locking suture from one end of the myoma bed to the other where it is anchored by a square knot. If the myometrial defect is small and adequate suture length still remains, the same suture is used to stitch the superficial myometrium and serosa up to the starting point of the first layer at the angle. While suturing the superficial layer it is extremely important to pass the sutures at an even distance and take almost same amount of tissue in each bite to give a neat look to the finished suture line. At the end of the suture line a good anchoring square knot is used and can be tied to the tail end of the first knot given at the start of the suturing. So, in this way, there is only one knot in the entire myoma bed. The amount of adhesions formed per suture line is directly proportional to the number of knots. Lesser the number of bulky knots, lesser the adhesion formation. Copious irrigation and lavage is done and complete hemostasis achieved. No adhesion barrier is used. About 2 liters of RL is left for hydrofloatation.

TIPS

When handling long suture lengths it is imperative that the suture be released inside the peritoneal cavity only slowly and passed in such a way that it does not appear much in the laparoscopic view. It is rather parked in the mid abdomen over the bowel and only necessary suture length is visible in laparoscopic view while suturing. Initially, it could be difficult to manage longer lengths but with more suturing experience gained especially for myomectomy it becomes much easier to suture the entire bed with one long suture and give only one knot on the surface.

CLOSURE OF VAGINAL VAULT AFTER TLH

Utilizing the technique of ipsilateral port and employing continuous curved needle suturing, closure of vaginal vault is the easiest form of suturing in gynae laparoscopic surgery. The closure is done in two layers starting on the right side of the patient for a surgeon standing on the left of the patient. The suture length used is about 40 cm, the suture material is polyglycolic acid 1-0 on a taper cut needle. A good bite is taken on the posterior vaginal wall at the angle, the needle is then passed into the anterior vaginal wall and an anchoring knot preferably an intracorporeal square knot is taken (Figs 8.7A to F). The tail end of the knot is left a little longer as it is used to finish the suture when we come back with the second layer. The first layer progresses in a continuous non-locking manner using two needle holders. After the angle stitch, a good bite of the right uterosacral ligament is taken and then we proceed up to the left angle passing bites successively through posterior and anterior vaginal walls, taking care to avoid the bladder coming in the suture. After this a bite is taken through the uterosacral ligament of the left side. I usually take the same suture to go back for the second layer. In the second layer (Figs 8.7G to L) anteriorly the pubocervical fascia and posteriorly the rectovaginal fascia is additionally incorporated in the suture line. Again it is important to take a through and through bite of adequate tissue that is neither too small nor too bulky, to give an anatomically aesthetic looking closure. The assistant's role is to apply adequate tension on the suture line and adjust the slack of the suture. Using two needle holders adds to the speed and comfort of closure. The second running layer is closed by anchoring a Square knot into the tail end of the knot of the first layer. At the end of the second layer we utilize the curve of the round body needle to make a knot known as the "half moon effect" or smiley needle. Towards the end when the remaining suture length is smaller it is advantageous to make the knot utilizing the curve of the needle. This adequate closure of vaginal vault provides all prophylactic measures for prevention of posthysterectomy vault prolapse and is thus an ideal method. If the patient has more slackness posteriorly then more bites are taken in uterosacral

Vault Suturing

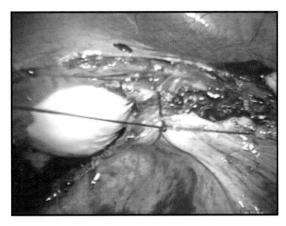

Fig. 8.7A: First knot tied

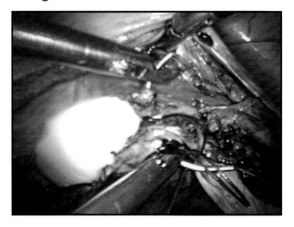

Fig. 8.7B: Needle passed through anterior and posterior vaginal wall

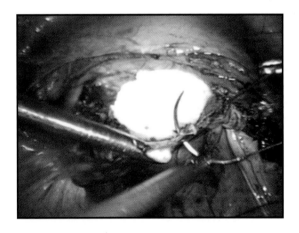

Fig. 8.7C: Needle passing through the posterior edge of vagina

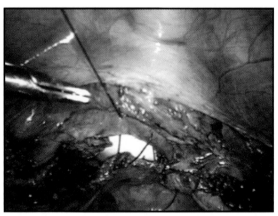

Fig. 8.7D: First layer in progress

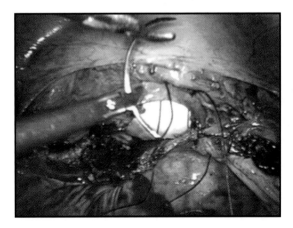

Fig. 8.7E: Needle is regrasped in correct alignment

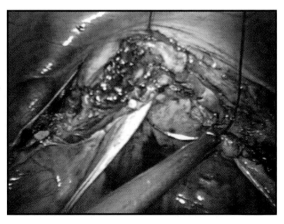

Fig. 8.7F: Needle passing through left uterosacral ligament

Vault Suturing

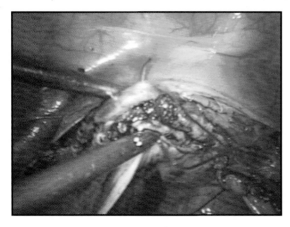

Fig. 8.7G: Second layer closure started

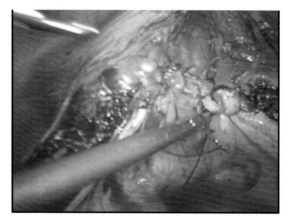

Fig. 8.7H: Second layer in progress

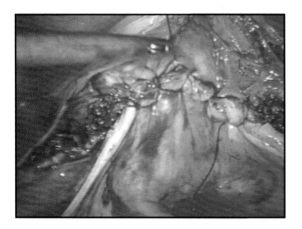

Fig. 8.7I: Second layer almost completed

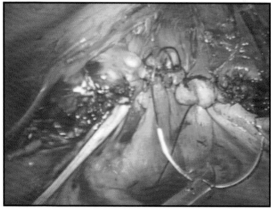

Fig. 8.7J: Holding needle in smiley position to close the continuous suture

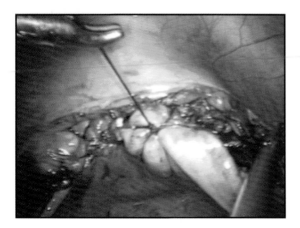

Fig. 8.7K: Securing the final knot

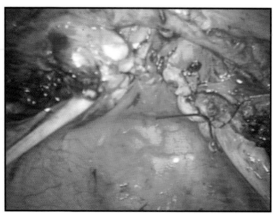

Fig. 8.7L: Completed vault repair with uterosacral ligament plication

ligaments to ensure proper support to vaginal vault.[21,22] So, through a combination of suturing in the vertical zone, employment of ipsilateral ports and use of two needle holders, very good suturing of the vault can be accomplished in a much shorter time without surgeon fatigue. And once again I stress, suturing of the vaginal vault is the easiest and, in fact, the best surgical area to practice continuous curved needle suturing.

Bladder Repair

Rather than intentional cystostomies gynecological laparoscopist would be suturing for too many unintentional, accidental bladder lacerations.[23,24] Bladder is easily injured in anterior dissections in patients with previous cesarean sections undergoing laparoscopic hysterectomy. Other vulnerable points of bladder injury are during entry, dissection and surgery in the space of Retzius. Prior surgery in this region compounds the risk to bladder. Rather than to panic, it is more important to recognize and adequately repair bladder injury laparoscopically. Bladder is our close neighbor and a "perfect gentleman". Wounds after bladder repair heal well if care is taken in suturing them laparoscopically on the same principles of suturing as described for myoma repair and vaginal vault repair. 3-0 vicryl on a small, curved, round body needle is utilized, ipsilateral port, placement and continuous curved needle closure is done in two layers without tension. The suture is usually started on the right side of the bladder laceration after ascertaining the position of the tringone and ureteric orifices the suture is anchored at the angle by a secure square knot. About 30 cm of suture length is employed (Figs 8.8A to F). After this point continuous curved needle suturing is done wherein adequate tissue bites are taken from the lower and upper edges of the bladder wall. Care is taken to grasp almost equal amount of tissue in each bite and to take the successive bites at most equal distance. This gives a very nice anatomical closure which heals well. The second layer of closure is started with the same suture after completing the first layer and it reinforces the first layer. It is important not to put too much tension on the suture by tying to make it watertight. Just adequate tension on the suture line ensures a good closure and good healing in postoperative phase. The completeness and adequacy of the closure is checked by inflating the bladder with about 150 ml of saline with methylene blue. After ensuring water tight closure a cystoscopy is performed to check the ureteric function on either side. The patient is put on continuous Foley's catheter drainage for seven days postoperatively.

Thus, again the message is, if one is adept at suturing, any complication can be managed laparoscopically without greatly altering the postoperative course and morbidity. Hence, the adage "Suture is Future"

Bowel Repair

Accidental enterostomy again could be a peril of more advanced laparoscopic procedures. Peritoneal entry in a patient with multiple previous laparotomies and management of advanced endometriosis are the two most frequently encountered modes of injury.[25–27]

The repair of bowel wounds laparoscopically is dependant, largely on two factors: Preoperative bowel preparation and Surgeon's suturing capabilities. It goes without saying that an adequately prepared bowel is the hallmark of successful outcome of primary laparoscopic repairs. A properly prepared bowel if injured by trocar or lacerated during adhesiolysis can be repaired transversely employing the ipsilateral port placement and curved needle intracorporeal suturing. This is accomplished by using 3-0 vicryl on a small curved needle, using 30 cm of suture length. Two layer closure is done, the important aspect being the tension free suture line (Figs 8.9A to F). The second layer reinforces the first layer and since it is done in a continuous manner the suture is closed at the end by taking a square knot. Mostly these wounds are small, about one to two cm and a laparoscopic closure can be easily done. Manual dexterity in laparoscopic suturing is important in completing this challenging task. The risk of litigation remains high in these unfortunate cases so it is extremely important that laparoscopic closure be done in a precise, tension free manner leading to good closure and healing in postoperative phase. After large bowel repair an underwater check for perfect closure is done by passing air through a Foley's catheter inserted in the rectum. If air bubbles come out from the suture site further reinforcing sutures are required.

Postoperatively patients are managed nil orally until bowel sounds appear and patient expresses a desire to accept by mouth. Prolonged IV supplementation and nasogastric suction is not required. Slowly the patient starts liquids and then progresses to a semi-solid and later a full diet.

Laparoscopic Management of Bladder Injury

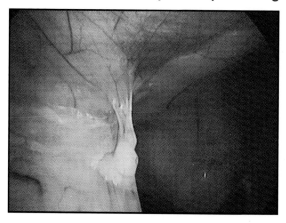

Fig. 8.8A: Omental adhesion to anterior abdominal wall in a patient of primary infertility with genital Koch's

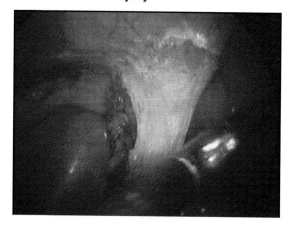

Fig. 8.8B: Adhesiolysis being done

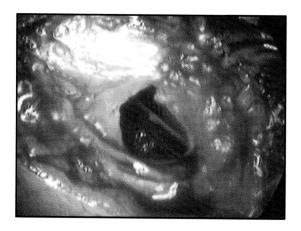

Fig. 8.8C: Appearance of bladder injury

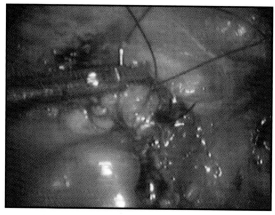

Fig. 8.8D: Beginning the curve needle suturing

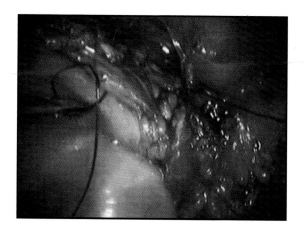

Fig. 8.8E: Continuous suturing in progress

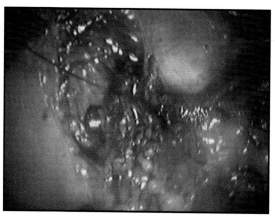

Fig. 8.8F: Final appearance of suturing

Laparoscopic Management of Rectal Injury

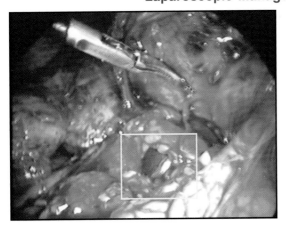

Fig. 8.9A: Rectal probe seen during laparoscopy

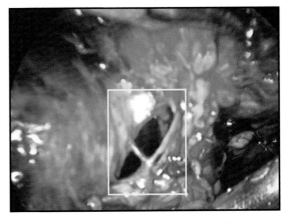

Fig. 8.9B: Appearance of rectal injury

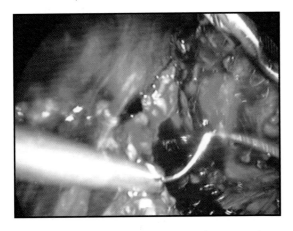

Fig. 8.9C: Starting the continuous two layer suturing

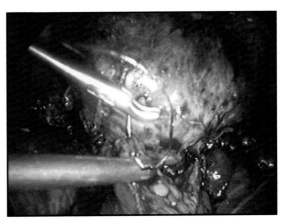

Fig. 8.9D: Suturing in progress

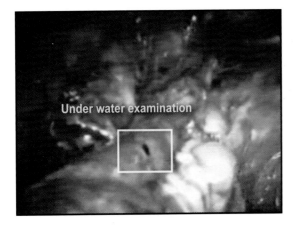

Fig. 8.9E: Under water examination showing a small rent with air bubbles coming out

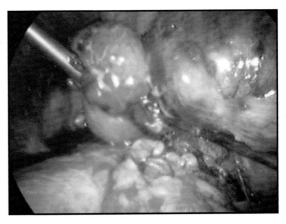

Fig. 8.9F: Final appearance after suturing

PELVIC RECONSTRUCTION

After having learnt and mastered suturing skills in easier applications like myoma bed and vault repair in laparoscopic hysterectomy, one is ready[28–32] to venture into complex and prolonged applications of suturing. High levels of skill and speed are required for total laparoscopic repair of enterocoele and other pelvic organ prolapse with or without an intact uterus. It is extremely important that the surgical anatomy of the pelvic floor and the support mechanism in a normal standing female be thoroughly understood before attempting a pelvic floor repair laparoscopically. Applications commonly required in pelvic organ prolapse:

1. Hi McCall culdoplasty with vault repair in laparoscopic hysterectomy
2. Uterosacral ligament plication for cervical descent not associated with significant rectocoele.
3. Posthysterectomy vault prolapse
4. Advanced degrees of pelvic organ prolapse with an intact uterus.

All the above applications are covered in various sections of this book. I shall just describe the technique of prolapse repair when uterus is intact in a younger patient still wanting child bearing. In the preoperative phase all defects are recognized and a careful note is made. Then during anesthesia the preoperative findings are reconfirmed and note made of any additional repair required other than the intended one. Port placement is same as in ipsilateral suturing with surgeon standing on the left of the patient. A vaginal probe is introduced in the posterior fornix which reduces the prolapse in the peritoneal cavity. A rectal probe is also inserted. Ureteric dissection is the first step before starting any dissection or suturing, ureteric dissection is done on both sides starting at pelvic brim right upto the base of uterosacral ligaments (Figs 8.10A to C). A transverse incision is given over the vaginal apex from one uterosacral ligament to the other. The vaginal walls are pushed anteriorly till the base of the uterus and posteriorly till the rectovaginal septum and fascia is exposed. A curved needle is passed through the lower port on the left side and is positioned and aligned by the needle holder in a smiley needle position held in the paraumbilical port on the left side. Two needle holders are used, the surgeon sutures with both hands. For prolonged suturing applications, being ambidextrous helps. I can suture with equal flair with both hands and this comes in handy whenever I need to change hands due to fatigue or better suturing application.

The first anchoring stitch begins by attaching the levator ani muscle to the mid vagina. This is secured by a square knot. Suture material used is 0-PDS, delayed absorbable. Thereafter the same, 45 cm long suture is used to approximate the redundant vagina anteroposteriorly. Series of sutures are passed from the base of the uterus up to the rectovaginal fascia. These series of tier sutures obliterate the potential hiatus from where prolapse occurs. After having achieved the levator stitch and the tier sutures on the right and left, we incorporate the uterosacral ligament an either side to this obliterated vaginal platform (Figs 8.10D to L). All this is done by continuous curved needle suturing employing suturing in vertical zone. Then the last step is the plication of uterosacral ligament. This is achieved by nonabsorbable suture 1-0 ethibond or 1-0 prolene. The exact technique requires taking successive bites in the uterosacral ligament starting at the level of the ischial spine. The ischial spine is palpated vaginally by the assistants or surgeon's finger and can thus be oriented laparoscopically. The successive bites of suture then pass at the base of the uterus or cervico uterine junction. This is tied extracorporeally using weston sliding knots (refer to chapter on sliding knots). The same is repeated on the contralateral side. At this point the surgeon examines from the vaginal end and if there is still redundancy or the cervix still shows at the hiatus or lower then the desired level, an extrastitch is taken with prolene from one uterosacral ligament and attached to a higher point between two uterosacral ligament at cervicouterine junction and then the same suture is passed on the contralateral uterosacral ligament. This is then brought back to the starting point by passing one or two sutures on the uterocervical junction and uterosacral ligament. This is then tied extracorporeally by a sliding weston knot. After passing this last suture the end result looks very neat as all the previous sutures get buried beneath this reinforcing suture and give extra support to uterus, cervix and vagina and brings the pericervical rim at the level of ischial spine. Anterior compartment repair is done by carrying out paravaginal repair (Figs 8.10M to O) and burch colposuspension in patients with SUI. A cystoscopy is routinely performed at the end of the procedure.

Laparoscopic Management of Prolapse Repair

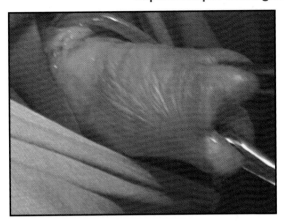

Fig. 8.10A: Prolapse uterus

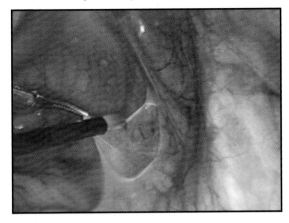

Fig. 8.10B: Starting ureteric dissection on the right side near the pelvic brim

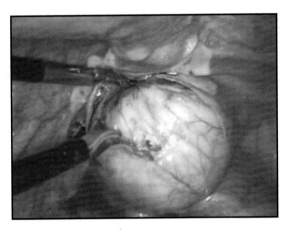

Fig. 8.10C: Transverse incision over the vaginal probe (probe placed in the posterior fornix)

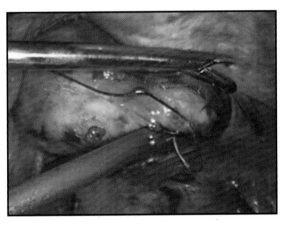

Fig. 8.10D: Vaginal probe in situ, passing a deep stitch through levator ani

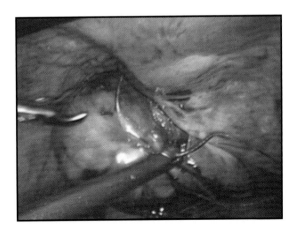

Fig. 8.10E: Attaching the levator to mid vagina

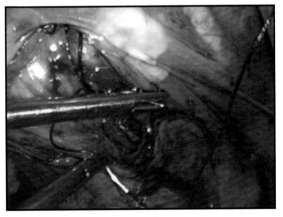

Fig. 8.10F: Passing suture to obliterate the vaginal hiatus

Laparoscopic Management of Prolapse Repair

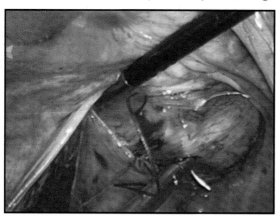

Fig. 8.10G: Passing similar suture on the left side

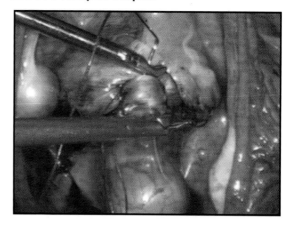

Fig. 8.10H: Passing suture between rectovaginal septum and upper end of vagina (rectal probe in situ)

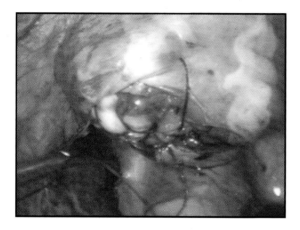

Fig. 8.10I: Vaginal hiatus completely obliterated by tier of sutures

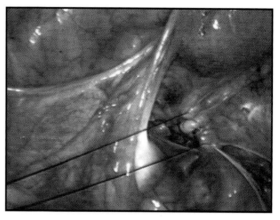

Fig. 8.10J: Plication of uterosacral ligament on right side

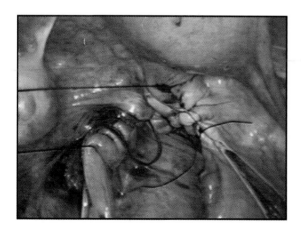

Fig. 8.10K: Passing uterosacral colposuspension suture on the left side

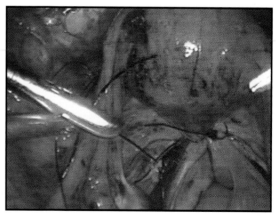

Fig. 8.10L: Final laparoscopic picture after prolapse repair

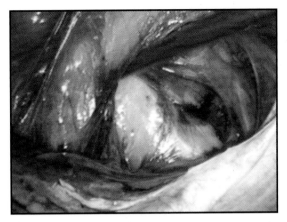

Fig. 8.10M: Dissection in the space of Retzius showing a wide Paravaginal defect. Bladder retracted medially by grasper

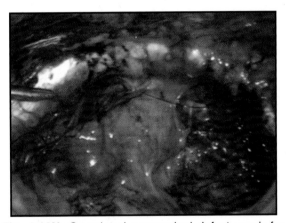

Fig. 8.10N: Completed paravaginal defect repair for anterior compartment repair. Four sutures passed on either side. Grasper pointing at Cooper's ligament

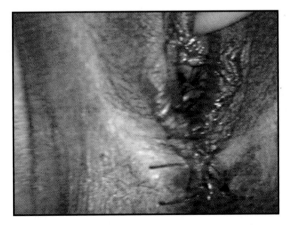

Fig. 8.10O: Final appearance of vaginal at end of prolapse repair

After the completed pelvic floor reconstruction, hospitalization is usually for 24 hours. Patients do not have any significant problem in the postoperative phase except at times for a dull backache for 2 to 3 weeks. Anatomical and functional correction utilizing this technique is excellent and patient satisfaction is almost 95 percent.

EXCISION OF RECTOVAGINAL ADENOMYOTIC NODULE

Endometriosis occurs in various grades of severity and causes severe symptoms to the patient mainly being pelvic pain, dysmenorrhea, dysparunia, dyschezia and rectal symptoms. A severe form of the disease is Adenomyosis of rectovaginal septum as defined by Donnez et al.[33–36] There are extensive adhesions in the cul-de-sac obliterating its lower portion and uniting the cervix or the lower portion of the uterus to the rectum, with adenoma of the endometrial type invading the cervical, uterine and probably also, but to a lesser degree, the anterior wall of the rectum. Cul-de-sac obliteration implies the presence of deep fibrotic rectovaginal adenomyosis beneath the peritoneum. The treatment options of this condition are at best surgical as medical suppressive therapy does not seem to work for the long-term pain relief.[37]

Surgical technique encompasses the radical resection of adenomyotic nodule. Patient's bowel is prepared in the preoperative phase and an informed consent obtained. A rectal probe, a vaginal probe and a good uterine elevator are put in situ after the patient is placed in semilithotomy position under GA. Strong uterine anteversion maintained and with rectal probe in situ a blunt scissor dissection is done between the back surface of uterocervical junction and the rectum. The dissection is carried out till complete rectal mobilization has been achieved upto the level of rectovaginal septum. Complete lateral clearing of all fibrotic adhesions and implants is done. Now after complete rectal mobilization and the adenomyotic nodule being fully exposed we put a sponge in vagina and prepare to excise the nodule in toto. Laser or monopolar hook can be used. All visible adenomyotic implants and nodule are excised along with at 5 mm disease free margin (Figs 8.11A to F). En-Bloc laparoscopic excision right upto vaginal wall is carried out and pneumoperitoneum is maintained by sponge in the vagina. The excised nodule is removed by a 10 mm claw forceps passed through a CCL extractor placed in the vagina. Colpotomy wound is closed laparoscopically employing 1-0 vicryl on curved needle (Figs 8.12A to F). After thorough

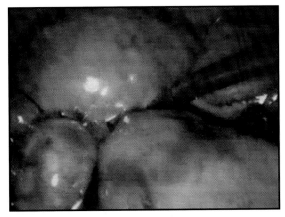

Fig. 8.11A: Total obliteration of pouch of Douglas

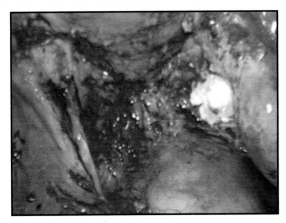

Fig. 8.11B: Rectum totally mobilized (rectal probe in situ) from the rectovaginal nodule

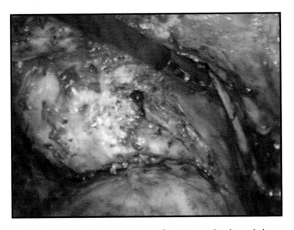

Fig. 8.11C: Appearance of rectovaginal nodule

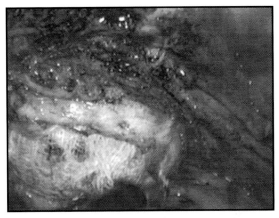

Fig. 8.11D: Incision by monopolar cautery for excision of adenomyotic nodule over a sponge in vagina

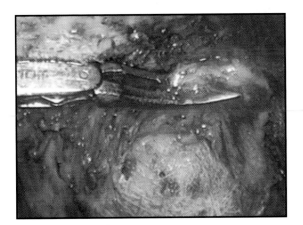

Fig. 8.11E: Continuing excision of adenomyotic nodule

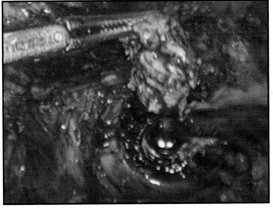

Fig. 8.11F: Complete excision and removal of adenomyotic nodule through CCL extractor and 10 mm claw forceps placed in vagina

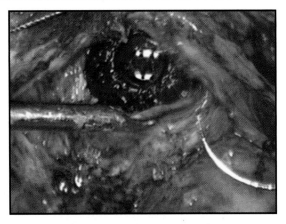

Fig. 8.12A: After rectovaginal nodule excision beginning curve needle suturing

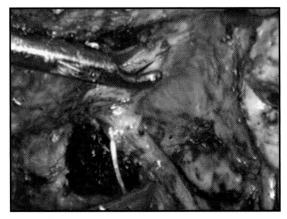

Fig. 8.12B: Passing the first suture through the lower and upper vaginal flap

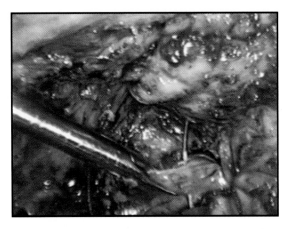

Fig. 8.12C: Progressive bite in the lower vaginal flap

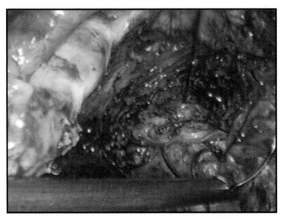

Fig. 8.12D: Continuous closure of colpotomy incision

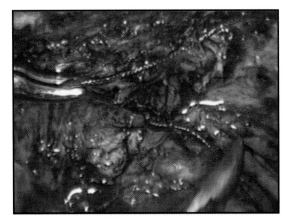

Fig. 8.12E: Tying the secure surgeons knot

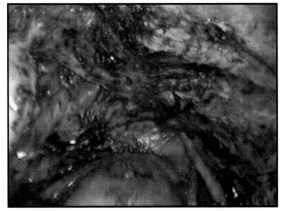

Fig. 8.12F: Final appearance of vaginal closure after rectovaginal nodule excision

suction irrigation and lavage a suture is passed through lower vaginal margin, then through the upper vaginal margin and the knot is secured by taking two throws of the suture. This is further reinforced by another knot by taking a single throw. Ipsilateral port placement works very well. A continuous closure from one end to the other is done and the hiatus closed completely. At end the suture is tied by utilizing the curve of the needle and taking two throws of the suture. The left needle holder then takes another single wrap and by pulling the sutures in opposite direction a secure surgeon's knot is completed. Two liters of fluid is left in the peritoneal cavity. A cystoscopy is performed at end of procedure to check the integrity of the ureters after such an extensive procedure. Postoperative recovery and pain relief are very good.

Several literature reports of rectovaginal nodule excision by various authors have appeared. Full thickness rectal lesion resections were carried out and repaired with suture in the series of Reich and associates.[38]

In Donnez series of 1125 cases[39] laparoscopic resection was performed successfully in all cases. Only seven cases of rectal perforation have been reported. All cases were diagnosed intraoperatively and repaired by colpotomy or laparotomy. Patients postoperative recovery and long-term pain relief has been reported good. In our cases we had one rectal injury which was repaired laparoscopically and patient fared well postoperatively.

In this chapter, the technique, concept and benefits of ipsilateral suturing have been discussed. The emphasis being on a stress free, comfortable surgical style which ensures optimum surgical performance and successful outcome. This technique pioneered by Dr Charles H Koh is ideal to be embraced by more and more laparoscopic surgeons in achieving excellence in suturing for optimizing precision in suturing applications.

REFERENCES

1. Semm K. Tissue puncher and loop-ligation-new ideas for surgical therapeutic pelviscopy (Laparoscopy) endoscopic intra-abdominal surgery. Endoscopy 1978;10:119-24.
2. Reich H, McGlynn F. Laparoscopic repair of bladder injury. Obstet Gynecol 1990;76:909-10.
3. Reich H, Clarke HC, Sekel L. A simple method for ligating with straight and curved needles is operative laparoscopy. Obstet Gynecol 1992;79:143-47.
4. Cuscheiri A, Nathanson LK. Instruments and basic techniques. In Cuschieri A, Berci G (Eds): Laparoscopic biliary surgery (2nd edn), Oxford; Blackwell Scientific Publication. 1992; 62-63.
5. Cuschieri A, Shimi S, Banting S, Vander Velpen G. Coaxial curved instrumentation for minimal access surgery. Endo Surgery 1993;1:30 3-35.
6. Koh CH, Janik GM. Laparoscopic microsurgical tubal anastomosis. In Adamson GD, Martin DC (Eds): Endoscopic Management of Gynecologic Disease. Philadelphia: Lippin Cott-Raven;1996;119-45.
7. Koh CH, Janik GM. Laparoscopic microsuturing techniques. St Louis: Medical Video Productions 1996.
8 Koh CH. Koh Ultramicro Laparoscopic Suturing System-Endo World, white paper Karl Storz Endosco.py-America, Inc 1995.
9. Endoscopic excellence by and for experts, 53rd Annual ASRM Meeting 18-22 October 1997;Cincinnati:Ohio. Sponsors 1998.
10. Advanced endoscopic surgery, AAGL and Ethicon Endo-Surgery, 21-2 August 1998; Cincinnati: Ohio, sponsors 1998.
11. Koh CH, Janik GM. Laparoscopic tubal reanastomosis. In: Endoscopic surgery for gynecologists (2nd edn). Tulandi, 1997.
12. Koh CH, Janik GM. Anastomosis of the fallopian tube, chapter. In Tulandi (Ed): Atlas of Laparoscopy and Hysteroscopy Technique (2nd edn). 1997.
13. Nezhat C, Nezhat F, Silfen S. Laparoscopic myomectomy. Int J Fertil 1991;36,275-80.
14. Hasson HM, Rotman C, Rana N. Laparoscopic myomectomy. Obstet Gynecol 1992;80,884-88.
15. Dubuisson JB, Chapron C, Mouly M. Laparoscopic myomectomy. Gynaecol Endosc 1993;2,171-73.
16. Miller C, Johnston M, Rundell M. Laparoscopic myomectomy in the infertile woman. J Am Assoc Gynecol Laparosc 1996;3(4):525-32.
17. Miller, CE, Davies S, Johnston M. Presented at the 27th Annual Meeting of the American Association of Gynecologic Laparoscopists, Atlanta, GA. November 10-15, 1998. Miller CE. Laparoscopic myomectomy with uterine reconstruction is a safe surgical procedure.
18. Dubuisson JB, Chapron C, Levy L. Difficulties and complications of laparoscopic myomectomy. Journal Gynecol Surg 1996;12(3):159-65.
19. Dubuisson JB, Chavet X, Chapron C, et al. Uterine rupture during pregnancy after laparoscopic myomectomy. Human Reprod 1995:10:1475-77.

20. Nezhat C. Laparoscopic myomectomy complications (Letter). Int J Fertil 1992;37:64.

21. Reich H. Laparoscopic hysterectomy. Surgical Laparoscopy and Endoscopy. Raven Press: New York 1992;2:85-88.

22. Reich H, McGlynn F, Sekel L. Total laparoscopic hysterectomy. Gynaecological Endoscopy 1993;2:59-63.

23. Lee CL., Lai YM, Soong YK. Management of urinary bladder injuries in laparoscopic assisted vaginal hysterectomy. Acta Obstet Gynecol Scand 1996;75:174.

24. Nezhat CH, Seidman DS, Nezhat F et al. Laparoscopic management of intentional and unintentional cystotomy. J Urol 1996;156:1400.

25. Nezhat C, Nezhat F, Ambroze W, Pennington E. Laparoscopic repair of small bowel, colon and rectal endometriosis. A report of twenty-six cases. Surg Endosc 1993;7:88.

26. Nezhat C, Nezhat F, Pennington E. Laparoscopic treatment of lower colorectal and infiltrative Rectovaginal septum endometriosis by the technique of video-laparoscopy. Br J Obstet Gynaecol 1992;99:664.

27. Redwine DB. Intestinal endometriosis. In Redwine DB (Ed): Surgical Treatment of Endometriosis. London: Dunitz, 2003;157-73.

28. Ross JW: Apical vault repair, the cornerstone of pelvic floor reconstruction. Int Urogynecol J 1997;8:146-52.

29. Ross JW. Techniques of laparoscopic repair of total vault eversion after hysterectomy. J Am Assoc Gynecol Laparosc 1997;4:173-83.

30. Miklos JR, Kohli N, Lucente V, Saye WB. Site specific fascial defects in the diagnosis and surgical management of enterocele. Am J Obstet Gynecol 1998;179:1418-23.

31. Lyons TL. Minimally invasive treatment of urinary stress incontinence and laparoscopicallly direct repair of pelvic floor defects. Clin Obstet Gynecol 1995;38:380-91.

32. Nezhat CH, Nezhat F, Nezhat C. Laparoscopic sacral colpopexy for vaginl vault prolapse. Obstet Gynecol 1994;4:381-83.

33. Donnez J, Nisolle M, Casanas-Roux F, et al. Laparoscopic treatment of rectovaginal septum endometriosis. In Donnez J, Nisolle M (Eds): An Atlas of Laser Operative Laparoscopy and Hysteroscopy. Carnforth, UK: Parthenon Publishing, 1994;75-85.

34. Donnez J, Nisolle M. Advanced laparoscopic surgery for the removal of rectovaginal septum endometriotic and adenomyotic nodules. Baillieres Clin Obstet Gynecol 1995;9:769-74.

35. Donnez J, Nisolle M, Casanas-Roux F, et al. Rectovaginal septum endometriosis or adenomyosis: laparoscopic management in a series of 231 patients. Hum Reprod 1995;10:630-35.

36. Donnez J, Nisolle M, Gillenot S, et al. Rectovaginal septum adenomyotic nodules: a series of 500 cases. Br J Obstet Gynaecol 1991;104:1009-13.

37. Donnez J, Nisolle M, Casanas-Roux F. Endometriosis-associated infertility: evaluation of preoperative use of danazol, gestrinone and buserelin. Int J Fertil 1990;35:297-301.

38. Reich H, McGlynn F, Salvat J. Laparoscopic treatment of cul-de-sac obliteration secondary to retrocervical deep fibrotic endometriosis. J Reprod Med 1991;36:516.

39. J Donnez, J Sqerifflet, M Smets. Laparoscopic treatment of rectovaginal septum adenomyosis. In Nutan Jain (Ed): State-of-the-art Atlas of Laparoscopic Surgery in Infertility and Gynaecology. New York, USA, McGraw-Hill, 2004,181-91.

Reich Modification of the McCall Culdoplasty to Prevent and/or Repair Prolapse during Total Laparoscopic Hysterectomy

HARRY REICH

IRIS KERIN ORBUCH

TAMER SECKIN

Chapter Nine

INTRODUCTION

Laparoscopic surgery provides excellent visualization and magnification of pelvic structures, decreased postoperative pain, and reduced hospitalization and recovery time. Laparoscopic vault suspension to restore Level I support can be attained by either the laparoscopic uterosacral ligament suspension techniques or via laparoscopic sacral colpopexy. The major drawback of the latter is the use of mesh. We prefer not using mesh.

Reich advocates doing a uterosacral ligament suspension as part of every total laparoscopic hysterectomy. Mesh is never used. The evolution from McCall's original culdoplasty to its laparoscopic counterpart will be described, including methods to lessen the effects of a high cystocele on urinary retention.

Various laparoscopic techniques are described to prevent prolapse at the time of hysterectomy and to repair prolapse occurring after hysterectomy (DeLancey Level I support), without using mesh.

In 1957 McCall described repair of an enterocele at the time of vaginal hysterectomy. McCall reported on forty-five patients in his landmark paper and described no recurrence of enterocele. His technique describes using *internal* and *external* sutures. The *internal* sutures are nonabsorbable (described as silk, cotton, or linen) to obliterate the enterocele sac by taking bites of both uterosacrals and posterior peritoneum. More specifically, his first suture takes the left uterosacral ligament, then the enterocele sac "at intervals of 1-2 cm" until the right uterosacral is reached. Next, the suture passes through the right uterosacral ligament. This suture is left untied to help guide more similarly placed sutures above the first suture. The number of internal sutures depends on the size of the enterocele sac. These *internal* sutures are not tied until the *external* sutures are placed. Three *external* sutures are then placed. McCall inserted a "No. 1 catgut suture from the vaginal side just right of the midline of the vagina about 2 cm above its posterior cut edge". Next the right uterosacral is taken, followed by the left uterosacral and out the vaginal wall at the same level as this suture was entered, but just left of the midline. The suture is not tied. Two more sutures are placed, each higher than the last. The top suture brings the vault to its highest level. Next the internal sutures are tied then the external sutures are tied. The peritoneum is closed in the usual fashion. McCall states that his method maintains vaginal length and does not narrow the vault as it obliterates the cul-de-sac.[1,2]

There have been several modifications to McCall's original technique. The Mayo Clinic version, pioneered by Richard Symmonds, described a modified endopelvic fascia repair. A wedge of vaginal mucosa is excised from both the anterior and posterior wall to allow access to the lateral vaginal supports. After the enterocele is excised, one to three *internal* McCall sutures are placed. Next, external sutures are placed incorporating the posterior vaginal wall, cul-de-sac peritoneum, and uterosacral-cardinal ligament complex. More external sutures can be placed based on the length of the vault.[3–5,15]

Cruikshank and Kovac showed in a prospective clinical trial that a modified McCall culdoplasty that reattaches the uterosacral ligaments to the apex of the vaginal is very effective at preventing future apical defects. At three years, the incidence of apical defects in the McCall group was 6 percent versus 30 percent in the control group.[6]

The McCall culdoplasty is a vaginal procedure (By today's terminology, culdoplasty is colpoplasty or culdoplasty). It was applied through an abdominal incision by Thomas Elkins with good results. Early experience with a total laparoscopic approach to hysterectomy was accompanied by various methods of cuff closure. These can be simplified into the traditional transverse cuff closure and the vertical cuff closure. The transverse closure should be accompanied by uterosacral ligament suspension on each side. The vertical closure almost always is done with a McCall type stitch, bringing the uterosacral ligaments together across the midline. We call this laparoscopic vertical closure a laparoscopic high McCall Culdoplasty.

Reich adapted the McCall culdoplasty to laparoscopic hysterectomy surgery after listening to a lecture by Thomas Elkins in 1992, soon after he developed the concept of total laparoscopic hysterectomy. This technique addressed posterior vaginal wall and vault support, but failed to mention the frequently occurring high cystocele in the anterior vaginal wall that often results in urinary retention. By 1994, the high McCall technique had undergone major modifications per Reich to include the anterior vagina.

He notes four laparoscopic operations using this technique or its modifications. The first two are done at the time of hysterectomy and the last two are for posthysterectomy vaginal cuff prolapse or possible pathology of the cuff:

1. Prophylactic technique to prevent prolapse at time of hysterectomy [(Laparoscopic high McCall (LHM)]
2. Repair of prolapse or occult prolapse with urinary retention (high cystocele) at time of hysterectomy (Reich modification of HM)
3. Repair of vaginal cuff prolapse after hysterectomy (Reich modification of HM)
4. Posthysterectomy excision of vaginal cuff scar (endometriosis or adhesions) followed by elevation onto uterosacral ligaments for pain and/or dyspareunia (Reich modification of HM).

Laparoscopic Technique to Prevent Prolapse at the time of Hysterectomy (TLH)

This procedure is indicated when minimal or no prolapse is present and the patient has no urinary complaints, especially retention related. It is considered a part of every total laparoscopic hysterectomy.

The vaginal delineator or a sponge packed in a glove is placed back into the vagina (Fig. 9.1) occluding it to maintain pneumoperitoneum for closure of the vaginal cuff. The uterosacral ligaments are identified by bipolar desiccation markings or with the aid of a rectal probe. The left uterosacral ligament is elevated and a 0-Vicryl suture on a CT-1 needle is placed through it using an oblique Cook needle holder (Fig. 9.2) . The suture is then placed through the left cardinal ligament, located at the posterolateral vagina just below the uterine vessels, then through the posterior peritoneum and rectovaginal fascia along the posterior vaginal epithelium, to and through the right posterolateral vagina and cardinal ligament to the right uterosacral ligament (Fig. 9.3). This suture is tied extracorporeally and provides excellent support to the vaginal cuff apex, elevating it superiorly and posteriorly toward the hollow of the sacrum. The rest of the vagina and the overlying pubocervicovesicular fascia are closed vertically with one or two 0-Vicryl interrupted sutures. In most cases the peritoneum is not closed (Figs 9.4 to 9.7) .

Cystoscopy is routinely done after vaginal closure to assure ureteral patency, 8-10 minutes after intra-

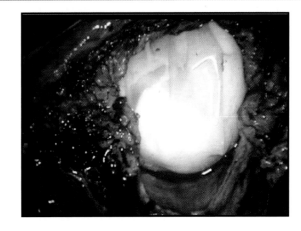

Fig. 9.1: A packed sponge in a glove was used to maintain pneumoperitoneum

venous administration of one ampule of Indigo Carmine dye. This is especially necessary when the ureter is identified but not dissected. Blue dye should be visualized through both ureteral orifices. The bladder wall should also be inspected for suture and thermal defects.

This technique for vaginal vault closure at the time of TLH has been used by Reich in all cases over the last 10 years, and no cuff prolapses have come to his attention.

Repair of Prolapse or Occult Prolapse with Urinary Retention (High Cystocele) at Total Laparoscopic Hysterectomy

Urinary retention may be present from a high cystocele adjacent to the cervix. The symptoms of urinary retention are seldom volunteered by the patient seeking hysterectomy and should be ascertained by the physician during the history. Many patients will, however, describe the improvement in micturition at their postoperative visit. The simple question is "Do you feel like you are completely emptying your bladder or do you feel that you still have to go after urinating?"

The technique to be described not only addresses the posterior wall, but the anterior wall as well. This method brings the anterior vagina much higher than the posterior wall. This procedure can be done during the same surgery following hysterectomy or in a patient with a previous hysterectomy. It is termed a "high McCall" suspension because after the first suture brings the uterosacral and cardinal ligaments

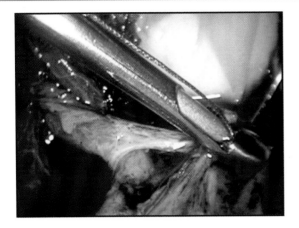

Fig. 9.2: The vaginal vault is closed with a series of sutures applied laparoscopically. 0-Vicryl on a CT-1 needle is placed through the left uterosacral ligament while the left ureter is visualized

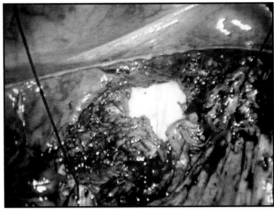

Fig. 9.3: The suture includes both uterosacral and cardinal ligaments on each side and the rectovaginal fascia

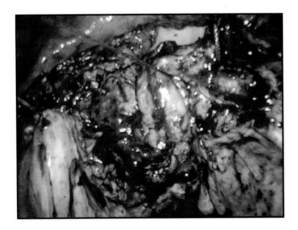

Fig. 9.4: The suture is pulled upwards. The uterosacral ligaments will be plicated and provide support to prevent postoperative vaginal vault prolapse

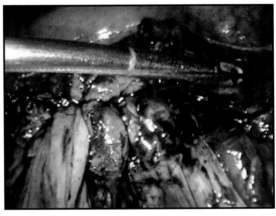

Fig. 9.5: The Clarke-Reich knot pusher secures the knot

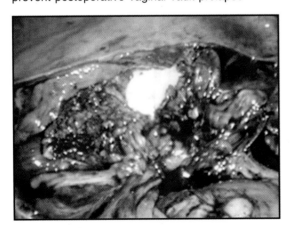

Fig. 9.6: The first suture is completed (High McCall Culdoplasty)

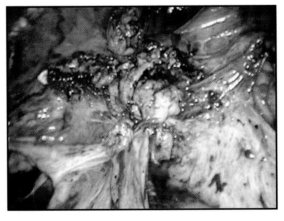

Fig. 9.7: A second suture completes the cuff closure. The vault is closed and hemostasis achieved

and posterior vagina together in the midline, subsequent sutures, bring the lateral and anterior vagina onto the uterosacral ligaments working progressively towards the sacrum.

At the time of hysterectomy, after the uterus is removed, a vaginal delineator or probe is placed in the vagina to maintain pneumoperitoneum. Vaginal hemostasis is obtained until complete, so as to not be dependant on compression by sutures. The left uterosacral ligament and posterolateral vagina are elevated. Going from left to right using the same 0-Vicryl suture, it is placed through the left uterosacral ligament, then through the left cardinal ligament followed by posterior vaginal tissue including the rectovaginal fascia but excluding vaginal epithelium. The suture exits near the midline, then back through rectovaginal fascia and vagina on the right followed by the right cardinal ligament and right uterosacral ligament. Extracorporeal knot tying is done, pulling up the vaginal apex and elevating it both posteriorly and superiorly towards the hollow of the sacrum. The first suture is placed below the level of the uterine artery pedicle as the cardinal ligament is identified as the thick band of connective tissue beneath the ligated uterine vessels.

The second suture is placed through the uterosacral ligaments closer to the sacrum and the endopelvic fascia just above the uterine vessel pedicle. The third suture is placed well above the cardinal ligament and through the uterosacral ligaments even closer to the sacrum resulting in vaginal vertical closure. All sutures after the first use 0-Ethibond. The last suture is usually placed into anterior vagina above the cuff at 12 o'clock to bring the anterior vagina much higher than the posterior wall. The last suture also is placed at the highest level toward the sacral area. As with any suspension, special care must be taken to ensure the integrity of the rectum and ureters. The sutures must not constrict the rectum, which is identified throughout the procedure with a rectal probe inside it. This suspension achieves a physiologic position of the vagina. In addition, it provides the vagina with good depth since the vagina can go high towards the sacral region where the uterosacrals originate. The closure of the vagina in a vertical fashion avoids the ureters as the sutures stay in the midline.[7,8]

Uterosacral ligaments are sometimes isolated before TLH by putting the flexed uterus on upward tension and placing a Vicryl suture around them near their sacral portion. These sutures can be left long to aid those surgeons more comfortable doing a LAVH. During LAVH, the suture can be pulled out with a finger and used with a free needle to attach the vaginal vault apex to the uterosacral ligaments.

Repair of Vaginal Cuff Prolapse after Hysterectomy (Reich Modification of HM)

Vaginal vault prolapse can usually be repaired by the technique described above.

Posthysterectomy Excision of Vaginal Cuff Scar (Endometriosis or Adhesions)

Followed by elevation onto uterosacral ligaments for pain and/or dyspareunia (Reich modification of HM).

Some patients present with pain and discomfort without obvious prolapse. If the cuff is excised and elevated, many patients experiences relief of pain. The exact mechanism is unclear.

CONCLUSION

There are many different methods to address vaginal vault prolapse and reduce its incidence at the time of hysterectomy and thereafter. Whichever method is employed, it is important to remember the principals of anatomy to guide reconstruction. In order to repair prolapse, the pubocervical and rectovaginal fascia must be reapproximated to each other and to the cardinal-uterosacral complex at the level of the ischial spine, hopefully at the time of hysterectomy. Reich's adaptation of the vaginal McCall culdoplasty addresses both the posterior and anterior wall near the vaginal apex. It brings the anterior vagina higher than the posterior wall. His application does not use mesh so as to minimize rejection and all the shortcomings of mesh. Although this chapter only addresses Level I DeLancey support procedures, it is important to understand that other compartment defects coexist (Level I support provides the most superior suspension of the vagina by the cardinal uterosacral complex). We understand the philosophy of Wattiez et al that a global approach to pelvic reconstruction must be instituted. In addition to Level I support defects, level II and III defects must also be addressed in the same procedure.[9] Thus, because multiple compartment defects coexist, and this occurs in the majority of cases, it is important to repair all the pelvic floor defects concomitantly. But the future of mesh remains to be determined, and time and reimbursement issues for multiple procedures during the same operation will limit this approach in the immediate future, at least in the USA.

REFERENCES

1. McCall ML. Posterior Culdoplasty. Surgical correction of enterocele during vaginal hysterectomy: a preliminary report. Obstet Gyn 1957;10;6:595-602.
2. Karram MM, Kleeman SD. Vaginal vault prolapse: In Te Linde's Operative Gynecology (9th edn): Lippincott Williams & Wilkins: Philadelphia 2003;999-1020.
3. Symmonds RE, Pratt JH. Vaginal prolapse following hysterectomy. Am J Obstet Gyn 1960;79;5:899-909.
4. Symmonds RE, Williams TJ, Lee RA, Webb MJ. Posthysterectomy enterocele and vaginal vault prolapse. Am J Obstet Gyn. 1981;140;8:852-59.
5. Lee AL, Symmonds RE. Surgical repair of posthysterectomy vault prolapse. Am J Obstet Gyn 1972;112:953-56.
6. Cruikshank SH, Kovac SR. Randomized comparison of three surgical methods used at the time of vaginal hysterectomy to prevent posterior enterocele. Am J Obstet Gynecol 1999;180:859-65.
7. Liu CY, Reich H. Correction of genital prolapse. J Endourol 1996;10;3;259-65.
8. Reich H, Vancaillie TG. Recent advances in laparoscopic hysterectomy and pelvic floor reconstruction. Surgical Technology International III.
9. Wattiez A, Mashiach R, Donoso M. Laparoscopic repair of vaginal vault prolapse 2003;15:315-19.

A Contemporary Approach to Laparoscopic Myomectomy

CHARLES EDWARD MILLER

Chapter Ten

Early in his neophyte career, a medical student learns that the most common tumor of the female reproductive tract is the uterine leiomyoma. While it is generally stated that 20 to 30 percent of women over the age of 35 have at least one myoma,[1,2] one study noted leiomyomata in 50 percent of females examined at time of autopsy.[3] Quite likely a genetic predisposition exists for myoma growth. Women of African descent have been noted to have a 3 to 9 times greater risk of possessing uterine fibroids then Caucasians,[4] who are more likely to have myomata than women of Asian ancestry.

Over the past century, the most common treatment for symptomatic uterine fibroids has been hysterectomy. More recently, however, there has been renewed interest in removal of the myoma alone, i.e. myomectomy. This is based in part on a desirable complication rate, necessity (delayed childbearing) and in part on choice; that is, many women prefer the more conservative procedure myomectomy, thus maintaining the uterus. Uterine preservation has not only focused attention on myomectomy, but myolysis,[5,6] cryomyolysis,[7] embolization[8, 9] and laparoscopic uterine artery ligation.[10]

Just as new procedures have come to the forefront in the treatment of symptomatic uterine leiomyomata, the technique of myomectomy has been vastly improved. With trends toward minimally invasive endoscopic surgery, procedures have been developed to accomplish a myomectomy via either a laparoscopic[11-15] or hysteroscopic route.[16-18] In this article, the author will present his technique for laparoscopic myomectomy. Technical variations described by other physicians will be noted. Also included will be discussions on patient profile, preoperative work-up, complication rate, risk of adhesion formation and subsequent pregnancy rate.

PREOPERATIVE EVALUATION

Due to the diminishment of tactile feedback, prior to laparoscopic surgery, it is imperative to know the size, location, and number of uterine leiomyomata. The physical examination determines whether the abdomen and pelvis are large enough, relative to the mass, to perform a laparoscopic approach. Relative size of abdomen and pelvis must be large enough for the ports to be placed above and lateral

to the total mass of myomas and it should be ascertained that if myomectomy is desired visualization is not compromised while dissection occurs. Having this information in hand lessens the risk of errant incisions, or overlooking significant deep intramural leiomyomata. Fibroid mapping can be performed via ultrasound (vaginal or abdominal) or MRI. In the author's experience, vaginal ultrasound allows adequate leiomyomata mapping in virtually all cases. In comparing the role of transvaginal ultrasound and outpatient hysteroscopy in the evaluation of patients with menorrhagia, Vercellini noted that transvaginal ultrasonography had 96 percent sensitivity, 86 percent specificity, 91 percent positive predictive value and 94 percent negative predictive value in the diagnosis of intrauterine abnormality.[19] Further evaluation of fibroid position can be ascertained via hysterosonogram, which better delineates a submucosal myoma.[20] Especially in cases where contradictions arise comparing previous ultrasound scans or when confidence in ultrasound technique is questioned, MRI can be utilized, as noted by Hutchins.[21]

It is important that the endometrial cavity be evaluated to rule out separate submucosal myomata, either prior to or at the time of myomectomy surgery. Preoperatively, the physician can choose hysterosonogram, hysterosalpingogram or hysteroscopy. At time of surgery, hysteroscopy or hysterosalpingogram can be performed.

Finally, prior to surgery, it is imperative that the patient's hematologic status be determined. A patient with normal hemoglobin levels should be given the opportunity to store autologous blood two weeks prior to surgery. If a patient's fibroids are causing anemia, a GnRH agonist can be utilized along with iron supplementation to raise preoperative hemoglobin levels.

Myomectomy via Laparoscopy—The Procedure

In order to enable adequate visualization, especially for posterior myomata, the author recommends using a carbon dioxide insufflation technique, rather than gasless laparoscopy. Proponents of gasless laparoscopy, however, such as Topel[22] and Maher[23] stress the advantage of using standard instrumentation in performing myomectomy.

As has become the standard for operative laparoscopy, the patient is intubated for the purpose of general endotracheal anesthesia. Once intubated, the patient is placed in the dorsal lithotomy position, prepped and draped. Dorsal lithotomy allows the uterus to be easily accessed for hysteroscopy and hysterosalpingogram. Moreover, once visualization of the endometrial cavity is complete, a uterine manipulator is placed inside the uterus to allow its mobilization and increase visualization.

Once the patient is placed in the dorsal lithotomy position, prepped and draped, and prior to pelvic examination, a catheter is placed inside the bladder. As these cases can be prolonged, especially when large or multiple fibroids are noted, having an indwelling catheter is advantageous. This can be placed either by the scrub nurse or the physician.

The patient is now examined under anesthesia. It is important to determine uterine size to correctly place ports. Moreover, position of the uterus (anteflexion, retroversion, etc.) is noted at this time to properly note uterine cavity orientation.

Unless previously performed, hysteroscopy is mandatory. In so doing, submucosal myomata can be noted and subsequently be removed via the hysteroscope under laparoscopic guidance. Moreover, impingement of intramural fibroids on the endometrium can be noted. Ultimately, however, hysteroscopic resection of uterine myomata, or endometrial ablation is not performed until the laparoscope is placed.

Once hysteroscopy (or intraoperative hysterosalpingogram) is complete, a uterine manipulator is placed. Various reusable or disposable cannulas are available. In order to maximize uterine mobilization, a portion of the cannula itself must pass into the uterine cavity.

Following placement of the uterine manipulator or prior to operative hysteroscopy or endometrial ablation, our attention is directed to laparoscopy. Figure 10.1 demonstrates proper positioning of surgeon, first assistant, scrub nurse, and anesthesiologist at time of laparoscopic myomectomy. The ability to manipulate the uterus is so important that the scrub nurse is positioned between the patient's legs to enable uterine manipulation throughout.

Generally, the laparoscope is placed through the umbilicus. However, if the uterus is greater than 18

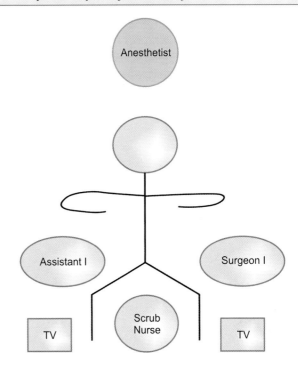

Fig. 10.1: Position of personnel for laparoscopic myomectomy

weeks size, or the patient is at risk of having periumbilical adhesions, an initial left upper quadrant incision is made per Bieber.[24]

For best visualization, a 10 mm laparoscope is utilized. Under direct visualization, secondary ports are placed. It is imperative that these ports be placed cephalad and lateral to the uterus. If ports are placed too medial and caudal, it is much more difficult to excise the myomata and repair the uterus; i.e. the "crossing swords" phenomenon.

Due to the risk of lateral port site herniation,[25-27] and to aid in postoperative recovery, the author utilizes secondary 5 mm ports. Because of this, morcellation and myoma extraction must be performed via the umbilical 10 to 12 mm port. In this scenario, a 5 mm laparoscope is placed through a secondary 5 mm port. When placed through a lateral port site at the level of the umbilicus, visualizing through a 5 mm laparoscope is not difficult.

Occasionally, when the uterus is truly large (20 weeks size or greater) all ports must be placed above the umbilicus. In this case, the left upper quadrant port is placed initially. The supraumbilical port and the right upper quadrant port can then be placed under direct visualization. Alternatively, one can start at the umbilicus and then place supraumbilical ports under direct visualization. Generally, once this is accomplished, the laparoscope is placed into the midline, supraumbilical port. It has been the author's experience that the midline port allows easiest visualization and ability to proceed with the intended surgery.

The patient at risk for periumbilical adhesions warrants further discussion. As mentioned, the author recommends initial insufflation and trocar and sleeve entry through the left upper quadrant. If periumbilical adhesions are noted, secondary ports are next placed to allow for instrumentation to lyse these adhesions. Now the umbilicus can be safely entered under direct visualization.

Once the sleeves for the laparoscope and secondary instrumentation is properly and safely placed, diagnostic laparoscopy can be performed. If adhesion, endometriosis or pathologic ovarian cysts are noted at time of pelvic inspection, these conditions must be treated accordingly.

Attention is now directed toward the uterus and the myomata. The major deterrence to myomectomy is blood loss. In order to minimize this blood loss, the myometrium around the myoma is infiltrated with a dilute vasopressin solution. Vasopressin causes vasoconstriction. Initially, one ampule of vasopressin was diluted in 20 cc of normal saline. Currently, the vasopressin is even more diluted, i.e. 30 mIU per 100 cc diluent. Although concern has been raised with pitressin usage as to the risk of delayed bleeding, the author has not noted this complication in well over 1,000 myomectomy procedures performed. Care must be taken to prevent vascular injection of vasopressin. Therefore, aspiration prior to slow injection is essential. Local injection of fluid also allows separation of the myoma from the myometrium; thus, allowing easier dissection.

In his classic description of the myomectomy procedure in 1898, W. Alexander recommended use of a single anterior incision into the uterus whenever feasible.[28] As many fibroids as possible are retrieved through this antro-placed incision. Uterine strength is less likely compromised, and the risk of adhesions is minimized. When fibroids are located posteriorly, a posterior approach is recommended.[4,29] While many experts, including the author, are in favor of a vertical incision on the uterus in order to stay away from the adnexa and thus decrease adhesion risk to the ovary and tube[3,29] others recommend a transverse hysterotomy incision.[30] Their contention is based on the fact that arteries and arterioles in the myometrium run in a horizontal direction.[31, 32]

Different energy sources have been utilized to perform the hysterotomy incision. These include use of monopolar electrosurgery,[33-35] carbon dioxide laser,[12,36] Nd:YAG laser,[17,37] KTP laser,[37] and the argon beam coagulator.[38] The author first presented the use of ultrasonic energy (Harmonic Scalpel®) for laparoscopic myomectomy at the 22nd Annual Congress of the American Association of Gynecologic Laparoscopists in 1993.[39] Subsequently, the utilization of ultrasonic energy for a laparoscopic approach to myomectomy has been also described by Stringer[40] and McCarus.[41] It would appear that myomectomy via this technique is safe even in patients interested in pregnancy.[15,43]

While initially utilizing the 5 mm hook blade of the Harmonic Scalpel® for myomectomy,[39] the author began to use the LaparoSonic Coagulating Shears® (LCS®) when the ultrasonic instrument was released.[43] Unfortunately, lateral 10 mm secondary incisions were required; along with this, the inherent risk of herniation was noted. Subsequently, the 10 mm LaparoSonic Coagulating Shears® was reduced to a 5 mm diameter. Currently, the ultrasonic instrument of choice for myomectomy is the Harmonic Scalpel Curved Blade®. It is a 5 mm diameter instrument, which enables rapid cutting and dissection.

In performing the hysterotomy incision, it is very important to incise through the fibroid's pseudo-capsule in order to make myoma dissection easy. This is especially important when the patient is pretreated with a GnRH agonist, as the pseudocapsule is often very thick. The author recommends incising until the surgeon sees the fibroid actually pushing up through the capsule. The dissection plane is now well visualized. Ultimately, in order to dissect out the myoma, energy may or may not be required. Regardless of energy use, strong and firm grasping equipment to dissect out and hold the myoma is a prerequisite (Fig. 10.5).

Although Dubuisson and Nezhat recommend the use of bipolar cautery to gain hemostasis on the myoma bed during the process of enucleation, the author stresses minimal use of bipolar energy. It is the author's contention that tissue destruction and necrosis secondary to the use of bipolar cautery has been an important factor resulting in subsequent fistula formation reported both by Nezhat and Dubuisson.[12,34,44-45] In contrast, the author has reported on 274 consecutive laparoscopic myomectomies without fistula formation.[46] Rather than obtaining hemostasis via bipolar cautery, the author recommends meticulous multilayer closure.[15,42] If the endometrium is violated, an interrupted closure of 3-0 PDS-II® is placed in the myometrium directly above the endometrium at 1 to 1.5 mm intervals (Fig. 10.8). If the defect is large, a purse-string suture of 2-0 or 3-0 PDS-II® is next placed in the myometrium (Fig. 10.9). Depending on the defect size, multiple purse-string layers or layers of mattress style suture of 2-0 or 3-0 PDS-II® may be necessary (Fig. 10.10). Finally, interrupted or continuous baseball style sutures of 3-0 or 4-0 PDS-II® are placed on the serosa (Fig. 10.11). Interceed® Adhesions barrier is then placed over the repaired uterine defect.

Unlike myomectomy via laparotomy, the fibroids must be evacuated from the pelvis as a separate step. In the past, most experts recommended posterior colpotomy incision for fibroid extraction.[12-14,33,35,46-50] Despite these views, the author has maintained the need to evacuate leiomyomata via the port sites. Concern about adhesion formation from the cul-de-sac to the uterus can be raised, particularly in the case of a posterior uterine incision.[42] Fortunately, this concern would appear to be a non-issue, given the ability to now use a power morcellator.[51] Carter and McCarus noted average time savings for all myomectomies using an electromechanical morcellator was 53 minutes.[52] The average time for reduction extraction of myomata less than 100 grams was fifteen minutes while 150 minutes was saved on average when myomata were in the 401 to 500 grams range.

While the author originally used the Steiner® electromechanical morcellator from Storz, currently the Gynecare® Power Morcellator is the instrument of choice. The Gynecare® morcellator has a larger diameter (15 mm versus 12 mm). Moreover, the sharp blade retracts to minimize risk. Finally, the Gynecare® morcellator has a valve to prevent loss of the pneumoperitoneum. The morcellator is placed through the 12 mm umbilical port under direct visualization of a lateral placed 5 mm laparoscope. Because the sharp blade of the Gynecare® morcellator retracts and the morcellator is equipped with an introducer, the 12 mm sleeve is removed from the umbilicus and replaced by the morcellator.

At times, the fibroid is so large that vision can be obscured in the process of dissecting the myoma from the uterus. In this case, morcellation is started during the process of enucleation. Thus, visualization is not compromised.

Laparoscopic Myomectomy— Advantages and Disadvantages

Laparoscopic myomectomy must be considered an advanced endoscopic procedure. As compared to laparotomy, four aspects of the laparoscopic approach make it technically more difficult.

Firstly especially if a myoma is deep in the myometrium, it may be difficult to locate. Therefore, proper fibroid mapping prior to the procedure, either via vaginal ultrasound or MRI is essential. Secondly, while myoma removal is generally a straightforward procedure via laparotomy, often enucleating is difficult in a laparoscopic setting. This is especially noted when the patient is pretreated with an GnRH agonist. In this case, the myoma softens, the pseudocapsule thickens and the resultant dissection planes are obscured. To make removal easier, one must cut through the pseudocapsule to the level of the myoma.[15]

Certainly, the major obstacle to a laparoscopic approach to myomectomy is the necessary multilayer uterine repair. Not only must the closure be hemostatic and minimize the risk of postoperative adhesions, it must also allow concomitant growth of the pregnant uterus. Whether intracorporeal or extracorporeal knot tying is performed, laparoscopic suturing is a tedious acquired skill. One can anticipate prolonged procedures as the surgeon crawls down the learning curve. To enable ease of suturing, suture devices, the Endostich® (USSC), and the Suture Assist® (Ethicon EndoSurgery) have been introduced. The 10 mm Endostich® has been utilized in laparoscopic myomectomy to close the uterus with interrupted and continuous locked sutures.[53] Accordingly, Stringer noted that the Endostich® shortened the operative time by approximately 40 minutes. The use of the Endostich® raises two concerns, however. Since the instrument's needle is

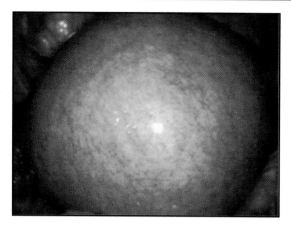

Fig. 10.2: Large fundal myoma is noted. One cannot visualize the uterine cornuae

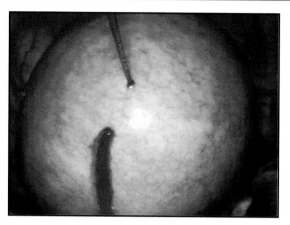

Fig. 10.3: Dilute Pitressin is placed via a trans-abdominal 18-gauge needle into the myometrium adjacent to the uterine myoma.

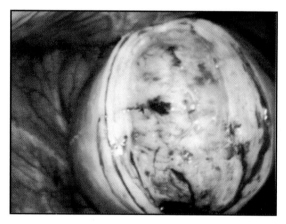

Fig. 10.4: A longitudinal incision is made with the curved blade of the Harmonic Scalpel™ through the serosa and myometrium down to the level of the myoma. Notice the minimal lateral distribution of energy

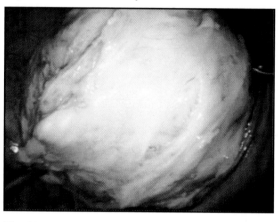

Fig. 10.5: Further dissection between the myometrium and myoma has occurred. This allows the myoma to be enucleated from the myometrium

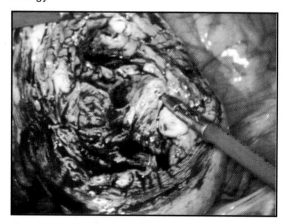

Fig. 10.6: The myoma has now been completely excised. The tip of the intrauterine cannula is at the end of the grasper to note the fact that the uterine cavity was not entered. Essentially, only the endometrium is in tact

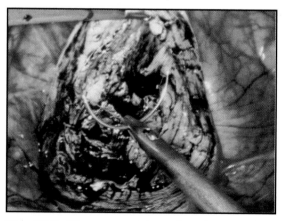

Fig. 10.7: The myometrium directly above the endometrium is closed with a running purse-string suture of 3.0 PDS-2.

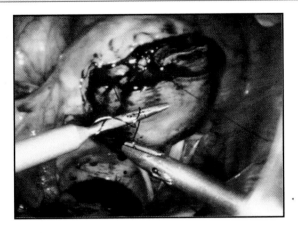

Fig. 10.8: The myometrium is then repaired with two more layers of running 3.0 PDS-2 in a baseball style fashion. Shown is the completion of the second baseball style closure of the myometrium

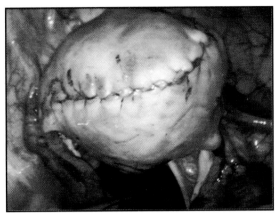

Fig. 10.9: A final running baseball style suture is placed closing the serosa

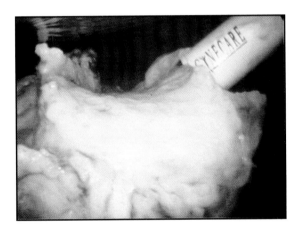

Fig. 10.10: The myoma is then morcellated via the umbilical port by placing the laparoscope through a lateral 5-mm port

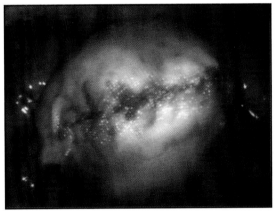

Fig. 10.11: Interceed ™ is placed over the repaired uterine defect

short, the ability to close the "dead space" of myometrium is hampered. Furthermore, the diameter of the Endostich® is 10 mm, thus the lateral port must be 10 mm or the instrument placed through the umbilicus. If the umbilicus must be used for the Endostich®, a lateral 5 mm port must hold the laparoscope. This makes suturing and visualization difficult.

Finally, myoma extraction from the pelvis must be performed at the time of the laparoscopic myomectomy. While many have advocated use of a posterior colpotomy incision,[3,17,18,20,21,23,25,29,42,62] the power morcellator has been noted to be fast and safe. In another way to ease the difficulty of suturing and

myoma extraction, Nezhat recommends laparoscopic assisted myomectomy.[54-56] This procedure is technically less demanding than time consuming. In this technique, myomata are enucleated via laparoscopy. The myomata are then evacuated from the pelvis, and the uterus repaired through a mini laparotomy incision. Even this procedure, however, is no easier for the posterior, deep myoma.[53]

These concerns posed by the technical difficulties of a laparoscopic approach to myomectomy have led to various recommendations based on myoma size and number as exhibited in Table 10.1. Parker recommended performing myomectomy via laparoscopy for myomata less than 6 cm in size.[57] Darai reserves laparoscopic myomectomy for patients presenting with no more than four myomas less than or equal to 7 cm.[54] According to Dubuisson in 1996, "Laparotomy must remain the approach for myomectomy whenever the fibroids are 8 cm or more in size and whenever it is necessary to remove more than two fibroids."[34] In his 1996 article for the Journal of the American Association of Gynecologic Laparoscopy, the author recommended a laparoscopic approach if the largest myoma was less than 10 cm in diameter or there were no more than 3 myomata greater than 5 cm.[53] However, with greater comfort gained in laparoscopic suturing, and the advent of the power morcellator, the author's exclusion criteria have indeed been relaxed. Over a 30-month time period, ending June 30, 1999, the author performed 259 myomectomies via laparoscopy. During the same time period, three myomectomies required laparotomy—patient 1 required concomitant bowel resection secondary to adhesions caused by two previous laparotomies for myomectomy, patient 2 had 92 fibroids removed, patient 3 had a 14 cm fibroid. Patient 3 had to be converted secondary to hemorrhage. The author performed laparoscopic myomectomies for cases with multiple leiomyomata above 5 cm and/or masses lesser than 10 cm.

In a second, now prospective, study from 8/99 through 9/04, 468 cases of laparoscopic myomectomy were evaluated by the author. Of the study population, complete data was compiled in 437 cases. One hundred and thirteen patients had the largest fibroid 8 cm or greater. This corresponds to 26% of the total case load. This includes four patients with 14 cm lead fibroids, six patients with 15 cm fibroids and one patient with a 17 cm fibroid. Table 10.2 shows the large uterine sites encountered and completed over a laparoscopic approach. Over ten percent of patients[49] had uterine sizes greater than or equal to 18 weeks size. Five or more fibroids were removed in 58 cases (13%). Three patients had 30, 34, and 43 fibroids excised respectively. In fact, while the patients having 30 and 43 fibroids removed did not attempt pregnancy, the patient who had 34 fibroids excised subsequently became pregnant and delivered via cesarean section.

Eighty-seven patients had fibroids weighing 250 grams or greater. This accounts for 28% of the study population. Eight percent (25 patients) had fibroids weighing 500 grams or greater. One patient's fibroids

TABLE 10–1			
Author	*Year*	*Recommendations and size*	*Number*
Parker	1995		< 6 cm
Darai	1996	4	< 7 cm
Dubuisson	1996	2	< 8 cm
Miller	1996	< 3, > 5 cm < 10 cm	

TABLE 10–2: Size of uterus (in weeks) at time of laparoscopic myomectomy	
18	21
20	15
22	5
24	5
26	2
30	1

weighed 1,220 grams, while another's weighed 1,359 grams.

Despite the increased technical difficulty of a laparoscopic approach to myomectomy and the potential for adding operative time,[40] a definite advantage exists in regards to postoperative convalescence. While the author routinely hospitalizes patients undergoing myomectomy via laparotomy for 3 to 4 days, virtually all patients in his study of 274 consecutive laparoscopic myomectomies were discharged within 23 hours of admission. In fact, most patients underwent outpatient surgery.[43] Other authors noted similar lengths in hospital stay.[12,57,13, 56, 58]

Finally, in an excellent prospective randomized study performed by Mais, twenty patients undergoing laparoscopic myomectomy were compared with a group undergoing myomectomy via laparotomy. The intensity of postoperative pain was lower in the laparoscopic group with a significantly higher proportion of patients analgesia free by day 2. Furthermore, the laparoscopic group had significantly more patients discharged from the hospital by day 3 and fully recuperated by day 15.

Complications with Laparoscopic Myomectomy

As stated by Wallach in Telinde's Operative Gynecology, myomectomy is generally considered more difficult and time consuming than hysterectomy.[3] He sights the potential for increased blood loss intraoperatively, with resultant postoperative anemia. Also mentioned is an increased risk of ileus.

Laparoscopic myomectomy has been noted to have low risk complications. Several studies are demonstrated in Table 10.3. In a study of 213 patients by Dubuisson, complications were noted in 1.4 percent (3 patients).[34] These patient's major complications were phlebitis, hepatitis, and uterine rupture. In Hasson's series of 56 patients undergoing laparoscopic myomectomy, no major complications were noted; 3 patients developed subcutaneous emphysema.[13] Nezhat noted two major complications in 154 women undergoing laparoscopic myomectomy (1.3%).[12] In a subsequent discourse, however, Nezhat reported a number of endometrial-serosal fistulas post-laparoscopic myomectomy.[45] Seinara reporting on 89 laparoscopic myomectomy procedures noted a 1.8 percent complication rate.[59] In the author's retrospective study of 274 consecutive laparoscopic myomectomies, three major complications were noted (1.1%). Two patients presented postoperatively with secondary port site herniation and bowel obstruction. A third patient underwent transfusion. No patients were noted to have postoperative ileus or pelvic inflammatory disease.

From August of 1999, through September of 2004, the author performed 468 laparoscopic myomectomies. Major complications were noted in 7 cases, while 37 patients had minor complications. Major complications included two postoperative bleeds, hernia (5 mm secondary port), pulmonary embolism, pelvic abscess, pelvic infection and an evulsed uterine artery while removing a large broad ligament myoma. There appears to be no correlation with complications based on size or number of myomata.

Laparoscopic Myomectomy and Uterine Rupture during Pregnancy

Uterine rupture post-laparoscopic myomectomy has been noted in several reports.[44,60-62] Dubuisson observed a single case of rupture at 34 weeks gestation. Interestingly, the uterus was repaired at the time of the original laparoscopic procedure. When a uterine fistula was noted at second-look laparoscopy, the defect was repaired with a single figures of eight suture. Dubuisson recently noted this single case of uterine rupture in a series of 97 patients

TABLE 10–3: Laparoscopic myomectomy: major complication rate (%)			
Author	*Year*	*Number*	*Complication rate*
Dubuisson	1996	213	1.4
Hasson	1992	56	0
Nezhat	1991	154	1.3
Seinara	1997	89	1.8
Miller	2004	468	1.5%

from 1989 through 1997.[47] Harris reported another case of uterine rupture at 34 weeks gestation following laparoscopic removal of a 3 cm fibroid. Although the uterus was repaired, Harris questioned both the suture technique as well as the use of electrocautery.[60] Pelosi and Pelosi described a uterine rupture at 33 weeks gestation after only a superficial myoma was removed.[61] Friedman noted a case of uterine rupture at 28.5 weeks gestation in a patient who previously had laparoscopic removal of a 5 cm intramural fundal fibroid with subsequent laparoscopic repair. In this case, the endometrial cavity had been violated.[62]

In contrast to the reports of uterine rupture in pregnancy post-laparoscopic myomectomy, studies by Hasson,[13] Ribiero and Reich,[55] Darai,[54] Roemich and Nezhat[63] and the author[15] revealed no uterine rupture either prepartum or intrapartum. Compiling these studies, a total of seventy-eight women delivered; a majority via cesarean section. In fact, because of the potential, albeit low risk of uterine rupture, the author recommends cesarean section for both laparoscopic and laparotomy approaches to myomectomy when intramural myomata are excised.[15]

Pelvic Adhesions Post-laparoscopic Myomectomy

The risk of adhesions post-laparoscopic myomectomy does not appear to be as severe as scarring following laparotomy. Hasson performed twenty-four second-look procedures in the 56 patients he treated via laparoscopic myomectomy.[13] Interestingly, the presence of adhesions noted at second-look laparoscopy was based on degree of adhesive disease at initial laparoscopy. Of the fifteen patients without adhesions at time of initial laparoscopic myomectomy, seven (46.6%) had no adhesions at time of second-look laparoscopy while eight (53.4%) had adhesions visualized (three minimal, five moderate to severe). On the other hand, only one of nine patients initially displaying adhesions at time of myomectomy was devoid of adhesions. Eight (89%) were noted to have adhesions (two minimal, six moderate to severe). Of the 24 patients undergoing second-look laparoscopy following a laparoscopic approach to myomectomy, eight (33%) had no adhesions, five (21%) had minimal adhesions and 11 (46%) had moderate or extensive adhesions.

Dubuisson et al performed a prospective study to assess the risk of adhesion post-laparoscopic myomectomy. Between October 26, 1990 and October 1, 1996, 45 patients underwent a second-look laparoscopy.[64] Seventy-two myomectomy sites were examined. Overall, postoperative adhesions were noted in 35.6 percent of patients. Adhesion rate per site was 16.7 percent. Again, the posterior incision and adhesions at initial surgery increased subsequent adhesion formation. The rate of adhesions on the adnexa postmyomectomy was 24.4 percent.

In a case-controlled study of 32 women (of which 28 women underwent second-look) on adhesion formation postlaparoscopic myomectomy and myomectomy via laparotomy, Buletti[65] noted significantly fewer patients with adhesions in the laparoscopic group. Moreover, degree of adhesions was also significantly reduced in the laparoscopy group.

Takeuchi H[80] published his study of adhesion formation postlaparoscopic myomectomy by second look microlaparoscopy. He opined there is increased adhesion risk with posterior incision and intramural myomas. Incidence of adhesion to adnexa was 17.6 percent and 9.8 per site. They conducted a prospective, nonrandomized study. Study group comprised of 115 laparoscopic myomectomy and 51 second look microlaparoscopy. In initial surgery fibrin glue gel was sprayed as anti-adhesion adjunct. Mean fibroids size was 6.1 ± 1.5 cm, mean number of fibroids, 3 ± 2.2 adhesion formation was noted on 152 myomectomy sites giving an incidence of 29.4 percent, 11.2 percent per myomectomy site.

Pregnancy and Delivery: Postlaparoscopic Myomectomy

In Table 10.4, pregnancy rates and delivery rates post-laparoscopic approach to myomectomy are noted. Of the 231 cases of myomectomy via laparoscopy, 127 achieved pregnancy (55%). Ultimately 46 percent (68) of the 150 patients exhibiting delivery data, achieved delivery. These rates are very favorable in comparison to pregnancy and delivery achieved post myomectomy via laparotomy.[2,4,6,8,34,35,47,74,75,83,84]

One must remember that laparoscopic myomectomy is generally performed in light of certain myoma size and number restrictions. For example, both the Dubuisson and Miller articles impose size and number restrictions for laparoscopy.[17,47] As more difficult procedures are performed via laparotomy, pregnancy rates are predictably compromised. On the other hand, it would appear that a laparoscopic approach to myomectomy can be utilized depending on surgeons' comfort and experience, in patients desire—some of pregnancy.

Seracchioli,[81] Human Reproduction 2000 compared fertility and obstetrical outcome after laparoscopic myomectomy versus abdominal myomectomy (Table 10.5).

Dubssion[82] in 2001 give data of 98 patients who had 145 pregnancies, 100 deliveries. They documented 3 cases of uterine rupture, 1 at incision site (1%) 72 patients underwent trial of labor, 58 (80%) delivered vaginally. There was no uterine rupture with trial of labor.

TABLE 10–4: Pregnancy rates and delivery rates post-laparoscopic approach to myomectomy						
Author	*Year*	*Number*	*Pregnancy*		*Delivery*	
Hasson	1992	17	71%	(12)	59%	(10)
Miller	1996	40	754%	(30)	65%	(26)
Dubuisson	1996	21	33.3%	(7)	33.3%	(7)
Ribeiro	1999	28	64.%	(18)	50%	(14)
Darai	1997	44	38.6%	(17)	25%	(11)
Dubuisson	1999	81	53.1%	(4)		

	N	Hgb drop	Hospital stay	Pregnancy rate	Ab rate	Preme
TABLE 10–5: Fertility and obstetric outcome-laparoscopic myomectomy vs abdominal myomectomy						
Laparotomy	65	2.17	142.8	55.9	12.1	20%
Laparoscopy	66	1.37	75.61	53.6	20	12%

Seracchioli. Hum Repro 2000;15(12):2663-68.

Recurrence

Various studies in the literature exist regarding recurrence rates after myomectomy. Long-term recurrence study by Rosetti[83] et al, 181 patients randomized between laparoscopic myomectomy and abdominal myomectomy. Follow-up period was 40 months. They found after abdominal myomectomy recurrence is 23 percent while with laparoscopic approach it is 25 percent. They opined, risk of recurrence is not related to myoma numbers, depth of penetration, myoma size. They noted risk of recurrence increased with preoperative GnRH agonist usage.

While Doriodot;[84] Y et al studied 196 patients over 47 months study period for recurrence after laparoscopic myomectomy. They defined recurrence as recurrence of symptomatology, recurrence at clinical examination and appearance of myoma 2 cm or larger on ultrasound examination. Recurrence rate noted was 22.9 percent (45 patients). Mean time of recurrence was 42 months 4.08 percent patients required a repeat surgery.

Nezhat FR[85] reported their study of 114 patients for recurrence rate after laparoscopic myomectomy. At 12 months recurrence reported was 10.6 percent at 36 months 31.7 percent and at 60 months 51.4 percent. In their study 38.6 percent required one more surgery.

LAPAROSCOPIC MYOMECTOMY UTILIZING ROBOTICS

Recently, the author has started to employ the DaVinci Robot® (Intuitive Surgical, Inc) for certain select cases of laparoscopic myomectomy. Even with the author's vast experience in performing laparoscopic myomectomy, robotics appear to offer advantages. Visualization is three-dimensional. As the gynecologist works comfortably at the surgeon's counsel, range of motion is not encumbered as in standard laparoscopy; the surgeon is able to turn his wrists as in standard suturing. Moreover, tremor can be negated.

Nevertheless, in its current state, there are pitfalls. At present, it is difficult to use a uterine manipulator secondary to placement of the robot between the patient's legs. Rather than 5 mm secondary ports, 8 mm ports must be utilized. Grasping equipment needs to be improved to allow for more aggressive fibroid dissection.

Advincula has exhibited excellent results in a pilot retrospective study.[86] He attempted 35 robot-assisted laparoscopic myomectomies in a university hospital setting with a conversion rate of 8.6%. There were a total of 48 myomas removed in 31 patients with completed robot-assisted laparoscopy. The mean number of myomas removed/patient was 1.6 (range 1-5). The mean diameter of myomas removed was 7.9 and 3.5 cm with the majority great than 5 cm. The mean myoma weight was 223.2 ± 244.1 g. Mean operating time was 230.8 ± 83 minutes. The average estimated blood loss was 169 ± 198.7 ml. One patient experienced cardiogenic shock from vasopressin, two developed postoperative infections, and one was found to have adenomatous adenomyosis instead of a leiomyoma. The median length of hospital stay was one day. Overall, robot-assisted laparoscopic myomectomy is a promising new technique that may overcome many of the surgical limitations of conventional laparoscopy.

SUMMARY

Although myomectomy via laparoscopy requires both skill and experience, it certainly must be considered a viable surgical procedure. Laparoscopic myomectomy has proven to be safe and cost effective. Moreover, the advantages to the patient are obvious.

Complications are low as is the subsequent adhesion rate. Moreover, pregnancy rates are consistent with myomectomy via laparotomy. The gynecologic endoscopist now has the instrumentation to allow a laparoscopic approach to myomectomy to be performed uneventfully in an outpatient arena.

REFERENCES

1. Robbins SC, Cotran RS. Leiomyoma (Fibromyoma). The Pathogenic Basis of Disease (2nd edn). Philadelphia: London, Toronto, WB Saunders Co, 1979;1271.
2. Novak ER, Woodruff JD. Myoma and other benign tumors of the uterus. Gynecologic and Obstetric Pathology (8th edn). Philadelphia: London, Toronto, WB Saunders Co 1979;260-62.
3. Wallach EE. Myomectomy. In JD Thompson, JA Rock (Eds): Telinde's Operative Gynecology (7th edn). JB Lippincott Company: Philadelphia 1992;647-62.
4. Buttram VC, Reiter RC. Uterine leiomyomata: Etiology, symptomatology and management. Fertil Steril 1981;36:433-45.
5. Goldfarb HA. Laparoscopic coagulation of myoma (myolysis). Obstet Gynecol Clin North Am 1995;22(4):807-19.
6. Phillips DR, Milim SJ, Nathanson HG, Haselkorn JS. Experience with laparoscopic leiomyoma coagulation and concomitant operative laparoscopy. J Am Assoc Gynecol Laparosc 1997;4(14):425-33.
7. Olive DL, Rutherford T, Zreik T et al. Cryomyolysis in the conservative treatment of uterine fibroids. J Am Assoc Gynecol Laparosc 1996;3(4, supplement):S36.
8. Goodwin SC, Vedanthan S, McLucas B, Forna AE et al. Preliminary experience with uterine artery embolization for uterine fibroids. J Vasc Interv Radiol 1997;8(4):517-26.
9. Hutchins FL Jr, Worthington-Kirsch RL, Popky GL. Uterine arterial embolization for the management of leiomyomas: quality of life assessment and clinical response. Radiology 1998.
10. Leroy Charles, Personal Communication.
11. Semm K, Mettler L. Technical progress in pelvic surgery via laparoscopy. Am J Obstet Gynecol 1980;138-71.
12. Nezhat C, Nezhat F, Silfen S. Laparoscopic Myomectomy. Int J Fertil 1991;36, 275-80.
13. Hasson HM, Rotman C, Rana N. Laparoscopic myomectomy. Obstet Gynecol 1992;80,884-88.
14. Dubuisson JB, Chapron C, Mouly M. Laparoscopic myomectomy. Gynaecol Endosc 1993;2,171-73.
15. Miller C, Johnston M, Rundell M. Laparoscopic myomectomy in the infertile woman. J Am Assoc Gynecol Laparosc 1996;3(4):525-32.
16. Neuwirth RS. Hysteroscopic management of symptomatic submucous uterine fibroids. Obstet Gynecol 1983;62:509-11.
17. Valle RF. Hysteroscopic removal of submucous myomas. J Gynecol Surg 1990;6: 89-96.
18. Corson SL, Brooks PG. Resectoscopic myomectomy. Fertil Steril 1991;55:1041-44.
19. Vercellini P, Cortesi I, Oldani S et al. The role of transvaginal ultrasonography and outpatient diagnostic hysteroscopy in the evaluation of patients with menorrhagia. Hum Reprod 1997;12(8):1768-71.
20. Goldberg JM, Falcone T, Attaran M et al. Sonohysteroscopic evaluation of uterine abnormalities noted on hysterosalpingography. Human Reprod 1997;12(10):2151-53.
21. Hutchins FL Jr. Uterine fibroids. Diagnosis and indications for treatment. Obstet Gynecol Clin North Am 1995; 22(4):659-65.
22. Topel, HC. Gasless laparoscopic assisted hysterectomy with epidural anesthesia. J Am Assoc Gynecol Laparosc 1994;1(4, Part 2):S36.
23. Hill DJ, Maher PJ, Wood EC. Gasless laparoscopy—useless or useful? J Am Assoc Gynecol Laparosc 1994;1(3):265-68.
24. Bieber EJ, Levrant S. The risk of anterior abdominal wall adhesions in patients with previous umbilical hernia repair. J Am Assoc Gynecol Laparosc 1994;1(4, Part 2):S4.
25. Boike GM, Miller, CE Spirtos NM, et al. Incisional bowel herniations after operative laparoscopy: A series of nineteen cases and review of literature. Am J Obstet Gynecol 1995;172(6)1726-31.
26. Kadar N, Reich H, Liu CY et al. Incisional hernias after major laparoscopic gynecologic procedures. Am J Obstet Gynecol 1993;168:1493-95.
27. Montz FJ, Holschneider CH, Munro MG. Incisional hernia following laparoscopy: A Survey of the American Association of Gynecologic Laparoscopists. Obstet Gynecol 1994;84,881-84.
28. Alexander W. Enucleation of uterine fibroids. Br Gynecol J 1898;14:47.
29. Verkauf BS. Myomectomy for fertility enhancement and preservation. Fertil Steril 1992;58,1-15.
30. Igarashi M. Value of myomectomy in the treatment of infertility (Letter). Fertil Steril 1993; 59: 1331.
31. Farrer-Brown G, Beibly JOW, Tabbit Mtl. The blood supply of the uterus. Arterial vasculature. J Obstet Gynaecol Br Commonw 1970;77:673-81.
32. Saeki M, Kotaki S. Vasculature of uterine myoma for myomectomy. Acta Obstet Gynecol Jan 1974;26:335.
33. Dubuisson JB, Chapron C, Levy L. Difficulties and complications of laparoscopic myomectomy. Journal Gynecol Surg 1996;12(3):159-65.

34. Dubuisson JB, Chapron C, Chavet X et al. Laparoscopic myomectomy: Where do we stand? Gynaecol Endos 1995;4:83-86.

35. Dubuisson JB, Chapron C. Uterine fibroids: Place and modalities of laparoscopic treatment. Eur J Obstet Gynecol Reprod Biol 1996;65(1):91-94.

36. McLaughlin DS. Metroplasty and myomectomy with the CO_2 laser for maximizing the preservation of normal tissue and minimizing blood loss. J Reprod Med 1985;30:1-9.

37. V Cecil Wright, MD. Clinical Professor, Dept of OB/GYN Univ of Western Ontario, London, Ontario. Laser Surgery in Gynecology: A Clinical Guide. WB Saunders Co: Philadelphia, PA. Chapter: CE Miller: Laser Laparoscopy: Fiber Lasers.

38. Daniell JF, Kurtz BR, Taylor SN. Laparoscopic myomectomy using the argon beam coagulator. J Gynecol Surg 1993;9:207-12.

39. Miller CE. Presented at the 22nd Annual Meeting of the American Association of Gynecologic Laparoscopists, San Francisco, CA. November 10-14, 1993. Miller CE. Laparoscopic Myomectomy Featuring the Harmonic Scalpel.

40. Stringer NH, Walker JC, Meyer PM. Comparison of 49 laparoscopic myomectomies with 49 open myomectomies. J Am Assoc Gynecol Laparosc 1997;9(4):457-64.

41. McCarus SD. Physiological Mechanism of the Ultrasonically Activated Harmonic Scalpel. J Am Assoc Gynecologic Laparoscopists. Vol #4;600-08:08/96.

42. Miller CE. Presented at the 22nd Annual Meeting of the American Association of Gynecologic Laparoscopists, San Francisco, CA, November 10-14, 1993. Miller CE. Myomectomy: A Treatment for Patients Desiring Fertility.

43. Miller CE, Davies S, Johnston M. Presented at the 27th Annual Meeting of the American Association of Gynecologic Laparoscopists, Atlanta, GA. November 10-15, 1998. Miller CE. Laparoscopic myomectomy with uterine reconstruction is a safe surgical procedure.

44. Dubuisson JB, Chavet X, Chapron C et al. Uterine rupture during pregnancy after laparoscopic myomectomy. Human Reprod 1995:10:1475-77.

45. Nezhat C. Laparoscopic myomectomy complications (Letter). Int J Fertil 1992;37:64.

46. Dubuisson JB, Lacru F, Foulet H et al. Myomectomy by laparoscopy: A preliminary report of 43 cases. Fertil Steril 1991; 86:827-30.

47. Dubuisson JB, Chapron C, Fauconnier A et al. Laparoscopic myomectomy and myolysis. Curr Opin Obstet Gynecol 1997;9(4):233-38.

48. Barau G, Larue L, Rizk K et al. Myomectomy using laparoscopy: 23 cases. Contracept Fertil Sex 1993;21(1):45-48.

49. Dubuisson JB, Chapron C. Laparoscopic myomectomy and myolysis. Baileres Clin Obstet Gynaecol 1995;9(4):717-28.

50. Dubuisson JB, Chapron C, Verspyck E et al. Laparoscopic myomectomy, 102 cases. Contracept Fertil Sex 1993; 21(12):920-22.

51. Steiner RA, Wright E, Tader V et al. Electrical cutting device for laparoscopic removal of tissue from the abdominal cavity. Obstet Gynecol 1993;81:471-74.

52. Carter JE, McCarus SD. Laparoscopic myomectomy: Time and cost analysis of power vs. manual morcellation. J Reprod Med 1997;42(7):383-88.

53. Stringer NH. Laparoscopic myomectomy with the endostich 10mm laparoscopic suturing device. J Am Assoc Gynecol Laparosc 1996;3(2):299-303.

54. Nezhat C, Nezhat F, Bess O. Laparoscopically assisted myomectomy: A report of a new technique in 57 cases. Int J Fertil 1994;39:39-44.

55. Nezhat C, Nezhat F, Luciano AA et al. Uterine surgery. Operative gynecologic laparoscopy: Principles and techniques. McGraw Hill. New York, 1995;205-38.

56. Nezhat C, Nezhat F, Silfen S. Laparoscopic Myomectomy. Int J Fertil 1991;36,275-80.

57. Parker WH. Myomectomy: Laparoscopy or laparotomy. Clin Obstet and Gynecol 1995;38(2):392-400.

58. Daniell JF, Gurley LD. Laparoscopic treatment of clinically significant symptomatic uterine fibroids. J Gynecol Surg. 1991;7;7:37-40.

59. Seinara P, Arisio R, Decko A et al. Laparoscopic Myomectomy: Indications, surgical technique and complications. Human Reprod 1997;12:1927.

60. Harris WJ. Uterine dehiscence following laparoscopic myomectomy. Obstet and Gynecol 1992;80(3);545-46.

61. Pelosi MA III, Pelosi MA. Spontaneous uterine rupture at thirty-three weeks subsequent to previous superficial laparoscopic myomectomy. Am J Obstet Gynecol 1997;177(6):1547-49.

62. Friedman W, Maier RF, Luttkus A et al. Uterine rupture after laparoscopic myomectomy. Acta Obstet Gynecol Scand 1996;75:683-84.

63. Roemisch M, Nezhat FR, Nezhat C. Pregnancy after laparoscopic myomectomy. J Am Assoc Gynecol Laparosc 1996;3:S42.

64. Dubuisson JB, Fauconnier A, Chapron C et al. Second look after laparoscopic myomectomy. Hum Reprod 1998 Aug; 13(8): 2102-06.

65. Bulletti C, Polli V, Negrini V et al. Adhesion formation after laparoscopic myomectomy. J Am Assoc Gynecol Laparosc 1996 Aug; 3(4):533-36.

66. Brown AB, Chamberlain R, Telinde RW. Myomectomy. Am J Obstet Gynecol 1956;71:759-63.

67. Ingersoll FM, Malone LJ. Myomectomy: An alternative to hysterectomy. Arch Surg 1970;100: 557.

68. Babaknia A, Rock JA, Jones HW. Pregnancy success following abdominal myomectomy for infertility. Fertil Steril 1978;30: 644-48.

69. Buttram VC, Reiter RC. Uterine Leiomyomata: Etiology, symptomatology and management. Fertil Steril 1981;36:433-45.

70. Berkely AS, DeCherney AH, Polan ML. Abdominal myomectomy and subsequent fertility. Surg Gynecol Obstet 1983;156:319-22.

71. Garcia CR, Tureck RW. Submucosal leiomyomas and infertility. Fertil Steril 1984;42:16-19.

72. Ribeiro SC, Reich H, Rosenberg J et al. Laparoscopic myomectomy and pregnancy outcome in infertile patients. Fertil Steril 1999; 71(3):571-74.

73. Reyniak JV, Corenthal L. Microsurgical laser technique for abdominal myomectomy. Microsurgery 1987;8:92.

74. Smith DC, Uhlir JK. Myomectomy as a reproductive procedure. Am J Obstet Gynecol 1990;162:1476-79.

75. Stark GC. CO_2 laser myomectomy in an infertile population. J Reprod Med 1988;33:134-37.

76. Verkauf BS. Myomectomy for fertility enhancement and preservation. Fertil Steril 1992;58,1-15.

77. Tulandi T, Murray C, Guralnick M. Adhesion formation and reproductive outcome after myomectomy and second-look laparoscopy. Obstet Gynecol 1993;82(2):213-15.

78. Gelbach DL, Sousa SE, Carpenter SE et al. Abdominal myomectomy in the treatment of infertility. Int J Gynecol Obstet 1993;40: 45-50.

79. Sudik R, Hüsch K, Steller J, Daume E. Fertility and pregnancy outcome after myomectomy in sterility patients. European J of Obstet and Gynecol 1996; 65: 209-14.

80. Takeuchi H. J American Association of Gynecological Laparoscopists (AAGL) 2002;9(4).

81. Seracchioli. Hum Repro 2000 15(12): 2663-68.

82. Dubuisson JB. Hum Reprod 20015(4): 869-73.

83. Rosetti A. Hum Repro 16(4):770-74.

84. Doridot Y et al. J American Association of Gynecological Laparoscopists (AAGL) 2001;8(4):495-500.

85. Nezhat FR. J American Association of Gynecological Laparoscopists (AAGL) 1998;5(3):237-40.

86. Advincula AP, Song A, Burke W, Reynolds, RK. Preliminary experience with robot assisted laparoscopic myomectomy J Am Assoc Gynecol Laparosc 2004;11(4): 511-8.

Laparoscopic Assisted Minilap Myomectomy

NUTAN JAIN

Chapter Eleven

Myoma uteri are the most common benign uterine tumors encountered in gynecological patients. The incidence now appears to be higher due to better diagnostic facilities like high resolution transvaginal ultrasonography, CT and MRI. Novak et al[1] reported an incidence of 20-25 percent of sexually active and 30-35 percent of all women irrespective of their age. Other studies indicate an even higher incidence, stating that 20-30 percent[2,3] women above the age of 35 have at least one myoma. Another study noted leiomyoma in 50 percent of the females examined at the time of autopsy. A genetic and racial predisposition also exists, women of African origin have 3 to 9 times greater risk of developing uterine fibroids than Caucasian women who are more likely to have myomas compared to women of Asian origin. Overall myomas are responsible for about one-third of all gynecological admissions to hospital services.[4]

Most common indications for removal of fibroids are menorrhagia, pain and infertility. Patients in the younger age group with infertility often present symptomatic or at times big myomas without any symptoms. Their reason for seeking gynecological consultation is only infertility and myomas are diagnosed during the course of investigations. Other patients may present menorrhagia, which could be worse with pain and clots, short cycles amounting to loss of work and affecting day-to-day activities. Yet another presentation would be pain due to pressure symptoms or degenerating myomas. Pressure symptoms develop due to large myomas and size of the myomas increases rapidly.[5] Earlier the only treatment for myomas was hysterectomy, but now more recently, there has been a shift towards preserving the uterus and removing only the myoma. This has been possible with the advent of newer technologies which target the destruction of the myoma alone like myolysis.[6,7] Cryomyolysis and embolizaiton[8,9] and laparoscopic uterine artery ligation.[10]

INDICATIONS

The most common indications of myomectomy appear to be:
1. Desire to conserve the uterus
2. Severe menorrhagia
3. Large myoma or multiple in number.
4. Pressure symptoms leading to abdominal pain.

5. Rapidly growing myomas.
6. Myomectomy for infertility in following situations.
   a. Altered tubo-ovarian relationship.
   b. Intracavitary fibroids
   c. Significantly large, multiple intramural myomas.
   d. Cornual fibroids, pressing upon the utero-tubal junction.
   e. As an opportunity to assess other coexisting pelvic factors like, endometriosis and PID.

Compared to open myomectomy the occurrence of postoperative peritubal adhesions has been found to be relatively low at 9.8 percent which shows that laparoscopic myomectomy or laparoscopic assisted myomectomy contributes to maintaining postoperative fertility. This along with the benefits of minimally invasive surgery are the main reasons for choosing them for the management of myomas.[11]

PREOPERATIVE EVALUATION

All patients must undergo a thorough sonography, which should be a combination of per abdomen, transvaginal and color Doppler sonography. It is mandatory to know the exact site, size, location and number of myomas. I attach so much significance to this that I always do it preoperatively myself to offset any chances of misdiagnosis between a myoma and an adenomyoma (Figs 11.1A and B)[12–15] I feel that preoperative workup before myomectomy is the single largest factor which determines the successful outcome of this technically demanding surgery. CT scan and MRI could be indicated in the face of multiple myomas to verify their location more precisely.

Size and number of myomas to be removed via laparoscopic route—laparoscopic myomectomy is definitely not for novices in the field of laparoscopy. It require greater skills and manual dexterity to complete a multi layer, sound anatomic closure of the myoma bed. For this reason alone, many authors have laid down guidelines regarding the size and number of myomas over which myomectomy should not be performed laparoscopically. All this appears due to the anatomical distortions provided by multiple fibroids and difficulty in suturing multiple myoma sites.[16] Though now several literature reports are appearing for laparoscopic myomectomy for large myomas.[17]

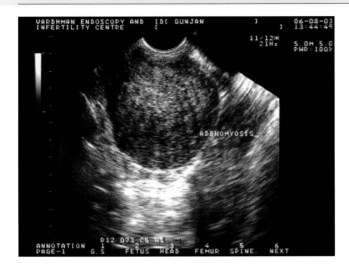

Fig. 11.1A: Adenomyosis

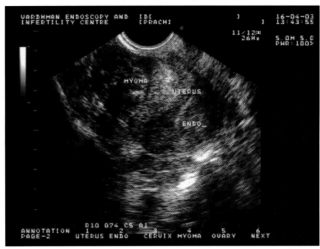

Fig. 11.1B: Myoma

Keeping in mind the technical difficulties in enucleating and removing large myomas and most importantly, suturing the multiple, large myoma beds with precision such that they can bear the stretch and tension of subsequent pregnancy and labor, the concept of LAM (Laparoscopic Assisted Myomectomy) has come.[18-22] When posed with large and multiple fibroids and a surgeon having lesser technical skills this hybrid surgery becomes a very feasible option. A 12 cm myoma could be within the suturing skills of one surgeon but for another it may become too large to enucleate, remove and suture. So the indications for LAM appear to be relative, according to the surgeon's expertise. By and large the indications for LAM are:

i. Uterus size more than 20-22 cm (Figs 11.2A and B).
ii. Multiple, large myomas
iii. Single, very large myoma
iv. Myomas in more technically demanding positions like very deep posterior myomas (Figs 11.3A and B).
v. Any time when a surgeon is less versed in suturing and does not have access to a morcelator, and then he may choose to remove myoma by minilap incision.

Pretreatment with GnRH agonists before myomectomy remains controversial. In a systematic review of randomized, controlled trials of the use of GnRH analogs before hysterectomy and myomectomy, it was found that preoperative and postoperative blood counts were improved by GnRH agonist therapy, uterine and myoma volume decreased, and operative time and blood loss were reduced.[23] Reduction in leiomyoma size makes the procedure less time consuming because a smaller uterine incision can be made and less morcellation is required. The individual myomas, however, are softer, which often results in the Lahey clamps tearing through the tissue resulting in the loss of upward traction. This can result in increased bleeding. We have never used GnRh analogs in our practice, as I believe that removing a 10 cm or a 14 cm myoma does not make any difference if we work in a correct anatomical plane with a sound surgical technique.

Procedure

Patient under GA, with nasogastric tube.
a. Modified lithotomy.
b. Primary umbilical port is shifted higher up anywhere between the umbilicus and xiphisternum according to the size of the myomas (Fig. 11.4).
c. All accessory ports (3-4 in number) made higher up to accommodate the large and multiple myomas and make the enucleation easier.
d. After entry, a thorough inspection of entire pelvis is done and the preoperative scan findings are validated. Exact size and site of myoma is documented. In an Infertility patient all attempts are made to do gentle adhesiolysis and normalize

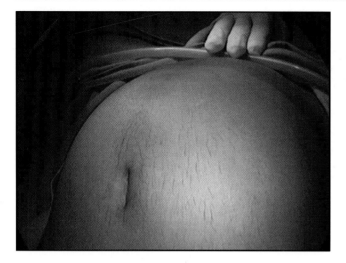

Fig. 11.2A: Per abdomen picture of 26 weeks size uterus

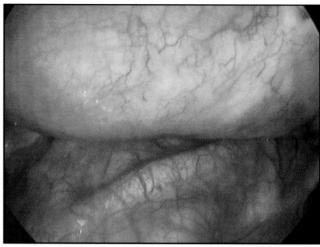

Fig. 11.2B: Big myoma overlying the aortic bifurcation

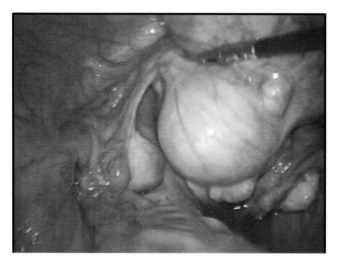

Fig. 11.3A: Deep posterior wall myoma

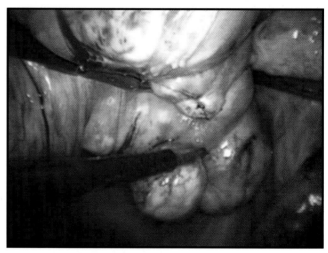

Fig. 11.3B: Multiple posterior wall myoma

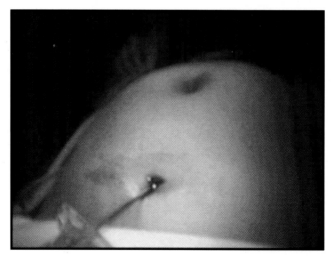

Fig. 11.4: Veress needle insertion just beneath the xiphisternum

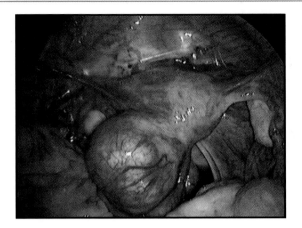

Fig. 11.5: Endometriosis of UV pouch with subserous myoma

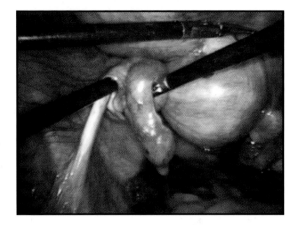

Fig. 11.6: Chromopertubation before myomectomy

the tube ovarian anatomy. Careful search is done to look for foci of endometriosis, which are fulgurated (Fig. 11.5). A chromopertubation is done to check for tubal patency (Fig. 11.6).

e. One ampoule of Pitresin diluted in about 100 ml of saline is injected subserosally in all the myomas.[24] It is important to enter the exact plane and inject a sufficient amount as pitressin acts not only by decreasing bleeding from myoma bed but also by developing a handy plane of cleavage between the pseudo capsule and myoma. Since in minilap there are usually too many and large myomas, we dilute 1 amp of pitressin in about 100 ml saline.

f. After injecting pitressin I proceed to do a diagnostic hysteroscopy, which provides sufficient time for the pitressin to be therapeutically effective. Hysteroscopy usually confirms the findings of prior transvaginal sonography.

SUBMUCOUS MYOMA

Fedele and colleagues[25] evaluated the accuracy of TVS in detection of small submucous myomas in patients who underwent both TVS and Hysteroscopy. The sensitivity and specificity of TVS and Hysteroscopy was same, TVS having sensitivity of 100 percent and specificity of 94 percent and Hysteroscopy having sensitivity of 100 percent and specificity of 96 percent. The predictive value of an abnormal scan was 81 percent while that of abnormal Hysteroscopy was 87 percent. TVS and Hysteroscopy have found to have such good correlation and from here comes the

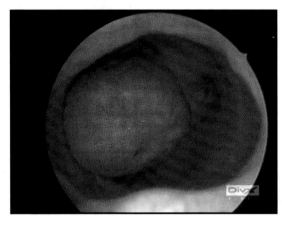

Fig. 11.7: Fibroid polyps

reliance on it as a useful[26,27] diagnostic tool in the preoperative assessment of endometrial cavity.

If there is any small polyp (Fig. 11.7), which was missed on the scan, it is removed. If there is a bigger myoma 3-4 cm then I prefer to leave it and remove it during the course of minilap myomectomy.

Laparoscopic Procedure

After injecting Pitressin and doing a hysteroscopy, we proceed to make a transverse incision on the biggest myoma. Transverse incision is usually preferred as it causes less blood loss since the incision goes in the line of radial arteries as they emerge from the uterine arteries (Figs 11.8A to F) A monopolar cautery hook or spatula is used to make and deepen the incision. Tissue harmonic scalpel can also be used. The myoma enucleation is started as soon as we reach the pearly white myoma. A myoma screw is applied

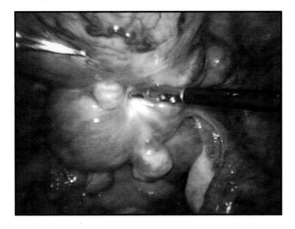

Fig. 11.8A: Initial appearance of myoma

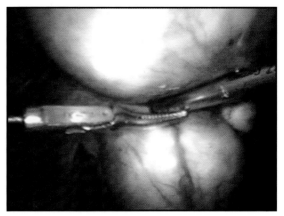

Fig. 11.8B: Injecting pitressin

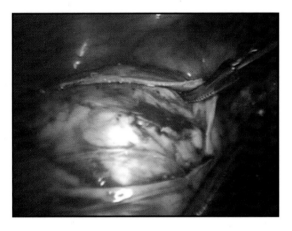

Fig. 11.8C: Transverse incision

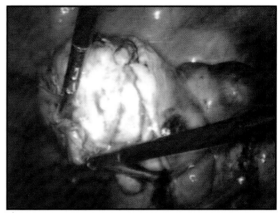

Fig. 11.8D: Enucleation of myoma

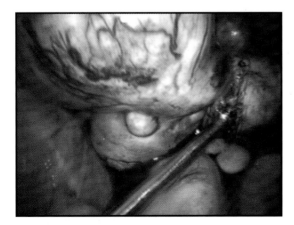

Fig. 11.8E: Myoma screw applied over the
posterior myoma

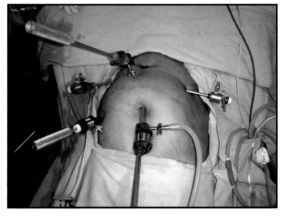

Fig. 11.8F: Placing two myoma screws, one over the
largest myoma through the suprapubic port and other
over the deepest posterior myoma through the left
paraumbilical port

over the most bulging part of myoma and enucleation progresses by means of sharp scissors dissection and preventive, prophylactic cautery by bipolar coagulation. This gives speed to the dissection. Thorough suction irrigation and lavage helps to keep the surgical field clear. Since now we will proceed for a minilap myomectomy it is not necessary to enucleate the entire myoma, it is rather much easier to let it remain attached to the uterus hooked by the myoma screw which makes it removal by minilap incision much easier and faster.

I personally prefer making incisions overall bulging myomas before proceeding for minilap myomectomy. Even a moderately deep, transverse incision made by monopolar cautery allows for a quick enucleation by a finger when mini lap incision is given. As the incisions are made by monopolar cautery in the exact cleavage plane after injecting pitressin, the incisions do not bleed. Hence, there is a no risk in giving incisions overall the myomas and then proceed for minilap incision.

Before proceeding to make a small 3-4 cm minilap incision, we ensure that, laparoscopically.

1. All myomas are conclusively located.
2. Their number is ascertained so that we can remove all.
3. All adhesiolysis, completed, chromopertubation done.
4. Biggest myoma is enucleated to some extent and myoma screw applied to it.
5. All other myomas have a transverse incision, which makes their location via minilap much easier and quicker, especially the deep posterior myomas.

Now with CO_2 pneumoperitoneum, a small 3 cm transverse incision is made just above the pubic hairline. The trick is to keep the skin incision smaller but to advance the rectus sheath incision 1-2 cm beyond the skin incision margins. This instantly gives a lot of space to work within. Some surgeons prefer to give a cruciate incision. Meaning thereby, that, the skin incision is transverse but the rectus sheath is opened vertically to a length of 6 cm by tunneling with a finger bluntly under the subcutaneous fat cranially towards umbilicus and caudally towards pubic bone. The myoma screw is already on the myoma so the peritoneum is incised vertically along it to quickly reach the largest myoma. Using a combination of vaginal manipulation, traction by myoma screw and surgeon's finger or knife handle, the myoma is enucleated . If it is too large we start reducing it piecemeal by cutting chunks of myoma using a conventional knife and keep removing them. Major debulking by cutting chunks of myoma tissue is done before removing a big myoma, so that the skin incision is not unduly widened. If we proceed patiently, it usually does not take too long, and adhering to the surgical plane causes hardly any bleeding. If at all the big myoma bed bleeds too much, then myometrial bed closure is done before proceeding to remove the other myomas. This is accomplished by using 1-0 vicryl on a curved needle. Very efficient closure can be done in two to three layers, starting from the base of myoma. Then the top most layer including subserosa and serosa is closed by 3-0 vicryl.

After making the peritoneal opening the CO_2 pneumoperitoneum is turned off. Now the procedure continues by the minilap route. One by one, all myomas are enucleated and removed by utilizing a tenaculum and surgeon's finger. After having first removed the biggest myoma, the smaller ones come out much more easily as the incision is widened by the removal of the first myoma. Irrigation and lavage continues by abdominal route. Suturing is done meticulously, trying to give a sound anatomic closure (Figs 11.9A to F), which will endure the stress of pregnancy and labor. All measures are taken to decrease adhesion formation like.

1. Minimal tissue trauma by gentle handling
2. Avoidance of tissue drying.
3. Decreasing blood loss by controlled preventive bipolar coagulation and working in correct tissue planes.
4. Thorough suction irrigation and lavage to keep field clear.
5. Meticulous closure and use of fine sutures over the serosa

I do not use any adhesion barriers and rely only on the above measures for postoperative reduction in adhesion formation.

After minilap, extraction of myomas and suturing is completed; (Figs 11.10A to C) we suture the small Pfannensteil incision and go back laparoscopically for a final inspection and clearing of the peritoneal cavity. All clots, fluids, debris and char is sucked out. All sutured myoma sites are visualized for any bleeding

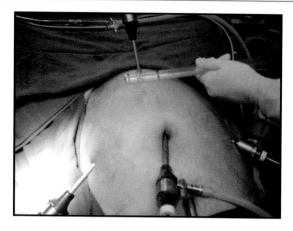

Fig. 11.9A: Marking the minilap incision

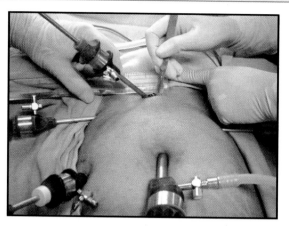

Fig. 11.9B: Giving the minilap incision

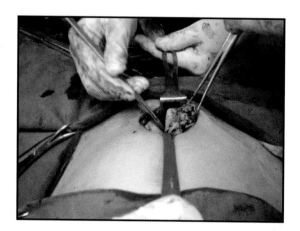

Fig. 11.9C: Enucleation of the myoma

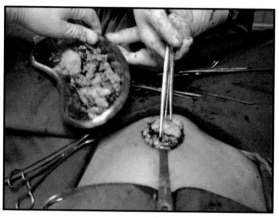

Fig. 11.9D: Removing the myoma piecemeal

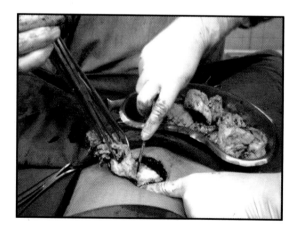

Fig. 11.9E: Cutting chunks of myoma using conventional knife

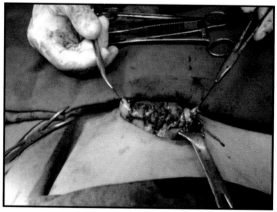

Fig. 11.9F: Completed suturing of myoma bed

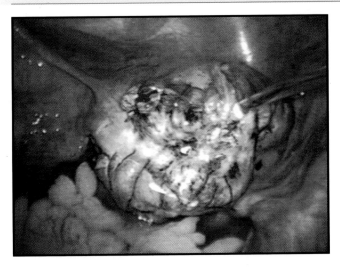

Fig. 11.10A: Uterus after completed myomectomy

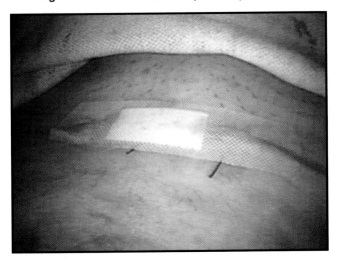

Fig. 11.10B: Final appearance of minilap incision

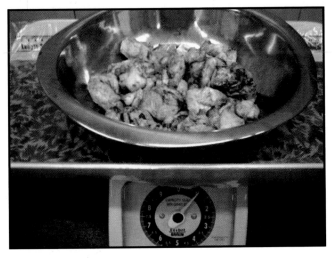

Fig. 11.10C: Weight of the myoma

point, which is coagulated by using a bipolar forceps. The magnification offered by operative laparoscopy and the wide field of vision is more superior to minilap, so we routinely spend time on improving the cleanliness of the surgical field by laparoscopic means. At end we instill 2 liters of ringers lactate into the peritoneal cavity. The hospitalization ranges from 24-48 hours during which the patients are fully ambulatory and comfortable. The postoperative course does not appear to differ too much from that of laparoscopic myomectomy.

OTHER TECHNIQUES OF LAM

With technological advancements coming in, minilap myomectomy is carried out with the help of atraumatic elastic retractors with or without laparoscopic guidance. A small 4-6 cm incision is given and the elastic abdominal retractor is put in place.

The benefit of elastic retractor is that it gives a rounded opening in anterior abdominal wall. The retractor is soft and atraumatic to the tissue of the abdominal wall while it keeps subcutaneous fat, muscles and peritoneum out of the operative field. This needs a 4-5 cm incision.[28]

The study by Glasser et al comprises of 139 myomectomies, mean wt of myomas removed is 275 (rage 30-975 gm), 137 where discharged in less than 24 hours. The mean operating time was 110 minutes (rage 44-260 min) EBL (No-200 ml) with mid in of 300 L. Three hysterectomy performed one for hemorrhage and two for recurrent myomas. Pelosi et al[29,30] have described their technique for myomas of extreme sizes. Hand assisted laparoscopic myomectomy (Figs 11.11A to D) fills the gap between conventional laparoscopic and laparoscopic assisted techniques and laparotomy for the massive fibroids. The ability to use an operative hand results in excellent laparoscopic exposure, effective myoma traction counter traction, digital feel and finer myoma enucleation, removal of myoma and suturing in full three layers. There are several hand assisted laparoscopic system available. They include the original Dexterity Pneumo Sleeve (Dexterity Surgical Inc., Rosewell, GA), Omniport (Advanced Surgical Concepts, Wicklow, Ireland), Gelport (Applied Medical, Randio Santa Margarita, CA) and the LAP DISC hand access device (Ethicon Endo-Surgery, Inc. Cincinnati, OH). The various systems available for

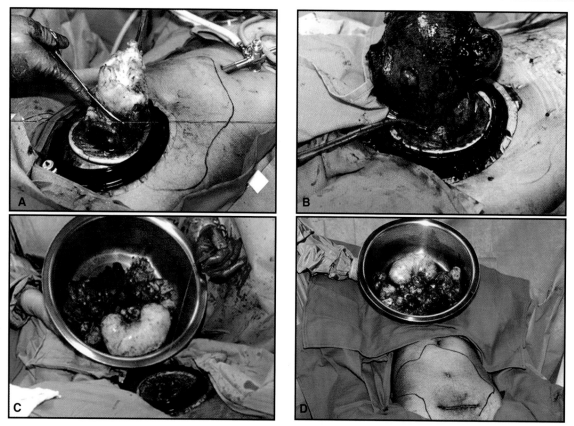

Figs 11.11A to D: Hand-assisted laparoscopic myomectomy. (A) Hand-assisted laparoscopic myomectomy results in a significant reduction in uterine size that allows partial exteriorization through the abdominal incision to continue the myomectomies. This creates a further decrease in uterine size, (B) The debulked uterus is then easily delivered through the incision to complete the myomectomies. A rubber hemostatic tourniquet is routinely used, (C) The uterus is reconstructed using a layered conventional suturing technique, (D) The laparoscopic and the hand-assisted laparoscopic incision are then closed. The total weight of the case example was 3,120 gm

hand-assisted laparoscopies are shown in Figure 11.12. They all provide extracorporeal extension of pneumoperitoneum and abdominal access for the surgeon during laparoscopic surgery, while maintaining constant peritoneal gas pressure.

Difficulties during Minilap Myomectomy

The most common problem that occurs lies in localizing the very deep posterior myomas. Due to the small incision the uterus cannot be hooked anteriorly to a great extent. In this situation, assistance can be taken from the vaginal manipulator but this may also not work at times. Once, I had to go back laparoscopically during a minilap myomectomy to make the incision over the deep posterior myoma. Enucleation and suturing was done by minilap incision. So the best technique is to localize all myomas laparoscopically and make an incision over them laparoscopically, before proceeding for minilap myomectomy,

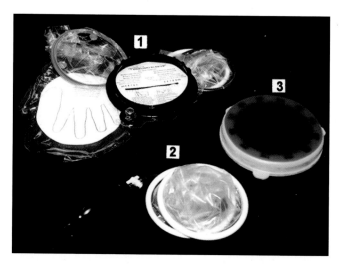

Fig. 11.12: Current hand-assisted laparoscopy systems. (1) Dexterity® Pneumo Sleeve (Dexterity Surgical Inc. Rosewell, GA), (2) Omniport (Advanced Surgical Concepts, Wicklow, Ireland), (3) Gelport (Applied Medical–Rancho Santa Margarita, CA)

more so for posterior and deep myomas. Anterior myomas are very easily accessible even when situated deep in the myometrium. The second difficulty usually arises with big (15-20 cm) myomas is in their piecemeal removal. With adequate surgical technique and patience there will be no need to widen the incision. It is best to keep tractions on the myoma by stout tenaculums and to keep cutting with a surgical knife whatever myoma is presenting in the minilap incision. Hurrying up this step may unnecessarily widen the incision while pulling out a big myoma.

Another problem could be lost myomas. During the laparoscopic phase of the surgery it is advisable to restrict oneself to only superficially enucleating the myomas and not entirely so that they are not lying free in the pouch of Douglas. While changing the patient's positioning from steep Trendelenburg to routine minilap, the myomas may get lost. So, it is advisable to keep track of the exact number of myomas: those seen initially, during surgery and those enucleated and removed.

Another difficulty could be bleeding. It is usually not excessive, it is simply that when large myomas are removed and till they are sutured the myoma bed may bleed. Many of these patients could be having a low hematocrit preoperatively on account of prolonged spells of menorrhagia. So compounded with low hemoglobin and relatively more blood loss, these patients may require blood transfusion. Hence, it is always good to have the patient's blood cross-matched and extra units kept ready.

Time spent on such surgeries where large size and large number of myomas are removed in combination to the laparoscopic and abdominal route is usually about 120-150 minutes. So the anesthetist, surgeon and surgical team should be prepared for a prolonged procedure. Surgical time can be reduced by adopting the laparoscopic route for inspection, adhesiolysis, myoma mapping, and chromopertubation and injecting pitressin. Making incision by monopolar cautery or harmonic scalpel over the biggest myoma and deep and posterior myomas and spending time only on more superficial enucleation which is enough to reach the definite plane of myoma, then attaching myoma screw on the myoma and quickly going over the minilap route rather than spending lot of time laparoscopically and then at the minilap. The end result is the same, so it is a better option to spend less time in enucleating the myoma during the laparoscopic phase of the surgery as we are actually converting an open laparotomy into a more feasible minilap procedure which will ensure a good outcome.

COMPLICATIONS

We have not encountered any complications and as such there does not appear to be any complications which could arise during a minilap procedure. Hemorrhage and blood transfusion are taken as acceptable for large and multiple myomas. Infection could arise; so prophylactic antibiotics are given at induction of anesthesia and two doses thereafter of third generation cephalosporin

RESULTS

Lap-assisted minilap myomectomy appears to be safer and relatively simpler procedure in the hands of experienced laparoscopists as well as novices since the much dreaded steps of myomectomy, i.e. suturing and morcellation can be completed by the minilap route. So, for the less experienced an 8 cm myoma can be dealt by minilap while an advanced endoscopist will resort to minilap for multiple and very big myomas. It appears to be a patient friendly procedure giving all the benefits of laparoscopy with the help of a small, 3-4 cm incision which heals well in the postoperative phase. We have done about 105 minilap-assisted lap myomectomies for myoma size ranging up to 23 cm and largest number of fibroids removed was 31 and weight of myomas ranging between 450-1100 gm. Mostly the indication is multiple 10-12 myomas and largest myoma being more than 15 cm. This is planned preoperatively, there is no sudden conversion on the table from laparoscopic myomectomy to laparoscopic assisted myomectomy. At least 10 patients required blood transfusion, which was anticipated preoperatively.

There has never been conversion to laparotomy and never a hysterectomy!. At our center, this procedure has been established with good surgical result in terms of reproductive out come. Pregnancy rates are very encouraging. Second look scopies performed in three patients revealed moderate, flimsy adhesions, showing the procedure to be less adhesiogenic. Most patients are delivered by cesarean section as the uterine cavity is usually opened in the face of multiple myomas. There has been no incidence of scar dehiscence during pregnancy or labor. Similar results have been found and published by several other surgeons. Nezhat et al[31,32] have compared all three groups, i.e. laparotomy, laparoscopic myomectomy (LM) and laparoscopic assisted myomectomy (LAM) and have found that adhesion score, postoperative recovery, hospital stay, blood loss and days for complete recovery are not statistically different in the groups of LM and LAM. Postoperative stay for LAM was 1.28 whilst .91 for LM, Blood loss was 267 ml in LAM and 143 ml in LM, Days to resume normal activity were 12.2 in LAM and 11.2 in LM. All these compared to laparotomy were less, blood loss 245 ml, postoperative hospital stay 3.3, days to resume normal work 39 days. Thus, it appears that LAM compares favorably with LM and empowers the surgeon to avoid the full laparotomic approach thereby giving patient all the benefits of minimally invasive surgery and good reproductive outcome.

So, in conclusion, LAM operation is safe, feasible, offers easy to perform minimally invasive myomectomy for deep intramural and multiple fibroids with all the benefits of laparoscopic surgery and good reconstructive and reproductive outcome.

REFERENCES

1. Novak ER, Jones GS, Jones HW. Myomes uterins. In Novak ER, Jones GS, Jones HW (Eds): Gynecologic Pratiquue. Paris: Editions maloine.1970;309-22.
2. Novak ER, Woodruff JD. Myoma and other benign tumors of the uterus. Gynecologic and Obstetric Pathology (8th edn). Philadelphia: London, Toronto, WB Saunders Co. 1979;260-62.
3. Wallach EE. Myomectomy. In JD Thompson, Ja Rock (Eds): Telinde's Operative Gynecology (7th edn). JB Lippincott Company: Philadelphia 1992;647-60.
4. Thompson JD, Rock Ja. Leiyomyomata uteri and myomectomy. In: Rock JA and Thompson JD (Eds): Te Linde's Operative Gynaecology. Philadelphia: Lipincott-Raen, 1992;371-69.
5. Reich H, Thompson KA, Nataupsky LG, Grabo TN, Sekel L. Laparoscopic myomectomy: an alternative to laparotomy myomectomy or hysterectomy? Gynecological Endoscopy 1997;6:7-12.
6. Goldfarb HA. Laparoscopic coagulation of myoma (myolysis). Obstet Gynecol Clin North Am 1995;22(4):807-19.
7. Philips DR, Milim SJ, Nathanson HG, Haselkorn JS. Experience with laparoscopic leiomyoma coagulation and concomitant operative Laparoscopy. J Am Assoc Gynecol Laparosc 1997;4(14):425-33.
8. Goodwin SC, Vedanthan S, McLucas B, Forna AE et al. Preliminary experience with uterine artery embolization for uterine fibroids. J Vasc Interv Radiol 1997;8(4):517-26.
9. Hutchins FL Jr, Worthington-Kirsch RL, Popky GL. Uterine arterial embolization for the management of leiomyomas: quality of life assessment and clinical response. Radiology 1998.
10. Leroy Charles, Personal Communication.
11. Takeeuchi H, Kinoshita K. Evaluation of adhesion formation after laparoscopic myomectomy b systematic second-look microlaparoscopy. J Am Assoc Gynecol Laparosc 2002;9:442-46.
12. Dodson MG, Pache TD. In Dodson MG (Ed): The Uterus in Transvaginal Ultrasound (2nd edn); New York, Churchill Livingstone 1995;56-60.
13. Fedele L, Bianchi S, Dorta M, Arcaini L, Zanotti F, Carineli S. Transvaginal Sonography in the diagnosis of diffuse adenomyosis. Fertil Streil 1992;58:94-97.
14. Fedele L, Bianchi S, Dorta M, Zanotti F, Brioschi D, Carinelli S. Transvaginal ultrasonography in the differential diagnosis of adenomyoma versus leiomyoma. Am J Obstet Gynecol 1992;167:603-06.
15. Scoutt LM, McCarthy SM, Moss AA. Computed Tomography and Magnetic Resonance Imaging of the Pelvis in Computed Tomography of the Body edited by Moss AA, Gamsu G, Genant HK (2nd edn), Philadelphia: WB Saunders 1992;3:1233-34.
16. Dubuisson JB, Chapron C, Chavet X et al. Laparoscopic myomectomy: Where do we stand? Gynaecol Endos 1995;4:83-86.
17. Tulandi T, Youseff H. Laparoscopy-assisted myomectomy of large uterine myomas. Gynaecol Endosc 1997;6:105-08.
18. Nezhat C, Nezhat F, Bess O. Laparoscopically assisted myomectomy: A report of a new technique in 57 cases. Int J Fertil 1994;39:39-44.
19. Nezhat C, Nezhat F, Luciano AA et al. Uterine surgery. Operative gynecologic Laparoscopy: Principles and techniques. New York: McGraw Hill 1995;205-38.
20. Nezhat C, Nezhat F, Silfen S Laparoscopic Myomectomy. Int J Fertil 1991;36,275-80.
21. Benedetti-Panici P, Maneschi F, Cutillo G. Surgery by minilaparotomy in benign gynecologic disease. Obstet Gynecol. 1996;87:456-59.

22. Nezhat C, Nezhat F, Fess O. Laparoscopically assisted myomectomy: a report of a new technique in 57 cases Intl J Fertil & Menop Studies 1994;39:39-44.

23. Lethaby A, Vollenhoven B, Sowter M. Efficacy of pre-operative gonadotrophin releasing hormone analogues for women with uterine fibroids undergoing hysterectomy or myomectomy: a systematic review. BJOG. 2002;109:1097-1108.

24. Fredrick J, Fletcher H, Simeon D. Intramyometrial vasopressin as a hemostatic agent during myomectomy. Br J Obstet and Gynecol, 1994;101:435-37.

25. Fedele L, Bianchi S, Dorta M, Brioschi D, Zanotti F, Vercellini P. Transvaginal ultrasonography versus Hysteroscopy in the diagnosis of uterine submucous myoma. Obstet Gynecol 1991;77:745-48.

26. Kurjak A, Kupesic S, Zalud I, Predanic M. In Dodson MG (Ed): Transvaginal Color Doppler. Transvaginal ultrasound. New York: Churchill Livingstone 1995;325-39.

27. Flesicher AC, Kepple DM, Entman SS. Transvaginal Sonography of uterine disorder. In Timor-Tritsch IE, Rottam S (Eds): Transvaginal Sonography (2nd edn). New York; Elsevier, 1991:109-30.

28. Mark H. Glasser minilap myomectomy: A minimally invasive alternative for the large fibroid uterus Journal of Minimally invasive Gynaecology 2005;12,275-83.

29. Pelosi MA III, Pelosi MA II. Laparoscopic-assisted transvaginal myomectomy. J Am Assoc Gynecol Laparosc 1997;4:241-46.

30. Pelosi MA II, Pelosi MA III. Hand-assisted Laparoscopy (handoscopy) for megamyomectomy. A case study. J Reprod Med 2000;45:519-25.

31. Nezhat C, Nezhat F, Bess O. Laparoscopically assisted myomectomy: A report of a new technique in 57 cases. Int J Fertil 1994;39:39-44.

32. Nezhat C, Nezhat F, Luciano AA et al. Uterine surgery. Operative gynecologic Laparoscopy: Principles and techniques. New York: McGraw Hill 1995;205-38.

Laparoscopic Paravaginal Repair and Burch Urethropexy

ROBERT D MOORE

JOHN R MIKLOS, NEERAJ KOHLI

Chapter Twelve

INTRODUCTION

Since the introduction of the retropubic urethral suspension in 1910, over 100 different surgical techniques for the treatment of genuine stress urinary incontinence (GSUI) have been described.[1] Many have been modifications of original procedures in an attempt to improve clinical outcome, shorten operative time, and reduce surgical morbidity. Despite the number of surgical procedures developed each year, the Burch colposuspension and pubovaginal sling operations have remained the mainstay of surgical correction for GSUI because of their high long-term cure rates. However, these procedures do not address the concurrent anterior vaginal wall prolapse often associated with GSUI secondary to urethral hypermobility. We present a laparoscopic approach to anterior vaginal wall reconstruction using the paravaginal repair and Burch colposuspension for treatment of cystocele and stress urinary incontinence, respectively, resulting from lateral vaginal wall support defects.

Emphasizing the principles of minimally invasive surgery, the laparoscopic approach has been successfully adopted for many procedures that previously relied on an abdominal or transvaginal route. First described in 1991, the laparoscopic retropubic colposuspension has rapidly gained popularity because of its many reported advantages, including improved visualization, shorter hospital stay, faster recovery, and decreased blood loss.[2]

Laparoscopy should be considered only as a mode of abdominal access and not a change in the operative technique. Ideally the indications for a laparoscopic approach to retropubic colposuspension should be the same as an open (laparotomy) approach. This would include patients with GSUI and urethral hypermobility. The authors believe the laparoscopic Burch colposuspension can be substituted for an open Burch colposuspension in the majority of cases. Factors that might influence this decision include any history of previous pelvic or anti-incontinence surgery, the patient's age and weight, the need for concomitant surgery, contraindications to general anesthesia, and the surgeon's experience. The surgeon's decision to proceed with a laparoscopic approach should be based on an objective clinical assessment of the patient as well as the surgeon's own surgical skills. Loss of the lateral vaginal attachment to the pelvic sidewall is called a paravaginal defect and usually results in a cystourethrocele and urethral hypermobility. If the patient demonstrates a cystocele secondary to a paravaginal defect diagnosed either pre- or intraoperatively, a paravaginal defect repair should be performed before the colposuspension. This approach combines the paravaginal repair with Burch colposuspension for treatment of anterior vaginal prolapse secondary to paravaginal defects and stress urine incontinence secondary to urethral hypermobility.[3–5] The paravaginal defect repair also places the anterior vaginal wall in its correct anatomic position, i.e. at the level of the arcus tendineus fascia pelvi prior to the Burch sutures being placed. This helps minimize the chance of overcorrection of the bladder neck with the Burch sutures because the paravaginal repair limits how much the Burch sutures can be tightened and only allows the bladder neck to be elevated approximately 1-2 cm above the level of the base of the bladder. This adjustment and limitation helps reduce the risk of postoperative voiding dysfunction.

We recommend that all patients have a modified bowel preparation consisting of a full liquid diet 48 hours before scheduled surgery and a clear liquid diet and one bottle of magnesium citrate 24 hours before surgery. This regimen appears to improve visualization of the operative field by bowel decompression and reduces that chance of contamination in case of accidental bowel injury. A single dose of prophylactic intravenous antibiotics is administered 30 minutes before surgery. Antiembolic compression stockings are routinely used. The patient is intubated, given general anesthesia, and placed in a dorsal lithotomy position with both arms tucked to her side. A 16 F 3-way Foley catheter with a 5 mL balloon tip is inserted into the bladder and attached to continuous drainage (Fig. 12.1).

Since Vancaillie and Schuessler[2] published the first laparoscopic colposuspension case series in 1991, many other investigators have reported their experience. Review of the literature reveals a lack of uniformity in surgical technique and surgical materials used for colposuspension. This lack of standardization is also noted with the conventional open (laparotomy) technique. Because of this lack of standardization and the steep learning curve associated with laparoscopic suturing, surgeons have

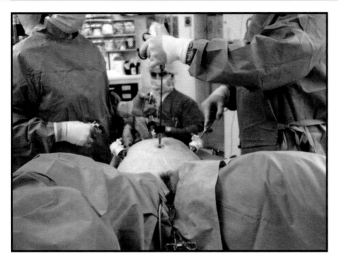

Fig. 12.1: Positioning. The patient is placed in dorsal lithotomy position in adjustable Allen stirrups. A 3-way Foley catheter is placed to be able to retrograde fill the bladder. The surgeon stands on the patient's left side and the assistant on the right side

attempted to develop faster and easier ways of performing a laparoscopic Burch colposuspension. These modifications have included the use of stapling devices, bone anchors, synthetic mesh, and fibrin glue.[6-8] However, we believe the laparoscopic approach should be identical with the open technique to allow comparative studies as well as to ensure the patient is receiving an identical procedure utilizing either approach. When conventional surgical technique is described and utilized, cure rates have been shown to be identical via a laparoscopic or open approach.[9-14] Advantages of the laparoscopic approach are improved visualization, decreased blood loss, decreased bladder/ureteral injuries and magnification of other pelvic floor defects that need to be repaired.[15-17] Other advantages include less postoperative pain, shorter hospital stays and shorter recovery time with faster return to a better quality of life.

The space of retzius is one of the most difficult areas to suture laparoscopically secondary to limited space and the angles required to place and retrieve sutures. We utilize one port to do all of our laparoscopic suturing and the surgeon is the only one passing and retrieving needles. Some authors recommend either using their assistant to load or retrieve needles or the surgeon changes sides of the table to suture on the patient's contralateral side. We feel this is not

necessary, nor is it efficient. Utilizing proper angles and needle placement, as well as utilizing the vaginal hand to elevate and manipulate the anterior vaginal wall, the surgeon can complete all suturing from one side of the table and utilize the assistant to hold the camera and retract only. We feel this helps improve efficiency, safety and optimizes the economy of motion of the procedure. There is no need for the surgeon or the assistant to change sides of the table.

Equipments and Sutures

Many different types of sutures and instruments have been described for use in laparoscopic paravaginal repair and Burch colposuspension. We feel that permanent sutures should be utilized in pelvic floor repairs and therefore utilize permanent sutures in laparoscopic Burch/PVR. Our suture of choice for pelvic reconstructive surgery is 2-0 Ethibond (Ethicon) on a SH needle, which is a braided permanent suture. To be able to tie extracorporeal knots when suturing in the space of retzius, it necessary to have a minimal suture length of 48 inches, therefore some sutures may need to be special ordered to obtain this minimal length. Since there is a limitation of space retropubically, we have found the ideal size of needle utilized should be no larger than an SH needle. CT-1 needles have been utilized, however we find these needles too large to manipulate in the space of retzius and feel there is more chance of injury to vascular and visceral structures. We utilize Gore-Tex permanent sutures on a CV-1 taper cut needle for the Burch portion of the procedure secondary to taking two passes through the pubocervical fascia. A double-pass allows us to get an adequate purchase of vaginal tissue and the nature of the Gore-Tex suture allows the suture to slide very easily through the tissue, even with a double-bite. Braided sutures such as Ethibond or Vicryl do not slide through the tissue like this and each throw through the tissue has to be taken separately which increases operative time. In paravaginal repair, only one pass is taken through the vagina and sidewall and therefore Gore-Tex (which is more expensive than Ethibond) is not necessary.

As stated above, the surgeon completes all suturing, retrieving of needles and knot-tying from one port on the patient's left side (if right handed). The assistant stands on the patient's right side and holds

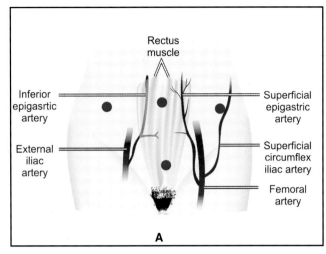
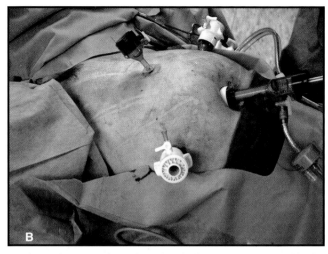

Figs 12.2A and B: Port Placement. Taut Adept ports are used throughout the procedure. A 10 mm balloon trocar is used in the umbilicus, as we complete open approach in all patients for safe access into the abdomen. Three other ports are placed, a 5/10 mm port in the left paramedian region which is used for all suturing, and two 5 mm ports placed in the suprapubic and right paramedian region. The suprapubic port is placed high, approximately 4 fingerbreadths above the pubic bone to be able to have access to the retropubic region

the camera with their left hand and uses their right hand to assist in the surgical field. The suturing port needs to a minimal of 10 mm to be able to accommodate passing the needle through the port. Secondary to multiple sutures being placed throughout a laparoscopic reconstructive procedure, it is not efficient to utilize other methods of needle placement into the abdominal cavity that may take several steps to try to utilize a smaller (i.e. 5 mm) port. We currently use the Adept (Taut) 5/10 mm port in the left lower quadrant that has a diaphragm designed to not leak gas when suturing and also allows up to a CT-1 needle to be passed easily in and out of the abdominal cavity. Two 5 mm ports are used as well. One is placed suprapubically that the surgeon utilizes with his left hand for a grasper to retrieve needles and the other is placed in the right lower quadrant that the assistant uses for retraction, suction/irrigation, etc. All sutures are thrown from the left to the right in the patient (Figs 12.2A and B and 12.3).

We utilize an Elmed needle driver for all of our laparoscopic suturing (Figs 12.4A to C). It is designed exactly like a traditional needle driver and also allows the needle to be placed with different angles and locked in these positions, which is important for suturing in the Space of Retzius. Self-righting needle drivers may be easier to use for beginners, however, they do not allow the needle to be at any other angle but 90 degrees, nor can the needle be leaned in or

out, again limiting your suturing abilities. The surgeon also utilizes an Access needle driver through the suprapubic port, however, it is used as a retriever/grasper and not a driver. We have found

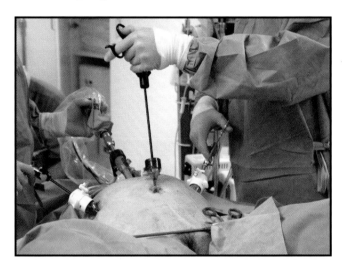

Fig. 12.3: Hand placement. The lateral ports are also placed up higher on the abdominal wall for easier access into the retropubic space and to be able to operate comfortably and ergonomically. The surgeon operates with both hands at all times. The left port is used to complete all suturing and the suprapubic port is used for grasping tissue and retrieving the needle. All knot tying is completed extracorporeally through the left paramedian port. The instrument used in the suprapubic port is held "backwards" which gives us much more range of motion with the instrument when rotating the wrist versus holding it the more "traditional" way

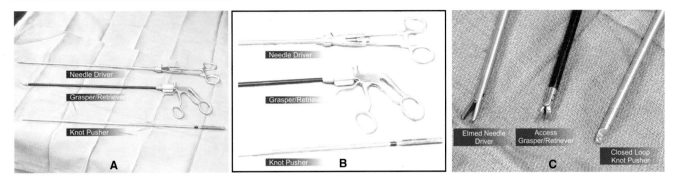

Figs 12.4A to C: Laparoscopic suturing instruments. The surgeon utilizes 3 instruments to suture. The needle driver is an Elmed needle driver, that is exactly the same as a traditional needle driver, however it is made longer for laparoscopic use. It is not self-righting as we need to place the needle at different angles at times when suturing and self-righting needle drivers do not allow you to do this. We utilize an access needle driver actually as our grasper and retriever as we find the jaws to be very precise to grasp as well as rotate fully and do not ratchet or lock down. The knot pusher is also manufactured by Access and is close-ended

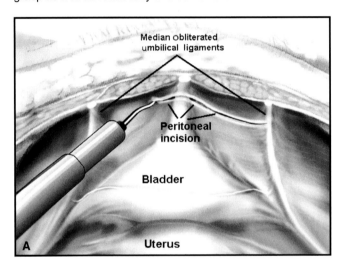

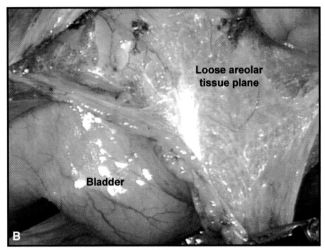

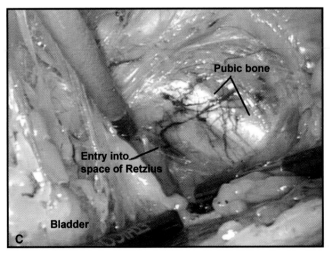

Figs 12.5A to C: (A) A transperitoneal approach is utilized to complete the procedure, this allows access to the remainder of the pelvis and to complete other reconstructive procedures as necessary. The bladder is retrograde filled with 200-300cc of sterile water solution through a 3-way Foley catheter. This allows clear visualization of the superior border of the bladder edge, which in some cases is above the level of the superior pubic symphysis. A harmonic scalpel is utilized to gain entry into the retroperitoneal space. An incision is made in the peritoneum approximately 3 cm superior to the dome of the bladder between the obliterated umbilical ligaments which can be clearly visualized in most patients, (B) Staying medial (inside) to the ligaments protects the surgeon from injuring the inferior epigastric vessels which run lateral to the ligaments. Identification of loose areolar tissue (white cob-web type tissue) confirms a proper plane of dissection, (C) After the space of Retzius has been entered and the pubic ramus visualized, the bladder is drained in order to prevent injury. Separating the loose areolar and fatty layers using blunt dissection develops the retropubic space. Blunt dissection is continued until the retropubic anatomy is visualized

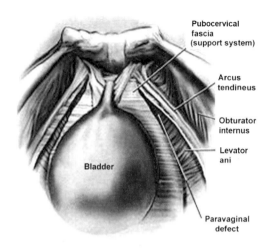

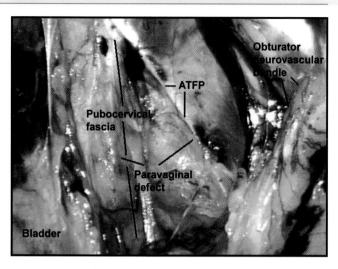

Figs 12.6A and B: Retropubic anatomy visualized after blunt dissection completed on patient's right side. A laparoscopic kitner (peanut) is used to gently clean off the pubocervical fascia. The pubic symphysis and bladder neck are identified in the midline and the obturator neurovascular bundle, Cooper's ligament and the arcus tendineus along the pelvic sidewall. Clearly visualized is the lateral margin of the detached pubocervical fascia and the broken edge of the white line, creating a paravaginal defect on this side.

The dissection is continued on the patient's left side and anatomy identified. The anterior vaginal wall and its point of lateral attachment from its origin at the pubic symphysis to its insertion at the ischial spine are identified

this to be an excellent needle retriever as it can be used as a grasper and has the advantage of slightly curved delicate jaws that can be rotated and does not lock down, therefore can also stabilize the needle in position in the tissue when necessary as well. We hold the Access "backwards" with our left hand, as this allows us almost 360° of motion with simple rotation of the left wrist. Sutures are tied extraporeally with a closed loop Saye/Reddick knot-pusher. Extracorporeal knot tying is much faster and more efficient than intracorporeal knot tying, again decreasing overall operating time.

POTENTIAL COMPLICATIONS AND INJURIES

Lower Urinary Tract Injuries

The most common reported complication of Burch and Paravaginal repair is injury to the bladder and/or the ureters. Lower urinary tract injuries have been reported to be as high as 4 percent in open proce-dures.[18,19] We have shown a much lower rate of injury with a laparoscopic approach,[17] however other reports have reported injury rates as high as 6 percent[20] and therefore one must be prepared to handle these complications. Clearly injury to the lower urinary tract is higher when there has been previous surgery in the space of retzius such as

previous Burch/MMK or retropubic sling procedure as the space will have extensive scar tissue in it and therefore risk of injury to the bladder or vasculature is much higher. We recommend only advanced experienced laparoscopic surgeons attempt dissection and repair in these patients. Again patient selection and surgeon experience are key determinants in minimizing risk of injury in advanced laparoscopic surgery.

Cystotomy is the most common bladder injury encountered and typically occurs during dissection into the space of Retzius. We recommend using a 3-way Foley catheter to retrograde fill the bladder with 250 cc of fluid prior to beginning the dissection into the Space. Once the bladder is filled, the superior edge of the dome of the bladder is identified and the incision made between the obliterated umbilical ligaments approximately 3 cm above this. After making the initial incision through the peritoneum, blunt dissection is used to find the loose aerolar tissue (cob-web like appearance) and then the dissection continued down to the pubic bone. Once the pubic bone is identified, the risk of bladder injury is minimal and therefore the bladder is emptied to have better visualization of the space. Blunt dissection is continued and then a laparoscopic Kittner is used to gently clean the fatty tissue off the pubocervical

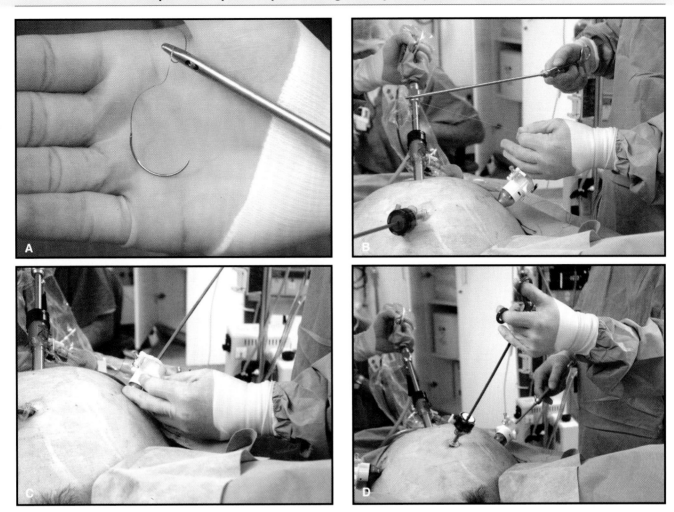

Figs 12.7A to D: Laparoscopic suturing technique. A 2-0 braided non-absorbable suture (Ethibond) on a SH needle is utilized for the paravaginal defect repair. The suture is grasped with the Elmed needle driver approximately 3 cm from the needle and is fed through the 5/10 mm Taut suturing port in the left paramedian region into the abdomen. The surgeon utilizes the Access needle driver in his left hand through the suprapubic port as a grasper/retriever during the suturing process (D). The assistant holds the camera and a grasper for retraction or suction and does not assist in any needle passage, retrieving, etc. The surgeon is self-sufficient and does all aspects of suturing from the left side with no assistance

fascia. A finger is placed in the vagina, to elevate the vagina up and the kittner (peanut) is then used to ensure the bladder is gently dissected medially off the lateral pubocervical fascia where sutures will be placed for the repair. As long the "white" pubo-cervical fascia can be visualized the risk of suture placement in the bladder is minimal.

If cystotomy occurs, it typically is during dissection and is at the dome of the bladder, far away from the ureters and typically is a very simple repair. Cystoscopy should be completed to ensure the ureters are not involved or close enough to the injury

that the repair would compromise them. The cystotomy should be repaired laparoscopically with interrupted sutures of 3-0 vicryl in two layers. Cystoscopy should be completed after repair to ensure water tight closure and ureteral patency. If the repair is close to one of the ureters, a ureteral stent should be placed during repair to ensure patency and to protect the ureter. Postoperative drainage for 7 days with Foley catheter is recommended following repair.

Postoperative cystoscopy is recommended for all patients undergoing Burch and / or paravaginal repair

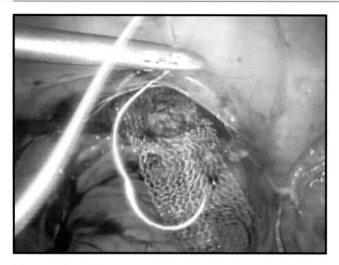

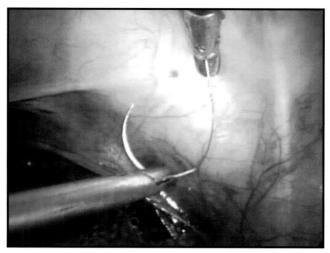

Figs 12.8A and B: Suture placement. Once in the abdomen, the surgeon regrasps the suture with the instrument in the suprapubic port with his left hand and allows the needle to dangle freely in the abdomen (A). The jaws of the grasper can then be rotated to place the needle in the proper position to be loaded in the needle driver in his right hand. The needle can also be gently laid on the sidewall to help in loading into a correct position as well (B)

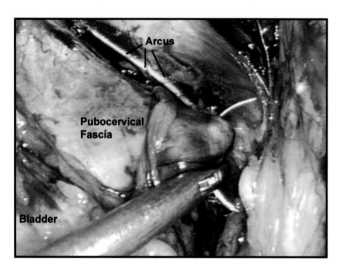

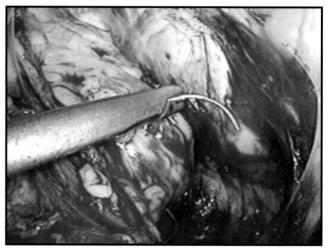

Figs 12.9A and B: Paravaginal defect repair, right side. The assistant lays an instrument across the bladder, opening the retropubic space for suturing. The surgeon places his left hand in the vagina and elevates the anterior vaginal wall up to place the first suture into the pubocervical fascia at the apex of the defect near the top of the vagina on the right side. The assistant retracts the bladder away from the pubocervical fascia and the surgeon then places the needle through the fascia (A). Maintaining the elevation of the vagina with his left index finger, the needle is then retrieved with the driver in his right hand, (B) and reset using both instruments if needed. Separate passes are always utilized for the vagina and the sidewall to ensure proper placement and adequate tissue bites

to ensure ureteral patency and that there is no injury to the bladder, or sutures in the bladder. An ampule (5 cc) of indigo carmine is given to the patient intravenously to ensure ureteral patency. If there is ureteral compromise, the sutures on that side must be removed. The most common suture that could cause ureteral obstruction is the highest paravaginal suture that is placed near the ischial spine and this is the first suture that should be released. If ureteral patency is still compromised, the next suture that should be removed is the Burch suture at the bladder neck. If the ureter is still not patent then all sutures on that side should be removed and a number 5 or 6 ureteral stent passed to assure patency. The stent

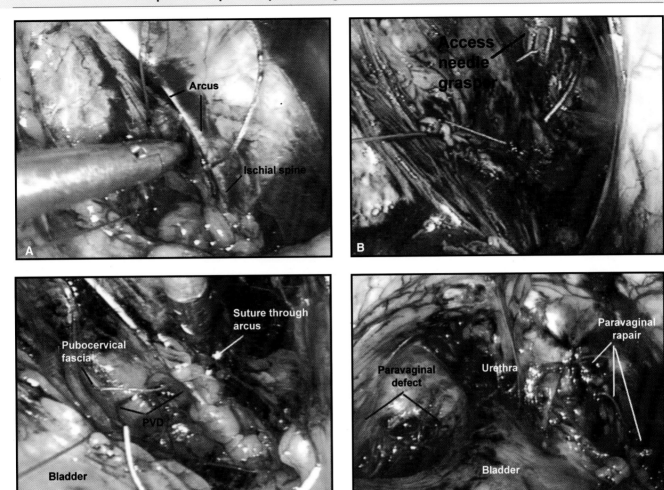

Figs 12.10A to D: Second needle pass, attachment to sidewall. Once the needle is reset, the surgeon then passes the needle through the ipsilateral obturator internus muscle and fascia around the arcus tendineus fascia at its origin 1-2 cm distal to the ischial spine (A). The assistant uses a grasper or retractor to keep the space open and extreme care must be used to identify and know the position of the obturator neurovascular bundle at all times. When placing sutures through the sidewall (on either side) the surgeon uses both hands, his right hand to drive the needle and his left hand with the Access grasper to retract if necessary and then retrieve the needle from the sidewall (B, C). The suture is then tied by the surgeon extracorporeally using the closed-loop knot pusher and 3-4 more sutures are placed with the same technique on this side for repair of the right sided defect (D).

should be left in place and the sutures replaced. As long as there is no evidence of ureteral injury (i.e. blue dye spilling into the space of Retzius), the stent can be removed immediately following the procedure. If a suture is seen penetrating the bladder on cystoscopy, it needs to be removed and replaced. There is no need for prolonged catheterization following removal of a suture from the bladder.

Vascular Injuries

The most common and devastating vasculature injury that can occur in the space of Retzius would be to the obturator neurovascular bundle. This should be one of the first structures visualized when entering the space and the surgeon must be aware of its location at all times throughout the procedure. Typically, injury to this structure occurs with the shaft of the needle (i.e. the back of it) when trying to manipulate the needle in the Space. If injury occurs to the obturator bundle, brisk bleeding will be encountered. Suction irrigation must be utilized immediately to try to obtain visualization and ultimately hemostasis. We recommend utilizing 10 mm hemoclips to obtain hemostasis laparoscopically, however, the

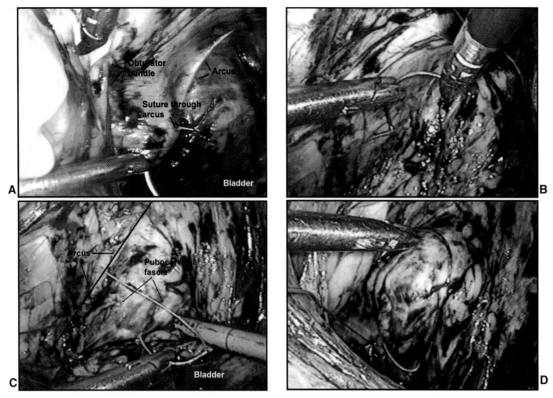

Figs 12.11A to D: Paravaginal Repair, left side. The repair on the left begins with placement of the first suture at the apex of the defect around the white line approximately 1-2 cm from the ischial spine (A). We always suture left to right and therefore on the left side, we go through the sidewall first and then through the vagina. Again, when placing the suture around the arcus, the surgeon utilizes both hands laparoscopically; the needle driver with his right hand, and the grasper/retriever with his left hand to initially retract, and then retrieve the needle from the sidewall (B). The needle is reset and then the vagina is again elevated up by the surgeon with his non-dominant hand, the bladder retracted off the pubocervical fascia by the assistant (C) and the suture placed through the vagina, and retrieved with the needle driver in the surgeon's right hand. Maintaining elevation of the vagina with the left hand, the surgeon has easier access to retrieving the needle (D)

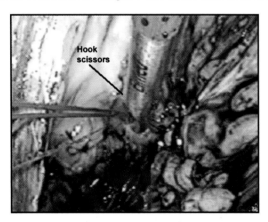

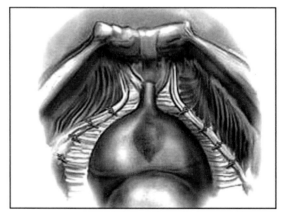

Fig. 12.12: Hook scissors to cut sutures. All sutures are cut by the surgeon with hook scissors. When tying the knot, the scrub technician places the hook scissors gently in the supra-pubic port, allowing the surgeon to cut the suture as soon as he is done tying the knot down. Hook scissors are much safer and can actually be used to "hook" the suture when its in a difficult position to cut, again maintaining a higher safety level

Fig. 12.13: Bilateral paravaginal defect repair

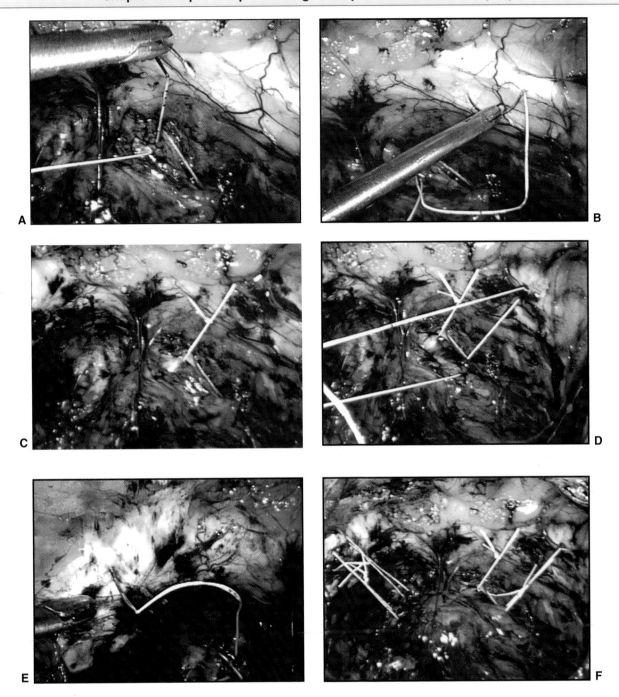

Figs 12.14A to F: Burch urethropexy is then completed in patients suffering from stress urinary incontinence. The urethrovesical junction is identified by visualization of the Foley catheter balloon. With elevation of the surgeon's vaginal finger, the vaginal wall lateral to the bladder neck is exposed on each side with the laparoscopic Kitner until glistening white periurethral tissue is exposed. Four Gore-tex sutures (CV-2) are utilized for the procedure. One suture is placed 2 cm lateral to the level of the midurethra and a second at the level of the urethrovesical junction on each side. A double bite is taken through the anterior vaginal wall and each suture is also passed through Cooper's ligament. Extracorporeal knot tying is utilized and a suture bridge is left to avoid excess elevation and tension

surgeon should be prepared to open immediately if hemostasis cannot be obtained. Blind placement of clips or the use of electrocautery is not recommended as this can compromise and/or damage the obturator nerve. Once hemostasis is obtained, the obturator nerve needs to be isolated to ensure that no clips have been placed across it. Another option is the use of Flow Seal, which is thrombin gel type agent that can be placed in the area of bleeding and has been shown to be able to seal off the vessels that are bleeding, even with arterial bleeding. We recommend having this agent available for immediate use in the operating room at all times. If the vessels retract into the obturator canal, obtaining hemostasis can be very difficult and it may be necessary to obtain vascular surgery consult and approach this through the groin.

CONCLUSION

Although there have been no studies regarding the long-term results of the laparoscopic paravaginal plus colposuspension procedure, one would assume that there is a higher cure rate for the paravaginal plus Burch colposuspension (8 to 12 sutures) compared with the Burch colposuspension only (4 sutures) for the treatment of stress urinary incontinence, because more sutures results in a greater distribution of force to the pelvic floor during episodes of increased abdominal pressure.

REFERENCES

1. Goebell R. Zur operativen beseillgung der angeharenen incontinence vesicae. Incontinentia Vesicae Gynakol Urol 1910;2:187-91.
2. Vancaille TG, Schussler W. Laparosocpic bladderneck suspension. J Laparoendosc Surg 1991;1:169-73.
3. Miklos JR, Kohli N. "Paravaginal Plus" Burch procedure: a laparoscopic approach. J Pelvic Surg 1998;4:297-302.
4. Kohli N, Miklos JR. Laparoscopic Burch colposuspension: a modern approach. Contemp Obstet Gynecol 1997;42:36-55.
5. Miklos JR, Kohli N. Laparoscopic paravaginal repair plus Burch colposuspension. Urology 2000;56:(suppl 6A)64-69.
6. Henley C. The Henley staple-suture technique for laparoscopic Burch colposuspension. J Am Assoc Gynecol Laparoscopists 1995;2:441-44.
7. Ou CS, Presthus J, Beadle E. Laparoscopic bladder neck suspension using hernia mesh and surgical staples. J Laparoendosc Surg 1993;3:563-66.
8. Kiilholma P, Haarala M, Polvi H, Makinen J, Chancellor MB. Sutureless colposuspension with fibrin sealant. Tech Urol 1995;1:81-83.
9. Liu CY. Laparoscopic treatment of genuine urinary stress incontinence. Clin Obstet Gynecol 1994;8:789-98.
10. Ross JW. Laparoscopic Burch repair compared to laparotomy Burch for cure of urinary stress incontinence. Int Urogynecol 1995;6:323-28.
11. Ross JW. Two techniques of laparoscopic Burch repair for stress incontinence: A prospective randomized study. J Am Assoc Gynecol Laparoscopists 1996;3:351-57.
12. Lam AM, Jenkins GJ, Hyslop RS. Laparoscopic Burch colposuspension for stress incontinence: Preliminary results. Med J Aust 1995;162:18-22.
13. Su TH, Wang KG, Hsu CY, Wei H, Hong BK. Prospective comparison of laparoscopic and traditional colposuspensions in the treatment of genuine stress incontinence. Acta Obstet Gynecol 1997;76:576-82.
14. Ross JW. Multichannel urodynamic evaluation of laparoscopic Burch colposuspension for genuine stress incontinence. Obstet Gynecol 1998;91:55-59.
15. Miklos JR, Moore RD, Kohli N. Laparoscopic pelvic floor repair. Obstet Gynecol 2002;14:387-95.
16. Miklos JR, Moore RD, Kohli N. Laparoscopic management of urinary incontinence, ureteric and bladder injuries. Curr Opinion Obstet Gynecol 2001;13:411-17.
17. Speights S, Moore RD, Miklos JR. Frequency of lower urinary tract injury at laparoscopic burch and paravaginal repair. Review of 171 cases. J Am Assoc Gynecol Laparosc 2000;7:515-18.
18. Harris RL, Cundiff GW, Theofrastous JP, et al. The value of intraoperative cystoscopy in urogynecologic and reconstructive pelvic surgery. Am J Obstet Gynecol 1997;177:1367-69.
19. Stevenson KR, Cholhan HJ, Hartmann DM, et al. Lower urinary tract injury during Burch procedure. Am J Obstet Gynecol 1999;181:35-38.
20. Paraiso MF, Walters MD, Karram MM, et al. Laparoscopic Burch Colposuspension versus Tension-Free Vaginal Tape: A Randomized Trial. Obstet Gynecol Surv 2005;60(3):166-67.

Laparoscopic Sacralcolpopexy and Enterocele Repair with Mesh

ROBERT D MOORE, JOHN R MIKLOS
NEERAJ KOHLI

Chapter Thirteen

INTRODUCTION

The anatomy, pathophysiology, and treatment of pelvic organ prolapse has significantly evolved over the last decade with increasing understanding of anatomy and development of minimally invasive surgical procedures. Although support for the pelvic viscera, the vagina, and neighboring structures involves a complex interplay between muscles, fascia, nerve supply, and appropriate anatomic orientation, the endopelvic fascia and pelvic floor muscles provide most of the support function in the female pelvis. Laparoscopic reconstructive pelvic surgery requires a thorough knowledge of pelvic floor anatomy and its supportive components before repair of defective anatomy is attempted. This chapter reviews the anatomy and laparoscopic repair of vaginal vault prolapse and enterocele with Y-mesh sacralcolpopexy.

ANATOMY OF PELVIC SUPPORT

Endopelvic Fascia

To understand the pelvic support system of the female pelvic organs, it is useful to subdivide the pelvic support system into three axes:
1. The upper vertical axis
2. The midhorizontal axis
3. The lower vertical axis.

    The endopelvic fascia—a network of connective tissue and smooth muscle—constitutes the physical matrix which envelops the pelvic viscera and maintains the integrity of the axes supporting the bladder, urethra, uterus, vagina, and rectum in their respective anatomic relationships.

    DeLancey further describes the three levels of support axes as follows: *level 1*—superior suspension of the vagina to the cardinal-uterosacral complex; *level 2*—lateral attachment of the upper 2/3 of the vagina; and *level 3*—distal fusion of the vagina into the urogenital diaphragm and perineal body.[1] In this support system, the endopelvic fascia system is thought to be continuous, extending from the origin of the cardinal-uterosacral complex to the urogenital diaphragm, providing structural support to the vagina and adjacent organs (Fig. 13.1). In this chapter we will be concentrating on Level 1 or apical support.

LEVEL 1—APICAL SUPPORT

The cardinal-uterosacral complex provides apical support by suspending the uterus and upper one

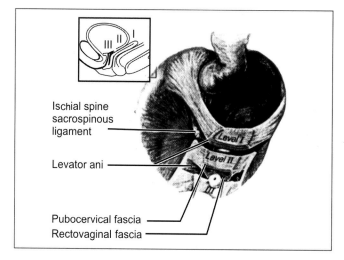

Fig. 13.1: Level 1 (apical suspension) and level 2 (lateral attachment). Level 1—paracolpium suspends the vagina apex from the lateral pelvic sidewall via the uterosacral-cardinal complex. Level 2—the anterior vaginal wall is attached laterally to arcus tendinous fascia pelvis and the posterior vaginal wall is attached laterally to the fascia overlying the levator ani muscle

third of the vagina to the bony sacrum. This complex can be described as two separate entities: the cardinal ligament and the uterosacral ligament. The cardinal ligament is a fascial sheath of collagen that envelops the internal iliac vessels and then continues along the uterine artery, merging into the visceral capsule of the cervix, lower uterine segment and upper vagina. The uterosacral ligament is denser and more prominent than the cardinal ligament. Collagen fibers of the uterosacral ligament fuse distally with the visceral fascia over the cervix, lower uterine segment, and upper vagina, forming the pericervical ring; proximally these fibers end at the presacral fascia overlying the second, third, and forth sacral vertebrae. This complex appears to be the most supportive structure of the uterus and upper 1/3 of the vagina. Disruption of the cardinal-uterosacral complex may result in uterine descensus or vaginal vault (apex) prolapse. Likewise, the most common cause of vaginal vault prolapse is previous hysterectomy with failure to adequately reattach the cardinal-uterosacral complex to the pubocervical fascia and rectovaginal fascia at the vaginal cuff intraoperatively.

    An enterocele is defined as a pelvic floor hernia where the parietal peritoneum comes into direct contact with the vaginal epithelium with no intervening fasica.[2,3] In normal pelvic supportive anatomy, the anterior pubocervical fascia, posterior rectovaginal fascia, cardinal-uterosacral ligaments and paracolpial fibers all converge, or fuse to form the pericervical ring. The integrity and continuity of these supportive tissues can be compromised in patients who have had a complete hysterectomy as previously described.[4-6] An enterocele is likely to be directly related to a disruption of the fusion of the proximal margins of the pubocervical and recto-vaginal fascia (Figs 13.2A to C). Although vaginal mucosa may cover this defect, it is not supportive, which greatly increases the likelihood that an enterocele will eventually develop within the vaginal cavity. Though it is possible to have an enterocele without concurrent vaginal vault prolapse, the two defects usually occur concomitantly. Although the depth and overall anatomic configuration of the cul-de-sac have been implicated in the development of the enterocele, it has never been proven to be the primary etiology.

LEVEL I SUPPORT—LAPAROSCOPIC APPROACH TO ENTEROCELE REPAIR AND VAGINAL VAULT SUSPENSION

Site-specific Enterocele Repair and Vaginal Vault Suspension

As previously mentioned, level 1 support involves the long paracolpial fibers which suspend the proximal vagina and cervicovaginal junction. The cardinal and uterosacral ligaments previously described merge with these fibers and attach to the pericervical ring. This network of connective tissue fibers and smooth muscle serves to prevent vaginal eversion. A disruption of the integrity of these fibers, as opposed to stretching, results in apical vaginal vault eversion. A disruption of the fascia at the vaginal cuff results in an enterocele formation.

Enterocele repair begins first by anatomically defining the fascia defect present that results in the herniation of peritoneum and bowel through the apex of the vagina. An enterocele is defined as a pelvic hernia where the parietal peritoneum comes into direct contact with vaginal epithelium with no inter-vening fascia. The development of an enterocele is likely to be directly related to a disruption of the fusion of the proximal margins of the anterior pubo-cervical fascia and posterior rectovaginal fascia or

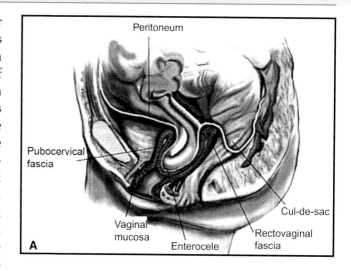

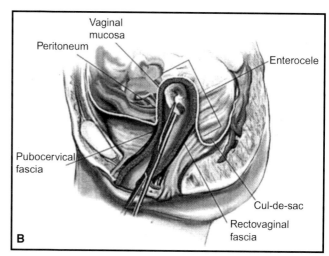

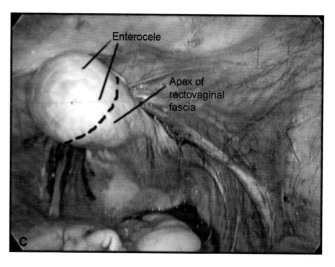

Figs 13.2A to C: An apical enterocele is encountered with vault prolapse (A). The vault is elevated up into the pelvis with an EEA sizer and the excess vaginal epithelium is identified

failure to surgically reattach these two fascial margins at the time of vaginal cuff closure following hysterectomy. It is possible that the surgeon may not incorporate the apex of the pubocervical and or the rectovaginal fascia at the time of closure of the vaginal cuff. Instead the surgeon may be only incorporating vaginal mucosa and unintentionally neglecting the reattachment of the supportive fascial layers. Poor surgical closure or disruption at the apex of the pubocervical and rectovaginal fascia results in parietal peritoneum in direct contact with vaginal epithelium. Chronic rises of intra-abdominal pressure will ultimately exploit this vaginal weakness with stretching of the peritoneum and vaginal mucosa and clinically evident symptomatic enterocele.

Laparoscopic Enterocele Repair

The technique of laparoscopic enterocele repair begins with identification of the vaginal vault apex, the proximal uterosacral ligaments and the course of the pelvic ureter. The identification of the vaginal vault and the delineation of the rectovaginal and pubocervical fascia are facilitated by the use of a vaginal probe. Using the vaginal probe (Fig. 13.2), traction is placed cephalad and ventrally, causing the uterosacral ligaments to stretch so they can be identified and traced backward their most proximal point of origin, lateral to the sacrum. In many cases the uterosacral ligaments are of very poor quality and/or very stretched out and therefore that is why we believe that the utilization of mesh to suspend the apex and ultimately assist in enterocele repair shows superior cure rates compared to trying to utilize ligaments that have already failed. The peritoneum overlying the vaginal apex is incised to expose the pubocervical fascia anteriorly and the rectovaginal fascia posteriorly. If the edge of the bladder is difficult to identify, the bladder is retrograde filled with sterile water to help identify the edge and then the bladder is dissected off of the anterior apical portion of the vagina. Likewise, if the rectovaginal space is difficult to identify, a rectal probe can be placed to identify the rectum and the peritoneum incised between the rectum and the vagina. The rectovaginal space can then be identified and the rectum dissected of the posterior wall of the vagina, almost all the way down to the perineal body. If the enterocele sac is large, it may be excised and the

apical edges of the pubocervical and rectovaginal fascia should be exposed (Figs 13.3A and B), otherwise the enterocele sac can be reduced by placing interrupted sutures from the pubocervical fascia anterior to the rectovaginal septum posterior. The enterocele repair is further supported by the placement of the Y-mesh over the apex of the vagina, as the anterior leaf goes approximately 1/3 of the way down the anterior vaginal wall and the posterior leaf, approximately 2/3 of the way down the posterior wall (ensuring attachment of the mesh to the pubocervical fascia anterior and the rectovaginal fascia posterior).

Laparoscopic Sacral Colpopexy

Abdominal sacral colpopexy remains one of the most successful operations for the treatment of vaginal vault prolapse with excellent results on long-term follow-up. If the surgeon utilizes laparoscopy as a means of surgical access and performs the sacral colpopexy in the same manner as in the open abdominal approach, operative cure rate should theoretically be equivalent.

The room setup and patient positioning is exactly the same as we described in the Laparoscopic Paravaginal Repair and Burch Urethropexy chapter. The patient is placed in dorsal lithotomy position with adjustable Allen stirrups. A 3-way 16-Fr Foley catheter is placed to gravity drainage. Inflatable sequential compression devices are placed on the patient's lower extremities for DVT prophylaxis. A 48 hour bowel prep is used for all of our laparoscopic patients. This helps decompress the bowel for better visualization and helps minimize risk of infection if bowel injury occurs. Two days prior to surgery the patient is placed on a full liquid diet (shakes, pudding, etc.), and the day prior to surgery only clear liquids are allowed. The afternoon prior to surgery the patient drinks 8 ounces of magnesium citrate to clean out the bowels. We also do not recommend the use of nitrous oxide for an anesthetic agent during laparoscopy because this can cause bowel distention during the case and increase risk of bowel injury.

Port placement is based on the surgeon's preference, skill and acquired technique. We place our ports in an identical fashion as was described in the Laparoscopic Paravaginal Repair and Burch Urethropexy chapter. Briefly, we utilize a 10 mm suturing port in the left paramedian region, and two five mm ports, one in the suprapubic region and the other in the right paramedian region. The surgeon stands on the patients left side and completes all needle passing, suturing, needle retrieving and knot tying by himself utilizing the left paramedian and suprapubic port. The assistant stands on the patient's right side and drives the camera and utilizes the right lower port for retraction, suction/irrigation, etc. Once the operative ports have been placed the vagina is elevated with an EEA sizer and the peritoneum overlying the vaginal apex is dissected posteriorly exposing the apex of the rectovaginal fascia. This dissection opens the rectovaginal space as described above and the dissection is taken down to within 3 cm of the perineal body (Fig. 13.4A). If bleeding is encountered it can be taken care of with bipolar electrocautery or surgical clips. Next, anterior dissection is performed to delineate the apex of the pubocervical fascia by dissecting the bladder off of the anterior apex of the vagina (Fig. 13.4B). If the edge of the bladder is difficult to identify secondary

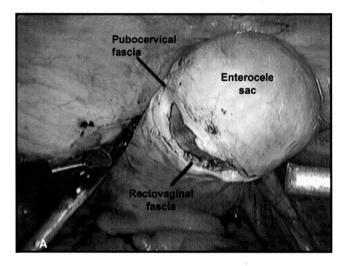

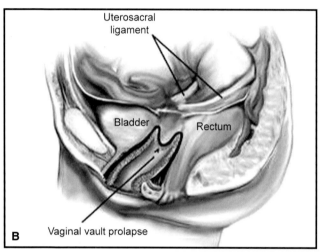

Figs 13.3A and B: The excess vaginal epithelium is excised to get down to the level of the pubocervical fascia anteriorly and the rectovaginal septum posteriorly. The cuff is then reapproximated with interrupted sutures. If the enterocele sac is smaller, the pubocervical fascia and rectovaginal septum can be re-approximated at the apex with plication sutures, therefore avoiding excision

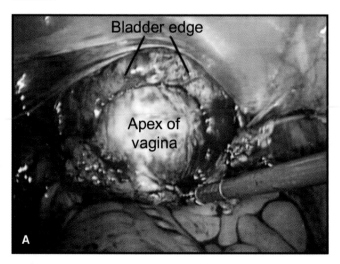

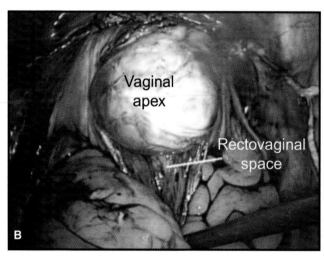

Figs 13.4A and B: The peritoneum and bladder is dissected off the anterior apical portion of the vagina (A). The bladder may be retrograde filled with fluid to help visualize the bladder edge if it is difficult to identify. The rectovaginal space is then entered and the peritoneum and rectum is dissected off the posterior apex and posterior wall of the vagina down towards the perineal body (B)

to scar tissue, the bladder can be retrograde filled through the 3-way Foley catheter with sterile water and then the bladder can be carefully dissected off the anterior segment. We take this dissection approximately 1/3 to ½ way down the anterior wall. A separation between the rectovaginal and pubocervical fascia confirms an enterocele at the apex. If a small enterocele is present it should be repaired in a site-specific fashion by imbricating the stretched vaginal epithelium between the apical edges of the pubocervical and rectovaginal fascia. Permanent suture can be utilized in a continuous purse-string fashion or in interrupted fashion. A large enterocele should be resected (Fig. 13.3A) and the cuff re-approximated with absorbable sutures so the

excessive vaginal epithelium is not utilized as a point of mesh attachment. Theoretically, suturing the mesh to the enterocele sac, instead of the more supportive pubocervical and rectovaginal fascia, may predispose the patient to an increased the risk of mesh erosion, suture pullout and/or surgical failure.

Attention is then directed to the sacral promontory and the presacral space. The peritoneum overlying the sacral promontory is incised longitudinally and this peritoneal incision is extended to the cul-de-sac (Figs 13.5A and B). A laparoscopic dissector is used to expose the anterior ligament of the sacral promontory through blunt dissection (Fig. 14.5C). The peritoneum on the sidewall is incised and freed up beneath the ureter so that the mesh

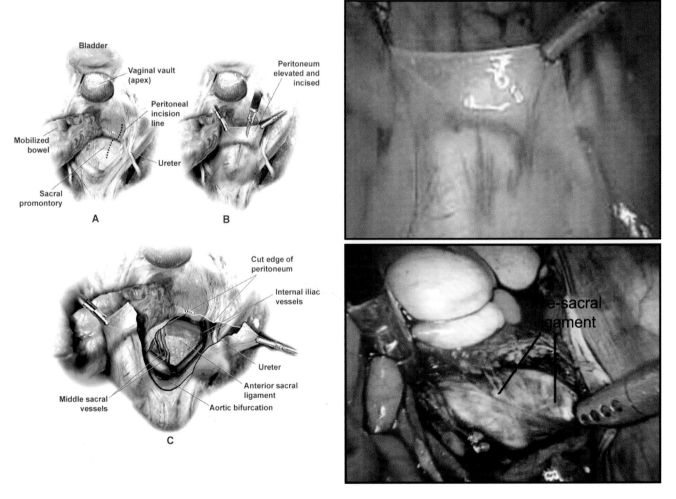

Figs 13.5A to C: Presacral space dissection: dissection of the presacral space exposes the anterior ligament of the sacrum and the middle sacral vessels. The incision is extended down the sidewall to be able to retroperitonealize the mesh at the end of the case

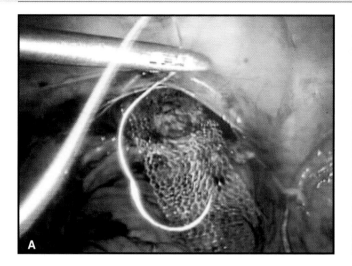 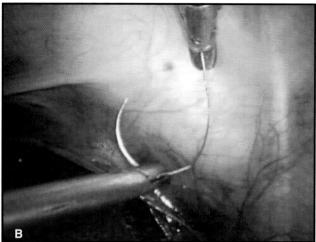

Figs 13.6A and B: (A) All sutures are brought in through the left 10 mm paramedian port with the needle driver. (B) The grasper/retriever is then used with the surgeon's left hand through the suprapubic port to help set the needle in the driver

can be retroperitonealized at the end of the case. Hemostasis is achieved using either coagulation or surgical clips. A 12 × 4 cm polypropylene mesh graft which is fashioned into a Y-shape, so there is an anterior and posterior leaf of the mesh. Typically, the anterior leaf is approximately 3 to 4 cm long and the posterior leaf is longer at 5 to 6 cm so that it can be brought down deeper into the rectovaginal space. The mesh is then introduced into the abdominal cavity through a 10 or 12 cm port (Figs 13.6A and B). The posterior leaf is sutured back to the tail of the mesh to keep it out of the way, as we suture the anterior leaf in place first. The vaginal apex is then directed anterior and cephalad exposing the pubocervical fascia for application of the surgical graft. The anterior leaf of the mesh is then sutured to the pubocervical fascia with three pairs of No. 2-0 nonabsorbable sutures beginning distally and working towards the rectovaginal fascia apex (Figs 13.7A to D). We utilize nonabsorbable sutures and tie extracorporeally with a closed loop knot pusher, which is time-saving and efficient. All suturing methods and equipment are described in detail in the Laparoscopic Paravaginal Repair and Burch chapter. We utilize the same techniques for suturing with enterocele repair and sacralcolpopexy. The first suture is placed through the mesh and then through the pubocervical fascia, being careful to avoid the bladder edge. Once the anterior leaf is sutured in place, the posterior leaf is then released and sutured in place in a similar fashion (Figs 13.8 to 11). We typically place the most distal suture through the

vagina first (being careful to avoid the rectum) and then bring the suture through the mesh and then tie it down into position (Figs 13.9A to D). The remaining sutures are taken through the mesh and the vagina, typically in one bite, and a total of 6-8 sutures are used to suture the posterior leaf into place (Figs 13.10 and 13.11). The surgeon should attempt to take stitches through the entire thickness of the vaginal wall, excluding the vaginal epithelium. If hysterectomy is completed at the time of the surgery, the cuff is reapproximated in the normal fashion prior to mesh placement and the procedure is then completed in the identical fashion as above. Some have suggested the use of a double layer closure of the vaginal cuff to help decrease rate of mesh erosion, however we do not routinely do this and we have seen no increase rate in cuff erosion. We do feel it is very important however to keep the sutures that are being placed to hold the mesh in place away from the vaginal cuff, as suturing the mesh right into the cuff can lead to extrusion in the suture line.

The vagina is then elevated into its normal natural position in the pelvis and the surgeon sutures the free end of the Y-shaped mesh to the anterior longitudinal ligament of the sacrum using two pairs of No. 0 nonabsorbable suture (Figs 13.13 to 13.16). The mesh should be attached with minimal tension on the vagina. In an attempt to decrease surgical time some surgeons have utilized Titanium bone tacks and hernia staplers for the mesh attachment to the anterior longitudinal ligament of the sacrum (Figs 13.15A and B). After reducing intra-abdominal pressure and

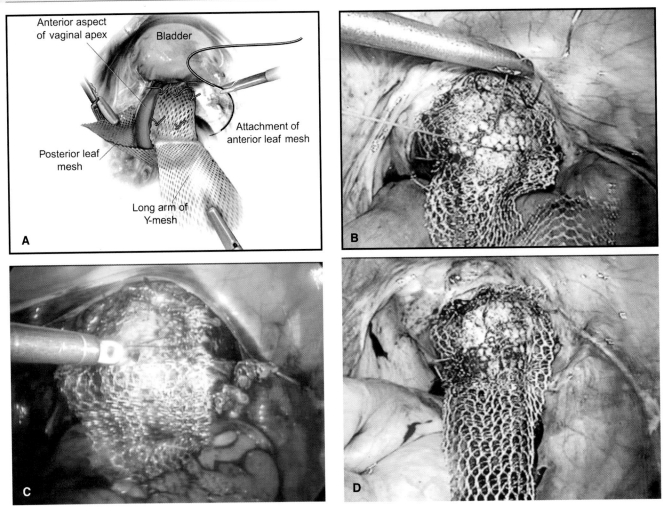

Figs 13.7A to D: Attaching the anterior leaf of the Y-shape polypropylene mesh. The anterior leaf of the mesh is placed first with two rows of three interrupted sutures to the anterior apex of the vagina. The distal sutures are placed first, being careful to avoid the edge of the bladder. The posterior leaf of the Y is tied back to the tail of the mesh to keep it out of the way

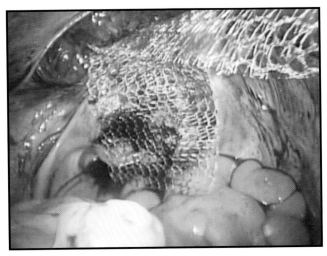

Fig. 13.8: The posterior leaf is then released to be able to suture it in place along the posterior wall

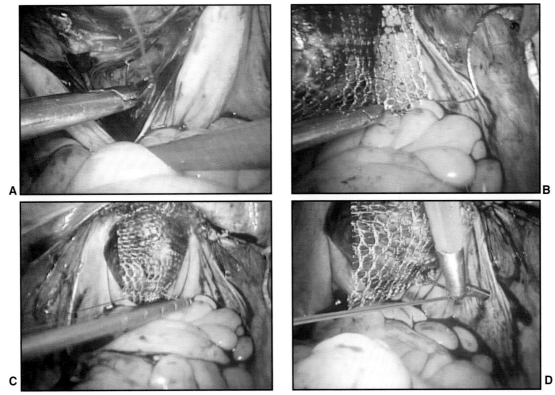

Figs 13.9A to D: Attaching the posterior leaf of the Y-shape polypropylene mesh. The vagina is tented up in the pelvis and the most distal suture (approximately 2/3 down the posterior wall) is placed through the posterior wall, fed through the mesh and then subsequently tied down with an extracorporeal closed loop knot pusher (A-C). Hooked scissors are used throughout the case as they can easily "hook" the suture and slide down to the point it needs to be cut. This helps protect surrounding visceral structures, by pulling the suture away from them prior to cutting the suture (D)

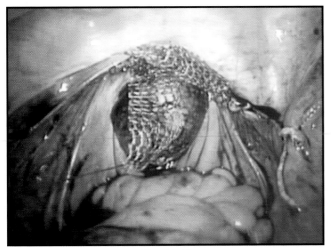

Fig. 13.10

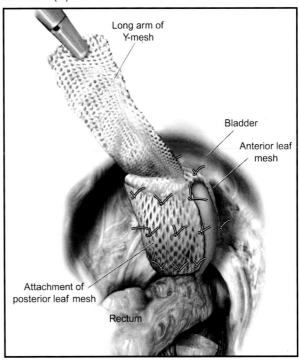

Fig. 13.11

Figs 13.10 and 13.11: The posterior leaf is attached with 6 to 8 sutures as it is longer than the anterior leaf. The final Y-shaped configuration is seen in Figure 13.11.

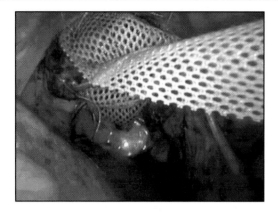

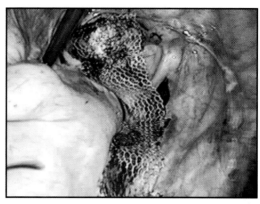

Fig. 13.12: This helps repair and prevent further enterocele formation at the cuff in addition to supporting the apex after attachment to the sacrum

Fig. 13.13: The apex of the vagina is then elevated into its normal anatomic position and the mesh is positioned in the pelvis for its attachment to the pre-sacral ligament. The mesh is positioned so that there is no tension on the vagina

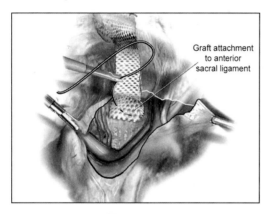

Graft attachment to anterior sacral ligament

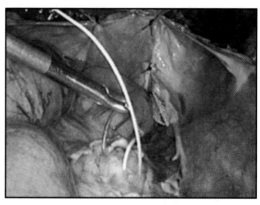

Fig. 13.14A

Fig. 13.14B

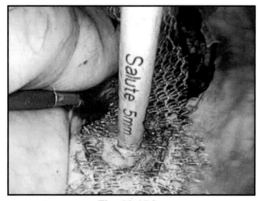

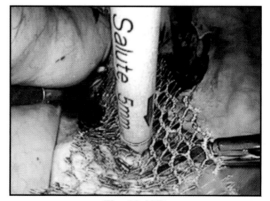

Fig. 13.15A

Fig. 13.15B

Figs 13.14A to 13.15B: Attachment of the long arm of the Y-mesh to the pre-sacral ligament. This can be accomplished with two permanent sutures (Figs 13.14A and B) or a device such as the wire loop hernia tacker (Figs 13.15A and B)

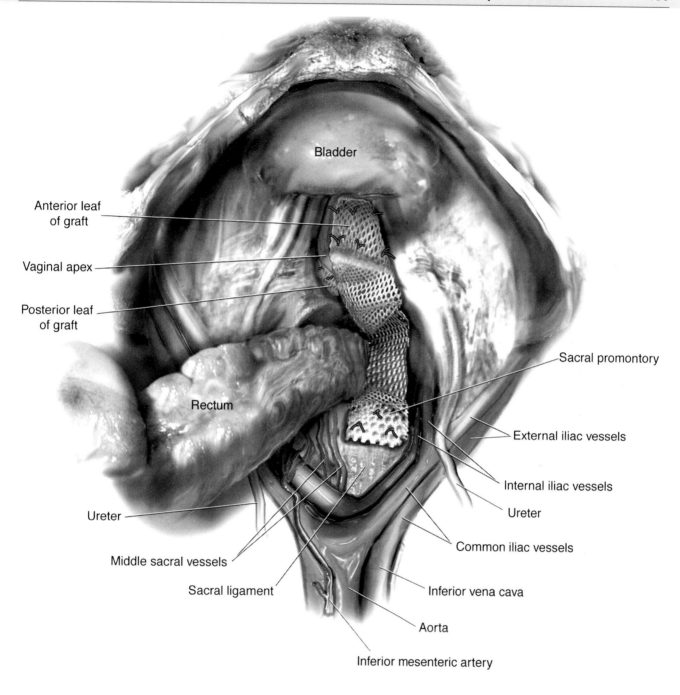

Fig. 13.16: Final position of the Y-mesh in the pelvis after sutured in place

inspecting the presacral space for hemostasis, the peritoneum is reapproximated with 2-0 polyglactin suture (Figs 13.17 and 13.18). We utilize a running suture starting at the level of the sacrum, down the sidewall, then up through the bladder peritoneum, then run it partially back up the sidewall to be able to tie easily near the starting point (Figs 13.17B to D). We feel the most important aspect of retro-peritonealizing the mesh is not necessarily to cover over all the mesh, but is to eliminate the open space

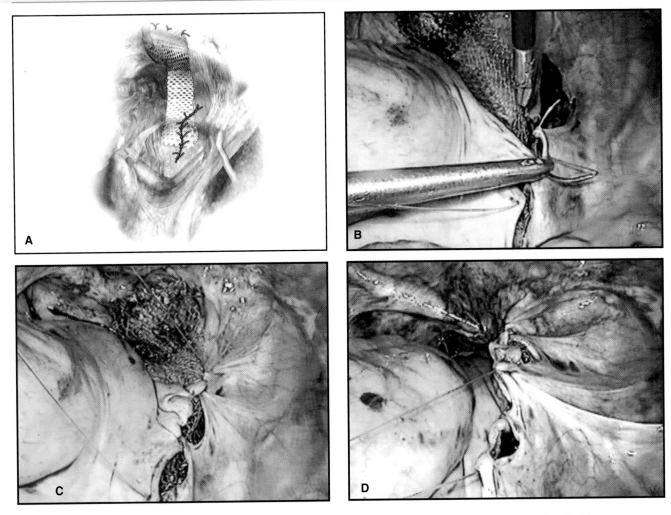

Figs 13.17A to D: Peritoneal closure. The mesh is then retroperitonealized utilizing an absorbable monofilament suture that "slides" in a running fashion with one suture

between the mesh and the right pelvic sidewall where bowel could potentially become entrapped and obstructed or ischemic.

Once the repair is completed, cystoscopy is completed to ensure ureteral patency and to ensure that there is no suture penetration into the bladder or damage to the bladder from dissection or suture placement.

Potential Complications and Injuries

Lower Urinary Tract Injuries

Potential injuries can occur to the ureters and or bladder during the repair. The ureters should be identified at the beginning of the case. Clearly the right ureter is at more risk of injury, secondary to the placement of the mesh on the sacrum on the right

side of the colon. The right ureter is identified at the pelvic brim prior to dissection down into the presacral space. As this space is opened and the incision is extended down into the pelvis on the right sidewall, the ureter should be clearly visualized throughout the dissection and is actually released away from the operative field with the dissection. The ureters could also potentially be compromised during suture placement of the mesh arms onto the anterior and posterior vagina, specifically the most distal lateral sutures on the anterior wall near the edge of the bladder where the ureters are entering into the bladder (a good dissection will help avoid this danger area) and the lateral sutures of the posterior leaf near the uterosacral ligaments. Cystoscopy is performed at the end of the procedure to ensure ureteral patency. If ureteral obstruction is

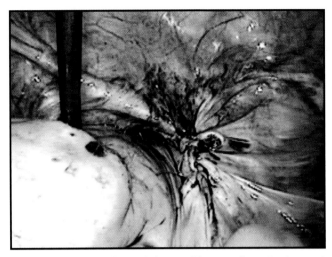

Fig. 13.18: Final peritoneal closure. The most important aspect of retroperitonealizing the mesh is to avoid having any open space between the graft and the right sidewall that bowel could potentially become entrapped in

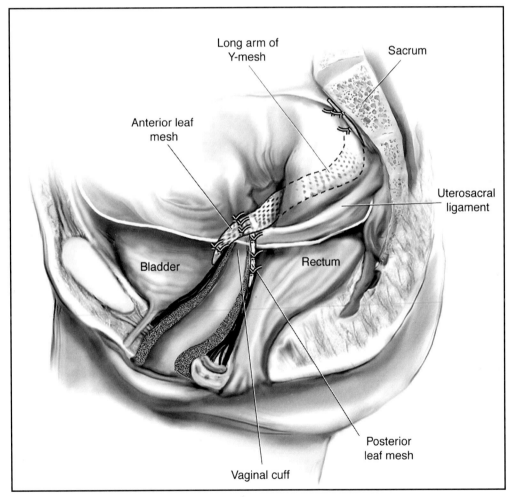

Fig. 13.19: Sacralcolpopexy sideview. Final positioning demonstrates the support of the apex with the graft going down the anterior and posterior walls attached to both pubocervical fascia and rectovaginal septum

identified, the suture causing this must be identified and removed and ureteral patency confirmed. If any evidence of compromise or injury is identified to the ureter, a ureteral stent should be placed and left in place for 14 to 21 days. If a suture is seen penetrating the bladder, it needs to be removed (laparos–copically) and replaced away from the bladder and no further treatment is necessary. If cystotomy occurs during the original dissection of the bladder off of the vagina, this should be repaired laparoscopically with a double layer closure with delayed absorbable sutures. The procedure can still be completed and mesh placed, however care should be taken to try to keep the mesh away from the suture line in the bladder. The bladder should be drained for an extended period of time with this type of an injury (7 to 10 days) to ensure proper drainage and healing. Overall, the risk of lower urinary tract injury is lower with sacralcolpopexy, than with other vault suspensions such as uterosacral ligament suspension.

Bowel Injury

The bowel can be injured with lysis of adhesions or with dissection of the rectum off of the posterior wall of the vagina. A proper 48 hour bowel prep described above is vital to help decrease the risk of bowel injury as this actually deflates the small and large bowel and makes it much easier to get the bowel out of the pelvis and have it stay in the upper abdomen and out of the surgical field. Additionally, the use of nitrous oxide should be avoided as well as an anesthetic agent as this will cause the bowel to become distended and inflated, increasing the risk of injury. If a small bowel injury occurs, we recommend primary repair laparoscopically and if a proper bowel preparation was completed, the mesh sacralcolpopexy can be completed, however antibiotic coverage should be completed for one week postoperatively. If the rectum or large bowel is injured during the dissection into the rectovaginal space, primary repair can be completed if proper bowel prep was completed, however we would not recommend mesh be placed following a large bowel injury. Certainly, antibiotic coverage is warranted postoperatively as well.

Vascular Injuries

As with any advanced pelvic surgical procedure, a thorough knowledge of the pelvic anatomy and vasculature is required prior to attempting laparoscopic sacral colpopexy. The overall risk for bleeding is actually quite low, however if it does occur, it can be a life threatening event. Our average blood loss in over 300 cases over the past two years has been less than 75 cc and we have not had to give any blood transfusions for intraoperative bleeding. We feel that the average blood loss for laparoscopic reconstruction is actually much less than with laparotomy secondary to more precise dissection and better visualization with laparoscopy and also eliminating the bleeding encountered with a large abdominal wall incision. There is actually minimal risk of bleeding or major vasculature injury with dissection of the vaginal cuff. This area can be quite vascular, especially down in the rectovaginal space, however it is typically venous in nature and can be easily controlled with cautery or surgical clips. Certainly, one should always identify and know the location of the ureters prior to any cauterization or clipping. However, dissection into the presacral space has the potential for catastrophic bleeding. We place the patient in deep Trendelenburg positioning with a left tilt so the bowel will be able to be placed in the upper abdomen and the rectum will fall off to the patient's left side. The right common iliac artery and vein are identified, as is the ureter. The peritoneum is tented up using fine graspers and the peritoneum incised over the sacral promontory. We then carefully dissect down into the presacral space until we reach the presacral ligament and carefully clean this area off with a laparoscopic Kittner until we see the white of the ligament. The middle sacral artery is identified and we ensure that we find a vessel free area to suture or attach the mesh. One must be careful as on occasion the left common iliac vein can traverse this area as well. If bleeding is encountered during the dissection or down in the sacral hollow, it can be life threatening and rapid conversion to laparotomy needs to be considered and prepared for. Bipolar electrocautery, surgical clips or hemostatic sutures may be utilized laparoscopically to try to control the bleeding, but again the position of the ureter needs to be identified to ensure it is away from the surgical field. Floseal (Cooper Surgical, USA), a thrombin gel agent, may be utilized laparoscopically and has been shown to be able to control both arterial and venous bleeding. We have utilized this material in several incidences and have had excellent clinical results and to date have not had to convert any patient to laparotomy. If bleeding cannot be controlled, conversion to laparotomy is required and packing/pressure should be placed immediately to control bleeding, restore volume and give the patient blood products if necessary. Thumb tacks with bone wax have been utilized in the sacral hollow to control bleeding vessels that have retract into the sacrum and again hemostatic agents such as thrombin gel may be utilized to help obtain hemostasis as well.

LEVEL 1 SUPPORT PROCEDURES: CLINICAL RESULTS

Richardson first described this anatomic defect for enterocele in 1995 in his landmark paper "The anatomic defects in rectocele and enterocele." Since that time, others have described laparoscopic surgical techniques which employ Richardson's anatomic theories in the treatment of enterocele and vaginal apex prolapse.[7-9] Recently Carter et al reported on 8 patients who underwent the Richardson-Saye laparoscopic vaginal vault suspension and enterocele repair technique with excellent results.[10]

There are no other reports in the literature that evaluate clinical results of the laparoscopic uterosacral ligaments suspensions and/or traditional types of enterocele repairs such as the Halban and Moskowitz procedures. However, some have described their surgical technique and/or complications. Lyons and Winer reviewed the technique and complications in 276 patients who had either a Moskowitz or Halban procedure.[11] The worst complications encountered in this series were port site infections. Koninckx et al emphasized using the carbon dioxide laser for vaporization of the enterocele sac, followed by uterosacral ligament shortening and suspension of the posterior vaginal wall.[12] A modified Moschowitz procedure with approximation of the posterior vaginal fascia to the anterior wall of the rectum has also been described laparoscopically. Despite the paucity of data regarding long-term cure rates, the uterosacral ligament suspension and site specific enterocele repair remains a mainstay in many surgeons armamentarium.

In 1994 Nezhat et al were the first to report a series of 15 patients who underwent laparoscopic sacral colpopexy.[13] They reported an apical vault cure rate of 100 percent on follow-up ranging from 3 to 40 months. In 1995, Lyons reported four laparoscopic sacrospinous fixation and ten laparoscopic sacral colpopexies.[14] Ross subsequently reported on 19 patients who underwent laparoscopic sacral colpopexy, Burch colposuspension and modified culdeplasty in 1997. The author reported seven complications including: three cystotomies, two urinary tract infections, one seroma, and one inferior epigastric laceration. Despite two patients being lost to follow-up, he reported a cure rate of (13/13) 100 percent for vaginal apex prolapse at one year.[8]

Cosson et al reported on their experience of feasibility and short-term complications in 77 patients who had undergone laparoscopic sacral colpopexies. Laparoscopy was actually performed on 83 patients with symptomatic prolapse of the uterus. Six cases required conversion to laparotomy because of technical difficulties. All of the remaining 77 patients underwent laparoscopic sacrocolpopexy. Subtotal hysterectomy was performed in 60 cases. Three patients required reoperations for hematoma or hemorrhage. Mean operative follow-up was 343 days. Three other patients required reoperation, one for a third-degree cystocele and two for recurrent stress incontinence. The surgeons concluded the sacrocolpopexy is feasible and the operative time, postoperative complications are related to the surgeons experience but remains comparable to those noted in laparotomy.[15]

Use of synthetic mesh for the treatment of vaginal vault prolapse has been performed since 1991 at The University of Auvergne, Clermont-Ferrand. At the University of Auvergne, more than 250 cases have been performed laparoscopically with an apical vault cure rate of approximately 92 percent.[16] Complications are rare with the most common being mesh extrusion (2%) and only in patients who underwent concomitant hysterectomy. Patients who had uterine suspensions or who have not had a concomitant hysterectomy have not experienced this complication. (Wattiez A, personal communication—International Society of Gynecologic Endoscopy—Berlin 2002). We have performed more that 300 laparoscopic Y-mesh sacral colpopexies with macroporous soft polypropylene mesh in the past two years and have had excellent clinical results with a very low rate of complications. Our cure rate is greater than 94 percent and we have had only two mesh erosions (0.6%) to date and both patients did have concomitant hysterectomy.

CONCLUSION

Laparoscopy should only be considered a mode of surgical access, which should not significantly change the technique of operative reconstructive surgery. Laparoscopy benefits the surgeon by improving visualization, decreasing blood loss and magnifying the pelvic floor defects which need to be repaired. Other advantages including less postoperative pain, shorter hospital stays, shorter recovery time and earlier return to a better quality of life have also been described in the literature. Disadvantages often cited in the literature include increased operative time and associated increased costs. The authors' personal experience is the operative time is similar and in many times reduced especially for patients with a high body mass index. However, complex operative laparoscopy is associated with a steep and lengthy learning curve after which operative time is can be significantly reduced based on surgeons experience and laparoscopy skills as well as the quality of the operative team.

A thorough knowledge of pelvic floor anatomy is essential before undertaking any type of reconstructive pelvic surgery, and advanced knowledge of laparoscopic surgery and suturing are essential to perform the surgical procedures discussed in this review. Despite the paucity in the literature, laparoscopic pelvic reconstructive surgery will continue to be driven by patient demands as well as surgeon preference. With increasing experience, greater data should support its continued use and favorable long-term outcomes.

REFERENCES

1. DeLancey JO. Anatomic aspects of vaginal eversion after hysterectomy. Am J Obstet Gyencol 1992;166:1717-24.
2. Richardson AC. The rectovaginal septum revisited: its relationship to rectocele and its importance in rectocele repair. Clin Obstet Gynecol 1993;36:976-83.
3. Richardson AC. The anatomic defects in rectocele and enterocele. J Pelvic Surg 1995;1:214-21.
4. Kauppila O, Punnonen R, Teisala K. Operative technique for the repair of posthysterectomy vaginal prolaspe. An Chir Gynaecol 1986;75:242-44.
5. Symmonds RE, Williams TJ, Lee RA, Webb MJ. Post-hysterectomy enterocele and vaignal vault prolapse. Am J Obstet Gynecol 1981;140:852-59.
6. Cruikshank SH, Kovac SR. Anterior vaginal wall culdoplasty at vaginal hysterctomy to prevent posthysterectomy anterior vaginal wall prolapse. Am J Obstet Gyencol 1996;174:1863-69.
7. Ross JW. Apical vault repair, the cornerstone of pelvic floor reconstruction. Int Urogynecol J 1997;8:146-52.
8. Ross JW. Techniques of laparoscopic repair of total vault eversion after hysterectomy. J Am Assoc Gynecol Laparosc 1997;4:173-83.
9. Miklos JR, Kohli N, Lucente V, Saye WB. Site specific fascial defects in the diagnosis and surgical management of enterocele. Am J Obstet Gynecol 1998;179:1418-23.
10. Carter JE, Winter M, Mendehlsohn S, Saye WB, Richardson AC. Vaginal vault suspension and enterocele repair by Richardson-Saye laparoscopic technique: description of training technique and results. J Soc Laproend Surg 2001;5:29-36.
11. Lyons TL. Minimally invasive treatment of urinary stress incontinence and laparoscopoicallly direct repair of pelvic floor defects. Clin Obstet Gynecol 1995;38:380-91.
12. Koninckx PR, Poppe W, Deprest J; Carbon dioxide laser for laparoscopic enterocele repair. J Am Assoc Gyencol Laparoscop 1995;2:181-85.
13. Nezhat CH, Nezhat F, Nezhat C. Laparoscopic sacral colpopexy for vaginl vault prolapse. Obstet Gynecol 1994;4:381-83.
14. Lyons TL, Winer WK. Vaginal vault suspension. Endosc Surg 1995;3:88-92.
15. Cosson M, Rajabally R, Bogaert E, Querleu D, Crepin G. Laparoscopic sacrocolpopexy, hysterectomy and burch colposuspension: feasibility and short-term complicaiotns of 77 procedures. J Soc Lap Surg 2002;6(2):115-19.
16. Wattiez A, Canis M, Mage G, Pouly JL, Bruhat MA. Promontofixation for the treatment of prolapse. Urol Clin N Amer 2001;28:151-57.

Laparoscopic Site Specific Repair of Vaginal Vault Prolapse

GREG CARIO

KEITH JOHNSTON

Chapter Fourteen

INTRODUCTION

Up to 50 percent of women over the age of 50 years have pelvic floor prolapse. Signs and symptoms in this group are present in about 10-20 percent [1-4] of cases. Vaginal vault prolapse is defined as a defect in the condensation of endopelvic fascia in the area of the vaginal apex after hysterectomy (Fig. 14.1). It has a reported incidence of 0.4-11 percent in post-hysterectomy patients.[5-8] This incidence translates to 2.0-3.6/1000 women years post abdominal or vaginal hysterectomy or 15/1000 women years post hysterectomy for prolapse. Although prolapse of the vaginal vault may be asymptomatic, many patients find it quite distressing, presenting with symptoms including a feeling of "something coming down", dragging, backache and sexual dysfunction. The close anatomical relationship of the urinary bladder, urethra and rectum to the vagina means that when vault prolapse occurs, in up to 72 percent of cases it is accompanied by anterior and posterior defects with associated urinary and bowel dysfunction. These symptoms include stress incontinence, difficulty-initiating micturition, postmicturition dribble, constipation, defecation difficulties and sexual dysfunction. An aging population with an ever-increasing demand for improved quality of life means that today's gynecologist will encounter pelvic floor prolapse with increasing frequency and be expected to manage it. Although vaginal vault prolapse can sometimes be managed conservatively with pessaries many patients will choose a more definitive surgical solution. We believe that the view of the pelvic floor anatomy offered by laparoscopy, together with advances in laparoscopic surgical skills, particularly curved needle suturing techniques allows a site specific minimally invasive approach to the correction of vaginal vault prolapse, with low morbidity, shorter hospital stay and improved results. Apical support is all about DeLancey's Level I and Level II supports, which we will discuss later. If you can identify these structures (which can only be done accurately at laparoscopy with its magnification), you can then identify the site specific defects and attempt to repair them.

Identifying these apical supports have been so difficult that the pericervical ring with its attached cardinal and uterosacral ligaments have been bypassed in many operative techniques. This is why the abdominal approach of sacrocolpoplexy is still considered the gold standard[9-13] as it attaches the prolapsed vagina itself to an easily identifiable and reproducible ligamentous structure. It in fact replaces the level I supports with a new support mechanism. This is major surgery however and carries with it all the morbidity associated with laparotomy. The traditional vaginal surgery for vault prolapse which was often associated with enterocoele was McCall's culdoplasty, posterior colporrhaphy and even Le Fort's colpocleisis. As well as the sacrocolpexy the abdominal approach included the Moschowitz, the Halban transverse obliterative procedure, wedge culdoplasty and the Zacharin's abdominoperineal procedure. Vaginal surgeons have found it very difficult to localize substantial support structures and in fact relied on endopelvic fascia for support which stretches and breaks and is unsuitable for long-term success. Beginning in the 1970's the vaginal approach to vault prolapse evolved with the sacrospinous fixation and then moved on with time to procedures like the intravaginal slingplasty, mesh sacrospinous vault suspension and other vaginal mesh suspensions. The results of vaginal surgery were still not as good as sacrocolpoplexy[14] and it was felt that abdominal surgery was too invasive.

Following on from the revolution in laparoscopic surgery and the early work on laparoscopic Burch's colposuspension, it became evident that there was a place for laparoscopic vault suspension. The laparoscopic approach to sacrocolpoplexy and other reconstructive techniques appear to have good results, and a recent paper by Ross et al reports an objective cure rate of 93 percent at 5 years.[15-17] Vaginal suspension to the uterosacral ligaments has also been shown to be an effective technique with good-long term results.[18,19]

Despite surgeons best efforts, prolapse recurs in upto 30 percent of patients and the problem often involves compartments of the pelvic floor, that were not repaired initially[25] as they were either not identified or not present at the time of surgery. As the laparoscope helps us better define site-specific defects, it also allows us to repair them and hopefully reduce the chance of recurrence.

Several techniques have improved the success of sacrocolpoplexy. These include the insertion of non absorbable sutures into the vaginal vault, keeping

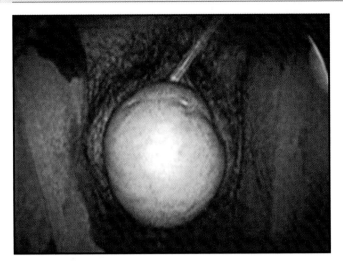

Fig. 14.1: Vaginal vault prolapse

the suspension tension free and the use of Mesh over a wide area of the vaginal apex. Posterior extension of the mesh to the perineal body has also been found to be beneficial in the prevention of posterior vaginal compartment prolapse.[12,13,22] A wide variety of meshes and synthetic materials have been used to the resuspend the vaginal vault. These include Gore-Tex, Marlex, Mersilene, Prolene, Polypropylene and Porcine Dermis. The commonest complications seen from sacrocolpoplexy with mesh are erosion problems, dyspareunia and bowel complications. Polypropylene and porcine dermis appear to have the best profiles for pelvic floor work. Vaginal mesh erosion has a reported incidence of 3 to 9 percent when used in sacrocolpoplexy.[23,24] The lessons from this experience have all been applied to the development of the laparoscopic approach.

This chapter will briefly review the anatomical basis of vaginal vault prolapse, our laparoscopic approach to its correction, through the repair of fascial defects and restoring ligamentous level I and II DeLancey's supports.

ANATOMY OF VAGINAL VAULT PROLAPSE

The pelvic floor is divided into three compartments. The anterior compartment contains the bladder and urethra. The middle contains the uterus and vagina and the posterior compartment contains the rectum. There are two components to the support of these compartments, the levator ani muscle and the endopelvic fascia. The levator ani muscles make up

the active component of pelvic floor support and the endopelvic fascia the passive component. At rest the levator ani muscles are contracted keeping the upper vagina, rectum and urethra elevated and closed by pulling them anteriorly toward the pubic symphysis.[20] In fact, in the upright position the upper two-thirds of the vagina are almost horizontal over the levator plate. Fascial condensations also offer support to the pelvic viscera. The fascial supports that prevent prolapse of the vagina are described below.

The vagina is a fibromuscular tube lined by stratified squamous epithelium approximately 10 cm in length, running antero-inferiorly from the cervix to the introitus. The apex of the tube (and uterus and cervix if present) is supported above the pelvic diaphragm at the level of the ischial spines by uterosacral-cardinal ligament complex. The uterosacral ligaments are paired crescent shaped folds or condensations of the endopelvic fascia and are described as a level É support by DeLancy. They arise from the anterior aspect of the sacrum and insert into the vagina, cervix and lower uterine segment forming the pericervical ring and they also insert into the fascia over the levator ani muscles with a fascial connection to the ischial spine. They are absolutely ideal for apical support and are easily identified laparoscopically.

Below the pelvic diaphragm are DeLancey's level II supports of the vagina. These run from the ischial spines to the urogenital diaphragm and are the composed of the pubocervical fascia anteriorly and rectovaginal fascia or septum posteriorly. These fascial layers insert directly and indirectly into the arcus tendinous ligament. These are of particular importance when describing site specific defects as loss of this support of the pubocervical fascia leads to anterior compartment defects and paravaginal defects. These are clinically evident as cystocele and urethroceles, which may result in possible hypermobility of the urethra and urinary incontinence.[21] Loss of rectovaginal fascia support, may result in posterior compartment defects, clinically evident as rectoceles or enterocoeles. The support for the distal end of the vagina is the Level III support as described by DeLancy where there is fusion between the urogenital diaphragm and the perineal body. The 3 levels of supports are demonstrated in

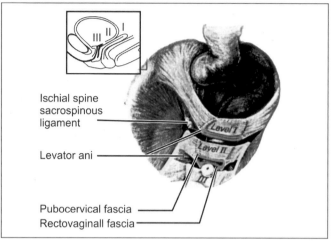

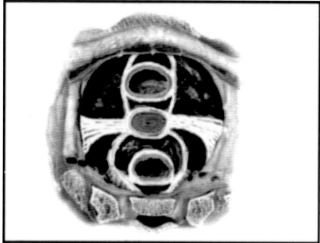

Figs14.2 and 14.3: Three levels of pelvic support

DeLancey's diagram above in Figures 14.2 and 14.3 shows pelvic compartment spaces.

SURGICAL TECHNIQUE

The author will only describe the two laparoscopic techniques in this chapter as many of the other procedures are described elsewhere in this book. The author will confine his description to vault prolapse and not include the operations, where the uterus is involved in the apical prolapse. These include uterine suspension to the uterosacral ligaments, the sacrospinous ligament and the sacral promontory—the laparoscopic sacrohysteropexy.

Laparoscopic uterosacral colpopexy. Author prefers this term rather than A High McCall's culdoplasty which is a vaginal procedure which only focuses on the uterosacral ligament close to the cervix rather than the sacral attachment which is far more robust and easily seen at laparoscopy. This is a simple procedure to perform once curved needle suturing is mastered. One usually needs to attend an intensive workshop, which focuses on this and spend many hours mastering the techniques on a pelvic trainer. At our workshops at the Sydney Women's Endosurgery Centre (SWEC), we teach this procedure during a one week training course and all the participants can take home a portable trainer with all the instruments, the sutures and a model of the uterosacral complex upon which to practice on for one month (Figs 14.4 to 14.6).

The procedure usually begins by dividing all the adhesions which can often be plentiful. It is absolutely

essential to restore normal anatomy before commencing this operation. The ureters are identified on each sidewall, and where they are not well clear of our surgical field we place relieving incisions medially to them, so that they may be protected and retracted laterally when suturing bulk bites of the uterosacral ligaments (Fig. 14.7). A probe is placed in the vagina to stretch the residual uterosacral ligaments and a probe in the rectum to retract the rectum to the contralateral side to help safely identify the sacral insertion of the ligament (Fig. 14.8). An O Ethilon (JNJ) or Monosoft (Tyco) on a CT-2 needle is used to take serial bites of the ligament and continue up onto the prolapsed vault in an inverted "J" shape ending on the contralateral lateral apex of the vaginal vault making sure that the bladder is not involved anteriorly. A modified Roeder's knot is tied extracorporeally and slide down using a Carlton-SWEC knot pusher. It is left loose and not tensioned until the same suture has been inserted in the other uterosacral ligament (Figs 14.9 to 14.11). The vault, may need to be separately purse-stringed using this nonabsorbable suture. Once the sutures are in position, they are tensioned so that the vault is elevated to the level of the ischial spines (Fig. 14.12). The ureters are checked to make sure they are not compromised and the procedure is complete if this is the only defect. This therefore approximates the pubocervical facia anteriorly which is picked up with the anterior vault stitches with the rectovaginal fascia posteriorly which is picked up with the posterior vault stitches and attaches them to the uterosacral ligament complex (Figs 14.13A and B).

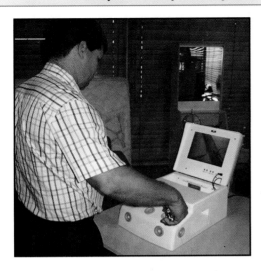

Fig. 14.4: Candidate practicing uterosacral plication on pelvic trainer

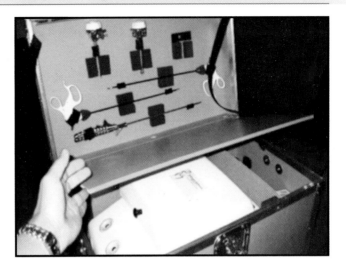

Fig. 14.5: Pelvic trainer and laparoscopic suturing instruments

As there is often a concomitant enterocoele or posterior compartment defect present the uterosacral colpopexy is often done at the end of a posterior paravaginal repair which involves opening the rectovaginal septum down to the perineal body and reconstructing the Level II supports from the fascia on the levator ani muscles and the endopelvic fascia so that they may be reattached to the Level I support formed from the uterosacral colpopexy. This repair may be augmented with mesh introduced laparoscopically or using a technique that we have just reported inserting the mesh through a small vaginal incision at the fourchette to make the dissection simpler and faster. It is also very common to require a high anterior paravaginal stitch or two just anterior to the ischial spines in the retropubic space suturing the anterolateral pubocervical fascia to the fascial white line with a secondary suspension to the Cooper's Ligament. This helps "square up" the vault anteriorly and guards against recurrence from anterior enterocoele. The details of these operations are not included in this chapter which is specifically directed to vault prolapse.

LAPAROSCOPIC MESH SACROCOLPOPEXY

This is a more complex procedure and one has to be an expert at curved needle suturing. The surgeon also requires an excellent assistant as retraction of the bowel can often be a challenge. There are various

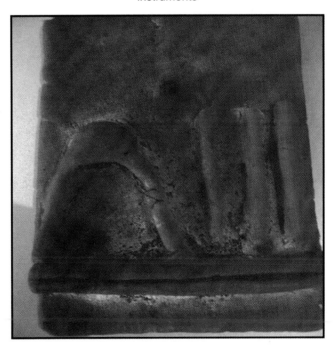

Fig. 14.6: Plastic mould of uterosacral ligaments to practice laparoscopic curved needle suturing

meshes available and some are custom built for this operation. The polypropylene meshes have to be fashioned at the time of the surgery and sutured externally into a "T" piece with an anterior pubocervical fascia process and a posterior rectovaginal fascia process as well as the longer sacral process (Figs 14.14 and 14.16). The operation begins once again

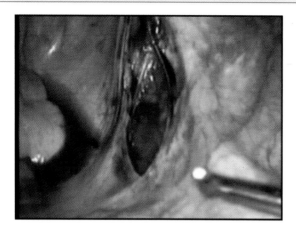

Fig. 14.7: Relieving incision on pelvic sidewall medial to ureter to allow safe placement of uterosacral plicating sutures

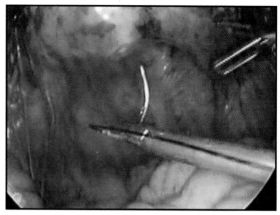

Fig. 14.8: Demonstration of uterosacral ligaments under tension with vaginal probe

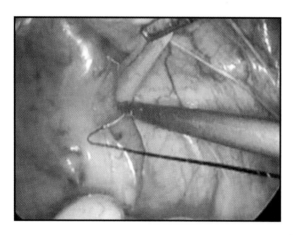

Fig. 14.9: Suturing of the right uterosacral ligament

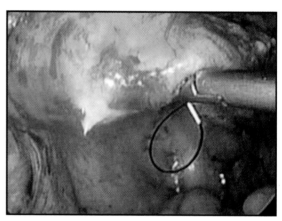

Fig. 14.10: Securing uterosacral ligament to the pubocervical fascia at the apex of the vaginal vault

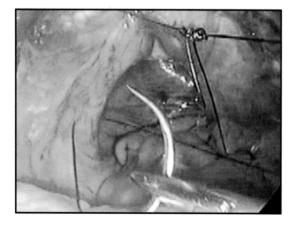

Fig. 14.11: Suturing of the left uterosacral ligament, note the modified Roeder's knot on the contralateral side is not tensioned until this suture is completed

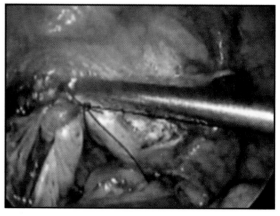

Fig. 14.12: Tensioning of plicating sutures with a Carlton-SWEC knot pusher

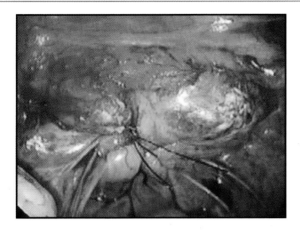

Fig. 14.13A: Vaginal vault is suspended at the level of the ischial spines

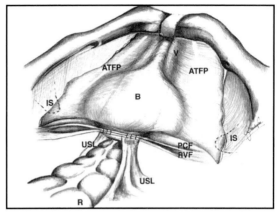

Fig. 14.13B: Intra-abdominal view following repair. ATFP, arcus tendineus fasciae pelvis; B, bladder; IS, ischial spines; PCF, pubocervical fascia; RVF, rectovaginal fascia; USL, uterosacral ligaments; R, rectum; V, vagina

with lysis of any adhesions and identification of the ureters laterally exactly as we have done above and once again we use relieving incisions medially to lateralize any drag on the ureters. The peritoneum over the vault probe is incised to identify the anterior limits of the pubocervical fascial defects and the rectal probe is used to enter the rectovaginal septum to identify the posterior limit of the defect which may involve only the upper third of the septum or may continue down to the perineal body. At the end of this step, we have fashioned our retroperitoneal prolapse cone ready for our mesh "cap" to be sutured to the vagina (Figs 14.17A and B).

We then move to the sacral promontory to prepare our sacral mesh attachment zone. It is necessary to get excellent exposure of the right paracolic gutter to keep the right ureter under vision laterally at all times and retract the sigmoid and mesocolon medially. The author often grab one of the sigmoid appendices and suture to the right paramedial quadrant peritoneum above my assistants' port site under little tension. This manoeuver usually gives excellent exposure of the target zone. We work in the right half of the sacral promontory and pick up the peritoneum and incise it to uncover the anterior longitudinal sacral ligament (Figs 14.18 and 14.19). This needs to be cleaned off to expose a 1-2 cm white area for mesh attachment. Once again the ureter needs to be visualized laterally and the sigmoid

mesentery with the median sacral vessel underneath medially and the left common iliac vein often above. We then take the peritoneal incision down the right paracolic gutter to connect with the right ureteric reeving incision and the vault dissection.

The mesh is then fashioned and placed over the vault. We begin by attaching the bladder flap going to the anterior limit of the dissection with 2 non-absorbable nylon sutures which again we tie extraperitoneally using a modified Roeder's knot slipped down with a Carlton SWEC knot pusher. Two more sutures are placed over the vault anteriorly before suturing the posterior mesh down to the base of the defect (Figs 14.20A to C). Once the mesh is attached to the prolapse cap we do not need to do any further fascial or ligamentous repair. The assistant now approximates the vault with a finger in the vagina to the level of the ischial spines and the length of the sacral process is determined so that the suspension is not under any tension. The sacral segment is then either sutured or tacked to the sacral zone on the anterior sacral ligament with 2 nonabsorbable sutures or tacks (Figs 14.21 and 14.22). The repair is now complete and the peritoneal defect is closed using either a continuous absorbable suture or a series of interrupted stitches (Figs 14.23 to 14.25). It is essential that there is no mesh exposed to stop adhesions and the mesh is not under tension.

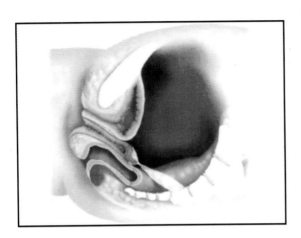

Fig. 14.14: Diagrammatic representation of mesh placement in sacrocolpoplexy

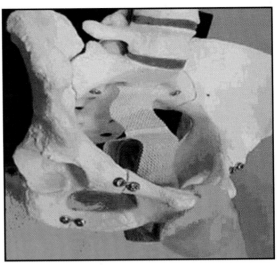

Fig. 14.15: Model demonstrating mesh placement in sacrocolpoplexy

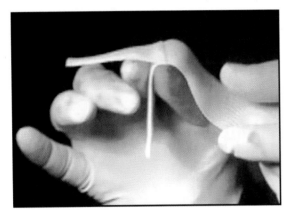

Fig. 14.16A: Fashioning of a "T" shaped mesh

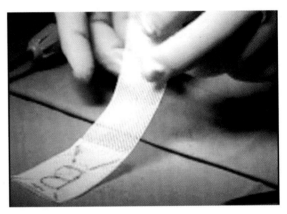

Fig. 14.16B: Labelling of anterior aspect of mesh "B" for intraoperative attachment to the pubocervical fascia

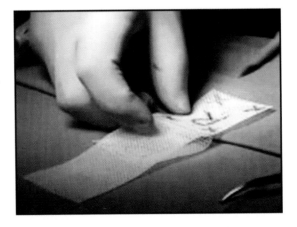

Fig. 14.16C: Labelling of posterior aspect of mesh "R" for intraoperative attachment to the rectovaginal fascia

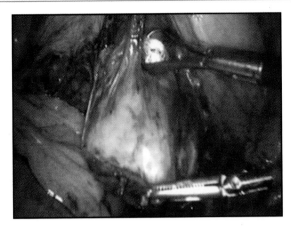

Fig. 14.17A: Dissection of bladder from anterior vaginal wall

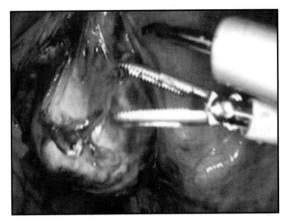

Fig. 14.17B: Dissection of the bladder off the vaginal vault exposing the pubocervical fascia for attachment of the mesh

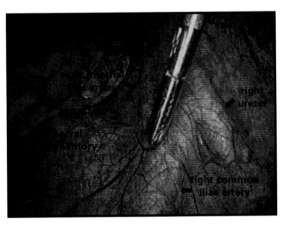

Fig. 14.18: Identification of the anatomy over the sacral promontory

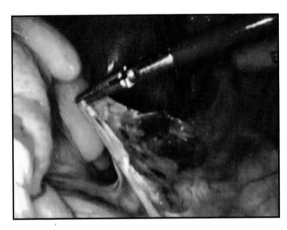

Fig. 14.19: Retroperitoneal dissection over the sacrum with ureter visible on right

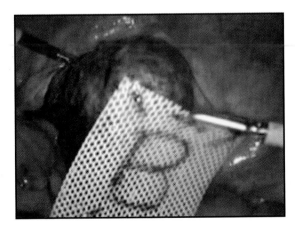

Fig. 14.20A: Placement of the mesh over the anterior aspect of the vault

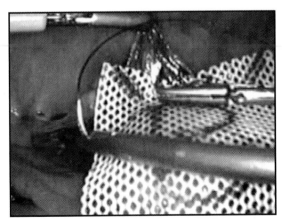

Fig. 14.20B: Suturing of the mesh to the pubocervical fascia

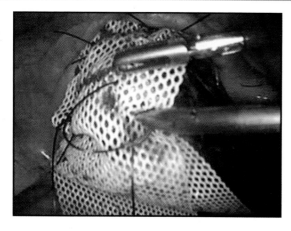

Fig. 14.20C:. Demonstrating placement of the mesh over the posterior aspect of the vaginal vault

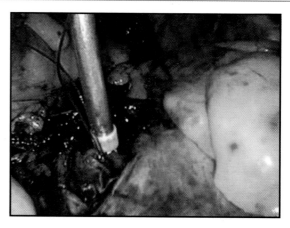

Fig. 14.21: "Straight In" Laparoscopic Sacral Colpoplexy System (American medical systems) fixing mesh to sacrum

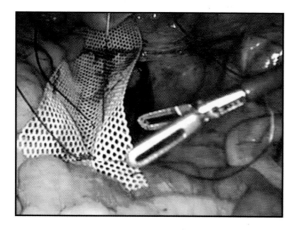

Fig. 14.22: Tension free fixation of mesh to the sacral promontory

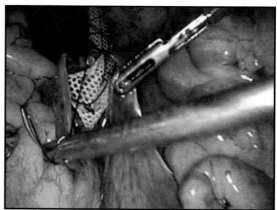

Fig. 14.23A: Re-peritonisation of the sacrum covering the mesh and separating it from the abdominal cavity

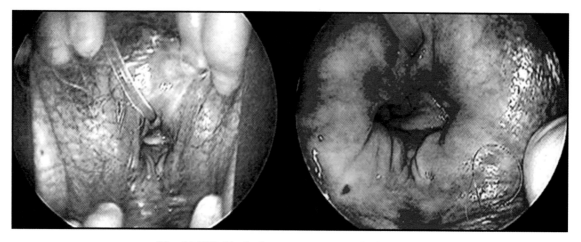

Fig. 14.23B: Vaginal appearance at end of surgery

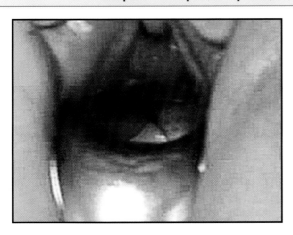

Fig. 14.24: Postoperative view of the resuspended vaginal vault

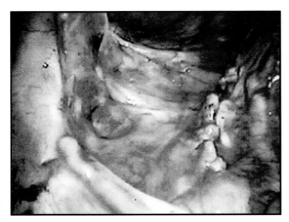

Fig. 14.25: Laparoscopic view of the reperitonised sacrum 1 year postoperatively

CONCLUSION

Vault prolapse involving Level I defects are common. They are often associated with multicompartment defects and often previous failed reconstructive surgery. Laparoscopy has enabled us to employ the abdominal approach and also the site specific approach very successfully to repair these defects. The complications of these procedures involve those of often-extensive bowel adhesiolysis and specific risks of bladder, bowel and ureteric injury with vascular injury to the median sacral vessels and rarely the left common iliac vessels. It demands an excellent knowledge of the pelvic anatomy and advanced laparoscopic skills. We still require objective outcome measures but the reports by Ostrzenski[27] (1998), Barber[19] et al (2000), Cook[28] et al (2004) Ross[15] (2005) and Higgs[19] et al (2005), are very encouraging with success rates ranging from 90-100 percent.

REFERENCES

1. Molander U, Milson I, Ekelund P, Mellstrom D. An epidemiological study of urinary incontinence and related urogenital symptoms in elderly women. Maturitas 1990;12:51-60.
2. Tapp A, Cardozo L. The effect of epidural anaesthesia on postpartum voiding. Neurourol Urodyn 1987;6:235-39.
3. Rush CB, Entman SS. Pelvic organ prolapse and stress incontinence. Med Clin North Am 1995; 79:1473-79.
4. Harris TA, Bent AD. Genital prolapse with and without urinary Incontinence. J Reprod Med 1990;35:792-98.
5. Delancy J. Anatomical aspects of vaginal eversion after hysterectomy. Am J Obstet Gynecol 1992;166:1717-28.
6. Karasick S, Spettel cm. The role of parity and hysterectomy on the development of pelvic floor abnormalities revealed by defecography. AJR 1997;169:1555-58.
7. Symmonds R, Pratt JH. Vaginal prolapse following hysterectomy Am J Obstet Gynecol 1960;79:899-909.
8. Marchionni M, Bracco G, Checcucci V, et al. True incidence of vaginal vault prolapse. J Reprod Med 1999;44;679-83.
9. Aurthure H, Savage D. Uterine prolapse and prolapse of the vaginal vault treated by sacral hysteropexy. Jobstet Gynaecol Br Emp 1957;64:355-60.
10. Baker K, Beresford JM, Campbell C. Colposacroplexy with prolene mesh 1990;171:51-54.
11. Addison W, Timmons MC. Abdominal approach to vaginal eversion. Clin Obstet Gynecol 1993;36:995-1004.
12. Timmons M. Addison WA, Addison SB, Cavenar MG. Abdominal sacral colpoplexy in 163 women with post hysterectomy vaginal vault prolapse and enterocoele. J Reprod Med 1992;37:323-27.
13. Brudbaker L. Sacrocolpolexy and anterior compartment: support and function. Am J Obstet Gynecol 1995;173:1690-95:discussion 1695-96.
14. Nichols D, Milley PS, Randall CL. Significance of restoration of normal vaginal depth and axis. Obstet Gynecol 1970;36:251-56.
15. Ross JW, Preston M. Laparoscopic sacrocolpplexy for severe vaginal vault prolapse: Five-year outcome. J Min Invas Gynecol 2005;12:221-26.
16. Ross J. Techniques of laparoscopic repair of total eversion after hysterectomy. J Amer Assoc Gynecol Laparosc 1997;4:173-83.
17. Nezhat C, Nezhat F, Nezhat C. Laparoscopic sacral colpoplexy for vaginal vault prolapse. Obstet Gynecol 1994;84:885-88.
18. Karram M, Goldwasser S, Kleeman S, Steele A. Vassallo B, Walsh P. High uterosacral vaginal vault suspension with fascial reconstruction for vaginal repair of enterocoele and vaginal vault prolapse. Am J Obstet Gynecol 2001;185:1339-43.

19. Barber MD, Visco AG, Weidner AC, Amundsen CL, Bump RC. Bilateral uterosacral ligament vault suspension with site-specific endopelvic fascia defect repair for the treatment of pelvic floor prolapse. Am J Obstet Gynecol 2000;1983:1402-11.

20. Delancy JOL. Anatomy and biomechanics of genital prolapse. Clin Obstet Gynecol 1993;36:897-909.

21. Delancy JOL. Structural aspects of the extrinsic continence mechanism.Obstet Gynecol 1988;72:296-301.

22. Snyder T, Kranz KE. Abdominal-retroperitoneal sacral colpoplexy for correction of vaginal vault prolapse. Obstet Gynecol 1991;77:944-49.

23. Visco AG, Weidner AC, Barber MD et al. Vaginal Mesh erosion after abdominal sacral colpoplexy. Am J Obstet Gynecol 2001;184:297-302.

24. Kohl N. Walsh PM, Roat TW, Karram MM. Mesh erosion after abdominal sacrocolpolexy. Obstet Gynecol 1998;92:999-1004.

25. Nygaard IK, Kreder KJ. Complications of colposuspension. Int Urogynecol J 1994;5:353-60.

26. Bump RC, Mattiasson A, Bo K, et al. The standardisation of terminology of female pelvic organ prolapse and pelvic floor dysfunction. Am J Obstet Gynecol 1996;175:10-17.

27. Ostrzenski A. New retroperitoneal culdoplasty and colpopexy at the time of laparoscopic total abdominal hysterectomy (L-TAH). Acta Obstet Gynecol Scand. 1998;77(10):1017-21.

28. Cook JR, Seman EI, O'Shea RT. Laparoscopic treatment of enterocoele: a 3-year evaluation Aust NZJ Obstet Gynecol 2004;44(2)107-10.

29. Higgs PJ, HL Chua, Smith ARB. Long-term review of laparoscopic sacrolcolpopexy. BJOG 2005;112;1134-38.

Laparoscopic Suturing of the Bowel

DAVID B. REDWINE

Chapter Fifteen

INTRODUCTION

During pelvic surgery, a gynecologist will most commonly encounter the intestinal tract in two clinical situations: dealing with endometriosis and dealing with adhesions. For a laparoscopic surgeon, a third possibility of encountering the intestinal tract is during trocar placement.

A surgeon treating intestinal endometriosis, will be performing some type of bowel resection, in which case, the injury to the bowel is intentional and part of the therapeutic effort. Unintentional injury to the bowel is possible when inserting laparoscopic trocars or performing enterolysis. Regardless of the mode of injury to the bowel, a surgeon must be adept at identifying bowel injury and judging whether it requires some type of repair, then either repairing that injury or have someone come to the operating room to repair it. The principles of bowel repair are similar regardless of whether the injury is intentional or unintentional: the bowel must not leak when the repair is done.

SURGICAL ANATOMY OF THE BOWEL WALL

The colon has four identifiable layers: serosa, outer longitudinal muscularis, inner circular muscularis, and mucosa. Beneath the peritoneal reflection of the cul-de-sac, the serosal layer is lost (Fig. 15.1), and above the cul-de-sac reflection, the serosa is essentially fused to the outer muscularis. Thus, the large bowel has three surgically useful layers—outer muscularis, inner muscularis, and mucosa. The wall of the small intestine is thinner and responds surgically as if it has only two layers: muscularis and mucosa. These separate intestinal layers have importance for both surgical treatment of intestinal endometriosis or unintended damage to the intestinal tract. These colonic layers can be peeled apart from each other like layers of an onion, which greatly facilitates endometriosis surgery. These layers can also delineate and limit the depth of unintended surgical injury. Many gynecologists think the bowel wall is as thin as a balloon and just as easily injured. The bowel is more surgeon-friendly than that. With experience, a surgeon will realize that the layers of the bowel wall allow a certain degree of intentional or unintentional injury to occur without necessarily penetrating into the lumen.

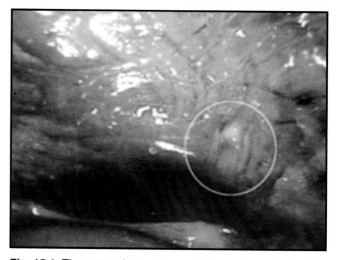

Fig. 15.1: The rectum is seen beneath the peritoneal reflection of the cul-de-sac, which has been resected to treat superficial endometriosis. Notice the longitudinal muscle fibers of the outer layer of muscularis. A small bowel burn is circled

With bowel adhesions following surgery or infection, the bowel wall beneath the adhesions is usually normal, although it is still possible to injure the bowel to some degree despite careful enterolysis.

Endometriosis of the bowel originates on the serosal surface and displays varying degrees of invasion into the muscularis. The disease rarely penetrates the bowel lumen, which is why colonoscopy is so frequently negative. Intestinal endometriosis occurs in well-identified recurring patterns, usually on the antimesenteric bowel wall in five possible sites in the following declining order of frequency of occurrence: sigmoid, rectum (identified as a rectal nodule associated with obliteration of the cul-de-sac), ileum, appendix, and cecum. Depending on the degree of invasion into the bowel wall and whether surgery is occurring on the colon or ileum, intestinal endometriosis may require one of four types of bowel surgery for its treatment:

1. Superficial resection of the serosa and a bit of outer muscularis.
2. Partial-thickness resection down to the inner circular muscularis or even deeper to the mucosa.
3. Full-thickness disk resection of the anterior bowel wall.
4. Segmental resection and anastomosis.

Complete obliteration of the cul-de-sac (Fig. 15.2) will require rectal surgery in most cases.[1] The specific morphology that will tell the surgeon if the rectal

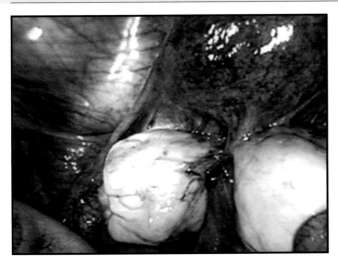

Fig. 15.2: Complete obliteration of the cul-de-sac is shown. The ovaries are adherent to their respective uterosacral ligaments. The rectum is adherent to the posterior cervix between the ovaries and is slightly rounded, indicating invasion of the muscularis by endometriosis

wall is involved by endometriosis in the "rounded rectum". This rounded appearance of the rectum at its point of adherence to the posterior cervix occurs because of fibromuscular metaplasia in a spherical shape in the bowel wall. In contrast, if the rectum is adherent to the posterior cervix but is flat, the rectal wall will be involved by little or no endometriosis.

Although laparoscopic segmental resection and anastomosis is feasible, this is done using surgical stapling devices rather than suturing, so this technique will not be discussed.

Avoiding Unintentional Bowel Injury during Surgery

Avoiding unintentional injury to the bowel is the best route to take, although even when the possibility of bowel injury is anticipated, it is not always possible to avoid it. Nonetheless, at each stage of a surgical procedure, there are certain steps which might help.

Insertion of Trocars

The rate of injury with trocar insertion ranges from 1/4448 (0.02%)[2] in one study to 10/32,205 (0.03%)[3] in another study, with the small bowel more commonly injured than the large bowel. These rates predict that most laparoscopists will never have an intestinal injury due to trocar insertion. Intestinal

injuries can be caused both by the Verres needle as well as by the primary trocar.

There are a variety of ways of inserting trocars, each with its champions as well as technical pros and cons.

Classic Technique

Classical teaching is to insufflate the abdomen with carbon dioxide delivered through a Verres needle before introducing the laparoscopic trocars. This has the immediately obvious disadvantage of requiring two blind insertions of potentially damaging surgical instruments: the initial needle insertion followed by the trocar insertion. Furthermore, if the insufflating needle were to penetrate a loop of bowel, then that loop would be inflated and present an even larger target for the insertion of the initial trocar, increasing the likelihood of injury. If the pneumoperitoneum is created correctly, the large bubble of gas within the abdominal cavity theoretically provides extra protection against bowel injury by the second trocar because the abdominal wall is elevated away from the posterior abdomen where the bowel is presumably resting peacefully due to gravity. However, the same elevation of the abdominal wall can be achieved mechanically by grasping the skin of the abdomen with fingers or towel clips on each side of the umbilicus while inserting the umbilical trocar with the insufflation port open.

Alternate Site Technique

In patients with previous laparotomy or laparoscopy, the possibility exists that a loop of bowel may be adherent to the abdominal wall at the umbilicus. Patients with previous laparoscopy, appendectomy, cholecystectomy or cesarean section will almost never have bowel adherent in the vicinity of the umbilicus.[4] If a loop of bowel is directly adherent to the abdominal wall beneath the umbilicus, then bowel injury will be virtually unavoidable. Fortunately, it is extremely rare for bowel to be so densely and confluently adherent to the abdominal wall at the umbilicus, even in patients with previous laparotomy. Nonetheless, to avoid this situation, some authors recommend a left upper quadrant location for initial Verres needle insertion followed by insertion of a 5 mm laparoscope in the same region in order to view the region beneath the umbilicus to determine if it is safe to pass a trocar in that location.

Open Technique

Using a scalpel to cut down through the layers of the umbilicus until the peritoneum is encountered and entered sharply is sometimes called open laparoscopy since the abdomen is opened (albeit through a very small incision) before the first trocar is inserted. When a special conical sleeve is sutured to the fascia to block the escape of pneumoperitoneum, this is termed the Hassen technique, after its originator, Harrith Hassen.

Trocar innovations have been introduced in an effort to reduce the rate of bowel injuries. Optical trocars allow a view of the area touching the trocar tip, theoretically allowing the surgeon to see a loop of bowel before injuring it. Radially expanding trocars have a small initial diameter which can be expanded when intraperitoneal placement has been confirmed.

An important variable in bowel injury by trocars is the sharpness of the trocar tip. A sharp tip is more likely to injure bowel than is a blunt tip. Disposable trocars, marketed in part because of their sharpness and ease of use, might be more dangerous than reusable trocars whose tips eventually get dull.

Preoperative ultrasound examination to detect visceral sliding against the abdominal wall has been proposed as a way to reduce trocar insertion injuries to the bowel in women with previous abdominal surgery.[4] When at least 1 cm of displacement or sliding of intra-abdominal contents against the abdominal wall was observed with deep inspiration and forced expiration, there was a 2 percent chance of bowel adhesions being present beneath the umbilicus as determined by subsequent surgery. When visceral sliding was decreased, there was a 54 percent chance of underlying adherent bowel. A previous vertical midline incision carried a 24 percent chance of underlying adhesions. In patients with previous vertical midline incisions, an alteration of initial trocar insertion should be considered, such as an open entry technique or alternate left upper quadrant site for initial trocar placement. It seems best for a surgeon to adopt a technique or two and become proficient in their use.

Direct Insertion Technique

I do not use needle insufflation to create pneumoperitoneum before trocar insertion, as I believe this introduces needless risk and time. Standing on the patient's left, I make a vertical incision within the umbilicus, starting at the bottom or lowest point where the abdominal wall is thinnest. The incision extends inferiorly for about a centimeter. With my left hand, I then grasp the skin of the abdominal wall to the left of the umbilicus, and the scrub nurse grasps the abdominal wall to the right of the umbilicus. Our hands elevate the abdominal wall as much as possible in an action which is a metaphor of the conduct of the rest of the surgery: whenever possible the surgical site is elevated away from underlying vital structures. With a reusable 10 mm trocar in my right hand, I insert the tip of the trocar within the umbilical incision. The insufflation port valve of the trocar is open, so that air will immediately be allowed to enter the abdominal cavity, theoretically allowing non-adherent bowel to drop away from the anterior abdominal wall. I visualize where the tip is aiming, my target being the center of the pelvis. Aiming in the direction of the uterine fundus would be another acceptable target (obviously the trocar should not extend entirely to the uterine fundus, which would be difficult to reach anyway). With the middle finger of my right hand alongside the shaft of the trocar sheath to act as a governor of depth insertion, I push the trocar through the umbilical incision with a slight twisting motion until I feel it pop through the fascia. When I remove the obturator of the trocar and pass the viewing laparoscope, I find that when the tip of the trocar has passed through the fascia, it has usually also passed through the peritoneum. In the rare case where the peritoneum has not been pierced, I frequently take my operating laparoscope and pass it down the sheath and, using 3 mm scissors, cut through the peritoneum under direct vision, mimicking the same action which is done at laparotomy.[5]

Most of my patients have had multiple previous laparoscopies or laparotomies. I usually do not alter my technique because of this. I find that the intestines are almost never adherent directly to the abdominal wall in the region of the umbilicus, although occasionally omentum may be adherent in this area.

I have only entered the bowel twice during initial trocar insertion in over 3,000 cases, and fortunately the injuries were immediately identified. In one of these patients, operated on early in my career, a general surgeon was called to help with the repair. Opening the abdomen with a laparotomy, he also entered the bowel lumen. In the other patient, I repaired the intestinal entry laparoscopically and proceeded with the intended surgery. The only time I alter my laparoscopic entry technique is when a vertical laparotomy incision extending around the umbilicus is present. In such a case, I will make my umbilical incision from the bottom of the umbilicus laterally toward the side opposite the laparotomy incision, my thought being that there may be a decreased chance for omental adhesions further away from the laparotomy incision. A previous low transverse laparotomy incision is no guarantee that periumbilical adhesions will be absent, since most commonly the peritoneum is opened vertically.

If it is possible to injure the bowel opening the abdomen at laparotomy, it is futile to think that the rate of bowel injury with Verres needle or trocar insertion during laparoscopy will ever be zero. A randomized controlled trial would require tens of thousands of patients to determine if there is any statistical difference between existing methods, all of which produce a very low rate of intestinal injury. Thus, it seems likely that the question will never be answered, so should it even be asked?

Enterolysis: Endometriosis versus Other Causes

Adhesions involving the intestinal tract may be due to previous surgery or from a pathological process such as endometriosis or ruptured appendicitis. Lysis of intestinal adhesions, or enterolysis, may require a different approach in some cases, based on the cause of the adhesions. The main difference is that endometriosis can invade the bowel wall, so intestinal adhesions in association with endometriosis may require some type of bowel resection rather than only an attempt at enterolysis, while adhesions due to previous surgery or infective inflammation typically do not require anything be done to the bowel proper. In fact, with this second type of adhesion, the surgeon will be actively trying to avoid damage to the bowel. Of course, since many patients with endometriosis will have undergone previous surgery, these patients may have both types of adhesions involving the intestines.

Adhesions involving the bowel have four main morphologic characteristics seen at surgery: confluency, density, vascularity and presence of a surgical plane (Table 15.1). Confluency refers to how much of the bowel wall is in direct contact with another structure. While no specific grading system for confluency exists, a surgeon will intuitively understand that bowel may be confluently adherent at a single point or area, or over a larger area. Density of adhesions is a subjective measure of the pliability or flexibility of adhesions. Dense adhesions are rather inflexible, while filmy adhesions are pliable, resembling cobwebs or wet glue.

These morphologic characteristics of adhesions may help the surgeon to correctly identify the cause of bowel adhesions which is very important for safe and complete treatment of pelvic pathology. The most important thing to distinguish is whether adhesions might be due to endometriosis because of the possibility of intestinal involvement by endometriosis. If the characteristics of adhesions due to endometriosis can be reliably identified, then all other types of adhesions are due to something else, such as previous surgery (Fig. 15.3). Intestinal adhesions due to endometriosis are sufficiently characteristic by their morphology that they can be

TABLE 15–1: Intestinal adhesion morphology by adhesion cause				
	Morphology			
Adhesion cause	*Confluence*	*Density*	*Vascularity*	*Surgical plane*
Previous surgery	Low or high	Low	Low or high	Usually present
Previous infection	Low	Low	Low or high	Usually present
Endometriosis	High	High	Low	Absent

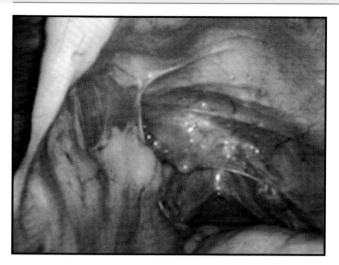

Fig. 15.3: Postoperative adhesions, such as those shown here, tend to be transparent, filmy, and are not confluent

reliably distinguished, as long as the surgeon takes the time to look and palpate and avoids classifying all adhesions as "just adhesions". Adhesions due to endometriosis are highly confluent, very dense to the point of lacking a distinct surgical plane, and are virtually avascular. Furthermore, intestinal adhesions due to endometriosis occur in only two areas:

1. Rectal nodules of endometriosis are associated with the rectum adherent to the posterior cervix, producing obliteration of the cul-de-sac (Fig. 15.2)
2. Sigmoid nodules of endometriosis may be adherent to the left ovary (or rarely to the right ovary).

Proper surgical treatment depends on accurate visual diagnosis at surgery. If obliteration of the cul-de-sac is present, but if the surgeon is thinking only about adhesions and not their cause, then the conclusion may be reached that "dense adhesions are present in the cul-de-sac or adense adhesions cause the rectum to be adherent to the posterior cervix". Strictly speaking, while such an observation is true, the surgeon may have missed an opportunity to make the correct pathological diagnosis. This is one of the many clinical mistakes which can result in incomplete diagnosis and treatment of endometriosis, which can lead to the repetitive surgeries which are the unfortunate hallmark of the modern treatment of this disease. With postoperative adhesions or adhesions due to infection or inflammation, putting the adhesions on stretch followed by simple enterolysis will suffice. When endometriosis is the cause of intestinal adhesions, the endometriosis must be treated.

Trocar Insertion as a Cause of Bowel Injury

Trocar injuries can be partial-thickness, full-thickness, or through-and-through. Partial-thickness injuries may go unnoticed since the injured loop of bowel may move away from its original position, and bleeding may be scant or absent. Full-thickness injuries may be diagnosed upon insertion of the optical laparoscope, whereupon the surgeon will be surprised to see intestinal mucosa instead of intra-abdominal contents.

Through-and-through injuries can occur either with the larger primary trocar or with smaller accessory trocars. To survey the abdominal cavity for this type of injury from the umbilical trocar, the viewing laparoscope should be rotated through a 360 degree field of view, searching for any loop of bowel which seems to head toward the anterior abdominal wall. If this is seen, then the viewing laparoscope and its sheath should be withdrawn slowly from the umbilical area, all the while watching for evidence of intestinal mucosa. A similar concept is useful after insertion of secondary trocars. The sites of entry through the abdominal wall should be observed after their insertion to ensure that no bowel has been impaled.

Enterolysis as a Cause of Bowel Injury

Simple Enterolysis

Simple enterolysis involves grasping an adherent portion of bowel with an atraumatic grasper and utilizing the age-old surgical principles of traction and countertraction. The grasper provides the traction and often the surface where the bowel is adherent provides sufficient countertraction to separate the bowel wall from the adherent surface and reveal a surgical plane. Even when the bowel appears initially to be confluently adherent, sometimes simple blunt adhesiolysis can be used to separate the bowel from the other surface. When adhesions can be put on stretch, they can be divided by sharp cutting, or cut with electrosurgery, laser or harmonic scalpel. Some adhesions are long enough that they can be cut at both points of attachment and removed by excision.

Enterolysis may result in partial- or full-thickness penetration into the bowel wall. Suture repair will be difficult or impossible until all of the adhesions are released in the area of injury. Otherwise, the needle will not have complete access to the area to be repaired. A hole in the bowel is not an absolute emergency that should bring an immediate halt to adhesiolysis if the injury is not in full plain view. Instead, continue the adhesiolysis until all adhesions in the vicinity have been released, then repair the bowel. Contents of the small bowel are not highly contaminated while contents of the large bowel are usually solid enough that extrusion of feces is unlikely to occur through defects smaller than about 2 cm in greatest dimension. If limited leakage or extrusion of bowel content occurs, it can be irrigated out, antibiotic coverage begun, and a drain left in place. Use caution when irrigating in the presence of a full-thickness defect in the colon since the irrigation fluid could cause some degree of liquefaction of colonic contents, which may increase the potential for contamination.

Laparoscopic repair of partial- or full-thickness bowel injuries resulting from enterolysis is identical to bowel repair following endometriosis surgery and will be discussed below.

Complicated Adhesiolysis Related to Endometriosis

"Complicated adhesiolysis" as used here refers to adhesions due to endometriosis. As indicated above, these adhesions are confluent, dense, avascular and may have no clear surgical plane of easy division, and a surgeon identifying only an adhesive process will completely miss major pathology. When such adhesions are present, there is a high probability of involvement of the bowel wall itself[6] so some type of bowel resection will be necessary. As such, the adhesions are of secondary importance to endo-metriosis as the surgical target. Treating the endometriosis will treat the adhesions.

Laparoscopic treatment of complete obliteration of the cul-de-sac by en bloc resection has been descri-bed in the literature[7] and represents a straight-forward comprehensive approach to the invasive nature of endometriosis found in this presentation of the disease. A greatly simplified synopsis of this technique follows: The normal peritoneum adjacent to the uterosacral ligaments is incised (Figs 15.4 and

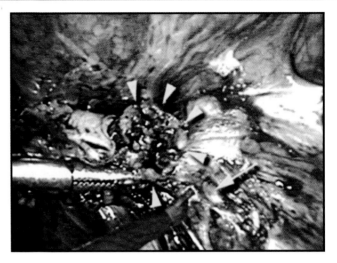

Fig. 15.4: This patient is undergoing laparoscopic treatment of complete obliteration of the cul-de-sac due to endometriosis. This morphologic manifestation of endometriosis indicates the presence of invasive disease of the uterosacral ligaments, cul-de-sac, and usually the anterior rectal wall as well. The right uterosacral ligament is demarcated by arrowheads. The 3 mm scissors are used with electrosurgery to incise normal peritoneum adjacent to the nodular disease of the ligament, isolating it from underlying normal retroperitoneal tissue. The right uterine artery is indicated by the arrow

15.5), then a transverse incision is created across the posterior cervix above the line of adherence of the bowel (Fig. 15.6). An intrafascial dissection down the posterior cervix shaves off the outer 2 mm or so of the cervix until the rectovaginal septum is encountered (Fig. 15.7) and developed bluntly. The cul-de-sac remains obliterated but is included in a mass of tissue on the anterior rectal wall. This tissue mass consists of the posterior cervix, uterosacral ligaments, and the obliterated cul-de-sac itself. The lateral fatty attachments of the lower rectosigmoid colon are severed (Fig. 15.8) to complete the isolation of the pathology. The surgery becomes bowel surgery at this point, (Fig. 15.9) with a partial- or full-thickness resection (Fig. 15.10) being done, depending on the size of the nodule and its depth of invasion.

When the sigmoid colon is adherent to the left ovary due to endometriosis, realization of a similar important endometriosis concept is useful. There frequently will be a nodule of endometriosis in the wall of the sigmoid at the point of attachment to the ovary. This can be identified by palpation. If a little of the ovary is resected and allowed to remain

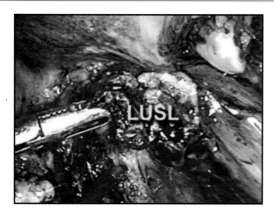

Fig. 15.5: This is the same patient shown in Figure 15.4. The left uterosacral ligament (LUSL) is being isolated by a peritoneal incision and retroperitoneal dissection performed bluntly and with electrosurgery

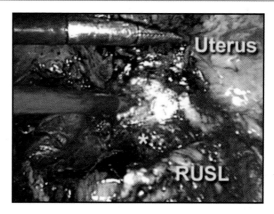

Fig. 15.6: A transverse incision is created across the posterior cervix above the adherent bowel. The cul-de-sac (asterisk) remains obliterated but is being separated from the cervix. The right uterosacral ligament (RUSL) will be transected by the transverse incision at its point of insertion into the posterior cervix

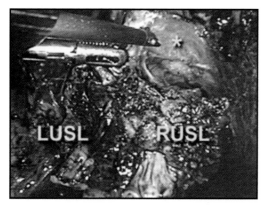

Fig. 15.7: The intrafascial dissection has proceeded posteriorly down the cervix until the areolar tissue of the rectovaginal septum (asterisk) is encountered. The nodular mass of the obliterated cul-de-sac which is composed of the right and left uterosacral ligaments (RUSL, LUSL), posterior cervix, and anterior rectal wall will be isolated onto the anterior bowel wall

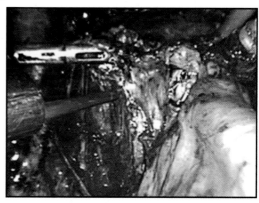

Fig. 15.8: The lateral fatty attachments of the rectum are severed by electrosurgery to complete the isolation of the nodule onto the anterior bowel wall

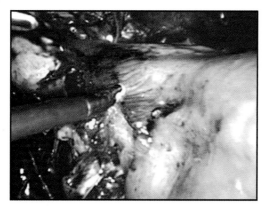

Fig. 15.9: The 3 mm scissors with 90 watts of pure cutting current are used to score the normal bowel wall proximal to the large nodule

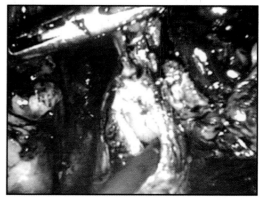

Fig. 15.10: Fibrosis associated with the nodule is dramatic, inevitably leading the scissors dissection into the bowel lumen

attached to the sigmoid, then the case becomes a bowel surgery case at that point.

Women with ovarian endometriomas have a higher chance of bowel involvement than endometriosis patients without ovarian disease.[8] Bowel involvement is also likely if obliteration of the cul-de-sac is present or if bowel involvement has been diagnosed at a previous surgery. Nodularity of the cul-de-sac or uterosacral ligaments also carries an increased chance of bowel involvement. Women with endometriosis of the posterior vaginal fornix carry a 71 percent chance that rectal surgery will be required.

Principles of Laparoscopic Bowel Surgery[9]

Energy Systems for Excisional Bowel Surgery: Electrosurgery versus Others

Laparoscopic excision of bowel endometriosis can be done with sharp dissection with scissors, or with monopolar electrosurgery. Electrosurgery carries some risk of lateral thermal spread which can be virtually eliminated if the surgeon understands its use. Low power settings are not necessarily safer and may be more dangerous than higher ones. Pure cutting current used at high current density with quick superficial strokes will result in a clean surgical cut with little or no lateral thermal spread. I use 90 watts of pure cutting current delivered through a 3 mm scissors passed down the operating channel of an operative laparoscope. By using the tip or edge of the scissors as a point electrode, extremely high current densities can be achieved. The electrode should be activated before touching tissue so that cutting will begin to occur immediately, avoiding pillowing of tissue around the electrode tip which will reduce current density, resulting in messy and dangerous coagulation effect instead of a quick cut. Another point of safety with monopolar electrosurgery is to use short bursts of power. Just as your hand can pass quickly through a flame with no injury, a quick burst of electrosurgery is less likely to produce unintended injury than several seconds of continuous use. The notion that electrosurgery is dangerous and should not be used laparoscopically is a falsehood generated either by those who do not understand its use or by those who seek to market another energy source. Any energy source can produce unintentional injury if used improperly.

Many energy sources can produce equivalent therapeutic endpoints if their use is understood. Thus, each type of bowel resection used to treat endometriosis can be accomplished using sharp dissection with scissor, or by electrosurgery, carbon dioxide laser, fiber laser, or harmonic scalpel. Monopolar or bipolar coagulation as a treatment of endometriosis violates one of the principles of safe surgery—the physical separation of target tissue from normal tissue before application of energy—since the action of coagulation occurs on peritoneum which is immediately adjacent to underlying vital structures. Furthermore, the details of electrocoagulation are too ill-described for electrocoagulation of endometriosis to be done in a standardized, reproducible fashion. Gynecological surgeons can reduce the potential for unintended bowel injury by abandoning electrocoagulation of peritoneal endometriosis, especially in the area of the cul-de-sac where the somewhat hidden underlying rectum can be injured.

It is fortunate that intestinal endometriosis typically occurs in recurring patterns on the anterior, antimesenteric surface of the bowel wall. Because the anterior surface of the bowel is in plain view during laparoscopy, this means that most cases of endometriosis will be easier to diagnose and treat than if disease occurred on the lateral or posterior sides. Since the same manifestations of intestinal disease will be encountered repeatedly, the surgical approaches which are necessary to treat these manifestations becomes rote, (Table 15.2) which is very reassuring to the surgeon caring for these patients.

Principles of Laparoscopic Suturing for Bowel Repair

The principles of bowel repair are the same whether the bowel is being repaired after endometriosis surgery or after unintended intestinal injury with a trocar or during adhesiolysis. The most important point is that if the lumen is opened, it must be closed. An important corollary is that if there is a possibility that the bowel lumen is open, this possibility must be investigated and proven or disproven. If it is unclear whether full-thickness injury has occurred, it would be safest to presume it had. If leakage of bowel contents occurs after the conclusion of surgery, the best that can happen is reoperation, sometimes

TABLE 15-2: Sites of intestinal involvement by endometriosis and type of surgical treatment, author's series

Site	Total cases	Type of resection required	Number of cases % of total
Sigmoid	439	Superficial	223
		Partial thickness	72
		Full thickness	67
		Segmental	98
Rectum	375	Superficial	77
		Partial thickness	70
		Full thickness	121
		Segmental	107
		Ileum	116
		Superficial	35
		Partial thickness	24
		Full thickness	25
		Segmental	50
Appendix	80	Appendectomy	80
Cecum	37	Superficial	12
		Partial thickness	6
		Full thickness	15
		Segmental	4

with a temporary colostomy. The worst that can happen is death of the patient.

The diameter of the bowel can be reduced if suture repair of a larger defect is done in the wrong direction. All suture lines, whether continuous (as is done on the mucosa) or interrupted (as is usually done on the seromuscularis) should start on the left or right side of the bowel and close the bowel from one angle to another (Fig. 15.11). The surgeon can be reminded of the correct orientation of bowel repair by looking down at the skin crease within his or her bent elbow. The orientation of the suture line in the bowel should look like that when finished. Placing sutures transversely across the large or small bowel will reduce the diameter of the lumen (Fig. 15.12).

Instruments Required for Bowel Suturing

Suturing will require a needle driver as well as a grasper to pick up and hold the needle and retrieve the needle after it is passed through tissue by the needle driver. It is helpful to avoid pop-off sutures because it is easier to remove a needle from the abdominal cavity when it has a length of suture on it.

Inserting and Removing Needles during Laparoscopy

Introducing and removing the needle can be done either through the main 10 mm or larger trocar sheath or through an accessory puncture site.

To pass a needle into the abdominal cavity through an accessory port site, a small (e.g. 5.5 mm) accessory sheath, which has already been inserted, is removed and held in the surgeon's hand. The needle driver is passed down through the sheath until the jaws are protruding. The suture is grasped in the jaws of the needle driver near the needle (Fig. 15.13) and then the needle driver is inserted back down the tract left in the abdominal wall by removal of the sheath. The suture will pull the needle through an arc as the needle passes through the abdominal wall (Fig. 15.14). Once the needle is in the abdominal cavity, the sheath around the needle driver can be advanced into the abdomen, thus re-establishing the utility of the secondary port site. After use of the needle, the suture can be grasped with the needle driver and then the sheath and needle driver are both pulled out of the abdomen simultaneously. The needle once again automatically travels in an arc as it exits the abdomen. Two or more needles can be removed in this way (Fig. 15.15). Small accessory punctures can become larger with repeated passage of a sheath, and annoying leakage of pneumoperitoneum around the sheath may result, so passage of the needle down the main sheath has an advantage.

Passing a needle into the abdominal cavity through the main trocar sheath does not require removal of the sheath. The arc of the needle must be small enough to pass down the sheath when held in the needle driver. The orientation of the needle is important as it is held in the needle driver (Fig. 15.16). If the arc of the needle is slightly too large to fit down the sheath, the needle can be straightened slightly.

Most packaged sutures are designed for use at laparotomy. As a result, they are too long for most laparoscopic uses. It is usually helpful to cut the suture before insertion into the abdominal cavity so that the proper length will be present (Table 15.3).

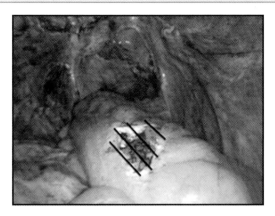

Fig. 15.11: Partial-thickness bowel resections result in defects of the muscularis, leaving the mucosa intact. The black lines indicate the proper placement of interrupted silk sutures to close the defect without reducing the bowel lumen

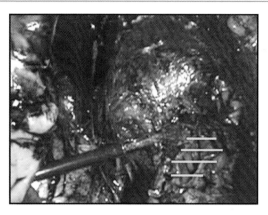

Fig. 15.12: The yellow lines indicate the incorrect placement of sutures to close a bowel defect. Such placement would significantly reduce the diameter of the bowel, possibly leading to partial obstructive symptoms

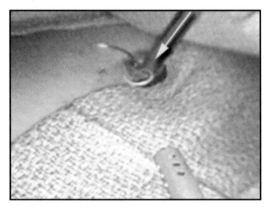

Fig. 15.13: The needle driver is passed down the accessory sheath (not shown) and has grasped the suture near the needle. The needle driver is being inserted into a 5.5 mm right lower quadrant accessory port site. Pushing the needle driver down in the direction of the arrow will pull the attached needle into the abdomen

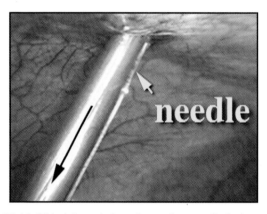

Fig. 15.14: This internal view shows the needle being pulled through the abdominal wall. After the needle and suture are inside the abdomen, the sheath will be advanced around the needle driver and into the abdomen

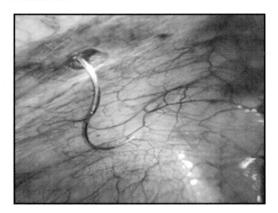

Fig. 15.15: One (or more) needles can be removed from the abdomen by grasping the suture near the needle(s), withdrawing the sheath (not shown) and pulling the needle(s) out by the suture

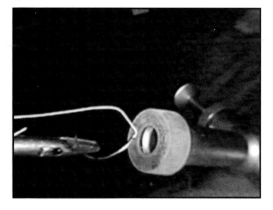

Fig. 15.16: To insert a needle down the 10 mm trocar sheath, it must be held in proper orientation in the needle driver. Notice that the sharp end of the needle does not lead the way inside the abdomen

TABLE 15–3: Cutting suture to length based on the task	
Task	*Suggested suture length*
Close a small seromuscular defect with a single suture	3-4 inches
Interrupted seromuscular sutures	3-4 inches
Purse-string sutures in seromuscular layer to bury mucosal corners	4-5 inches
Closing mucosa	6-8 inches
Suspending lateral angle for full-thickness repair	full length

Intracorporeal Knot-tying

Intracorporeal knot-tying is easier if two key points are kept in mind:

1. A suture loop is created toward the tying instrument so that the instrument may be easily inserted through the loop during knot-tying
2. The free end of the suture is placed on a tissue surface nearby for easy pickup (Fig. 15.17). Square knots are theoretically preferable, but in actual practice, four or more sequential overhand throws in the same direction (also known as a Granny knot) can be used.

Superficial Bowel Resection for Endometriosis/ Partial-Thickness Intestinal Injury

When endometriosis involves the serosa and outer muscularis of the colon, the lesions are frequently less than 5 mm in greatest dimension and can be removed by superficial resection done with scissors or electrosurgery. The lesion is circumscribed with lines of incision into the outer layer of muscularis, then undermined and removed. While very shallow defects may not need suture, I recommend that such defects be reinforced with suture. A laparoscopic surgeon should take every opportunity to practice intracorporeal suturing. Repairing superficial defects in cases where the result of the repair is inconsequential will train the surgeon for the time when an excellent repair is vital.

Superficial bowel resections or unintended seromuscular lacerations can be repaired with interrupted 2-0 silk or a similar size of absorbable suture. Silk suture is the classic suture used by general surgeons to repair the seromuscularis of the bowel and does not have much memory, allowing it to lay in place for easier tying. I use 2-0 silk because it does not break as easily as the smaller 3-0 silk. I

try to avoid penetrating the intact mucosa with the needle and stitch, although this is not a problem if it occurs. A small defect less than 5 mm across may be closed with a single stitch (Figs 15.1, 15.18 and 15.19).

Larger defects (Fig. 15.20) will require multiple stitches. Place the first stitch on one lateral edge of the defect (Fig. 15.21), then place the second stitch on the opposite lateral edge. The advantage of this is that the lateral corners of the defect can sometimes become hidden if suturing begins in the middle of the defect and then proceeds laterally. The remainder of the seromuscularis can be closed with interrupted sutures placed between the lateral angles (Fig. 15.22).

"Mucosal Skinning" for Endometriosis

When endometriosis involves both layers of muscularis, dissection is begun into the normal bowel wall adjacent to the nodule and the nodule is circumscribed, working just in the muscularis at first. As the nodule is progressively isolated to the center of the dissection, an attempt is made to find a surgical plane between the soft bowel wall and the firmer nodule. The dissection will often lead deeper until the mucosa is encountered. If there is no significant submucosal fibrosis, the nodule within the muscualris can be dissected away from the underlying mucosa by pulling them apart with two blunt grasping forceps. Circumscribing the nodule with a seromuscular incision is important in limiting the extent of mucosal skinning. Otherwise, the muscularis can be separated from the mucosa so easily that the dissection can go too far past the nodule, leaving a larger defect than is necessary. The seromuscularis is repaired as for a partial-thickness bowel resection, described immediately above.

Full-Thickness Disc Resection for Endometriosis

Full-thickness bowel resections are those that have penetrated into the bowel lumen. It is common to encounter hypertrophy of an appendix epiploica adjacent to the nodule of endometriosis in the sigmoid colon. This is a normal response of the body to the irritative effects of the endometriosis, as the fatty tissue tries to cover the diseased area. These hypertrophied areas of fat must be cleared away sufficiently to expose normal bowel wall on all sides of the nodule, and this is most easily done before the nodule is removed. Proper exposure of normal

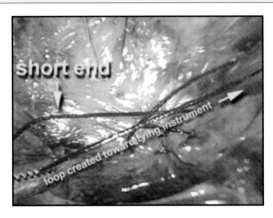

Fig. 15.17: The two rules of easy intracorporeal tying: 1. Create a loop of suture pointed toward the tying instrument (the needle driver); 2. Leave the short end of the suture nearby for easy pickup by the tying instrument

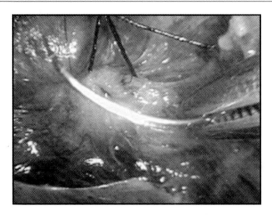

Fig. 15.18: The small, superficial burn of the rectum seen in Figure 15.1 is being repaired with a figure of 8 suture with 2-0 silk

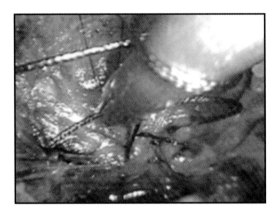

Fig. 15.19: The tying instrument (the needle driver) has inserted itself around and within the loop and is about to pick up the free end of the suture which was laid nearby

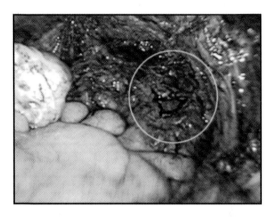

Fig. 15.20: A partial-thickness defect of the bowel wall resulting from difficult enterolysis is circled

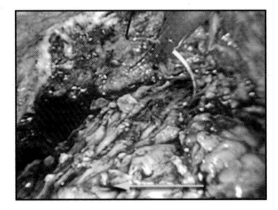

Fig. 15.21: Suture repair with 2-0 silk begins here on the right side of the defect. The needle will pass through normal outer muscularis, then pass through the muscularis to exit near the deepest part of the distal edge of the defect which is marked by the arrow

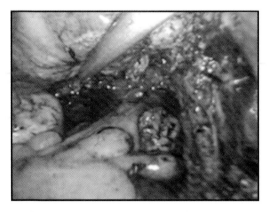

Fig. 15.22: The defect shown in Figure 15.20 has been completely repaired

bowel wall is important for suture repair of the bowel, otherwise the sutures may not be placed properly, increasing the chance for a postoperative bowel leak. These fatty appendages often have a robust blood supply and bleeding will commonly be encountered which can be controlled by electrocoagulation.

When a bowel nodule of endometriosis is spherical and larger than about 1 cm in diameter, submucosal fibrosis will often be present. During an attempt at mucosal skinning, this submucosal fibrosis may lead the dissection into the bowel lumen. This is not a surgical error but represents a surgical inevitability. If the nodule has been previously circumscribed, the dissection can proceed through the mucosa around the nodule, then cut back out through the muscularis until the initial circumscribing incision is encountered.

One of the interesting features of intestinal endometriosis is that a bowel nodule gathers together a certain length of muscularis along the anterior bowel wall. This means that when the nodule is removed, the defect that is left will be about three or four times longer than the diameter of the nodule. For example, a 1 cm nodule may leave a surgical defect 3 cm in greatest dimension. There will come a point where increasing size of a nodule will leave such a large defect that the surgeon will decide to perform a segmental resection rather than a disc resection. For me, that size is about 2 cm, which will leave a defect up to 8 cm in greatest longitudinal dimension. Another surgical finding that may prompt a decision to perform a segmental bowel resection is if there are several nodules close to each other along a length of bowel. Individual excision of each nodule will leave multiple coalescing defects which would be highly problematic to repair.

Full-thickness resections (Fig. 15.23) can be closed in one or two layers, although I prefer a double layer closure. A double layer closure begins with a running suture closure of the mucosa using an absorbable suture such as 3-0 vicryl. The free end of the suture adjacent to the first knot should be left fairly long so the lateral edge of the mucosal closure can be easily found. One intracorporeal knot can be eliminated by tying a stopper knot (Fig. 15.24) in the end of the suture before it is placed inside the abdomen. As at laparotomy, it is easier to sew toward oneself (Fig. 15.25). Stitches are placed about 5 mm apart. The final knot on the ending lateral side should be cut so

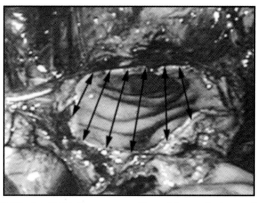

Fig. 15.23: A full-thickness resection of the anterior rectal wall was required for treatment of the rectal nodule seen in Figures 15.4 to 15.10. The arrows indicate the proper direction of sutures to close the bowel without reducing the diameter of the lumen

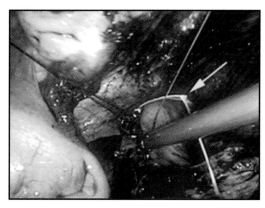

Fig. 15.24: The bowel has been suspended by traction sutures of 2-0 silk placed at each angle. The mucosal closure is begun at one angle. A stopper knot (arrow) near the suture end has been tied before the suture was inserted into the abdomen, eliminating the need for one intracorporeal knot

that the free end of the suture is long, again for identifying the lateral edge of the mucosal repair (Fig. 15.26).

The seromuscularis can now be closed with 2-0 silk or vicryl suture in an interrupted fashion. A purse string suture (Fig. 15.27) can be placed around each lateral edge of the mucosal suture line, allowing each end of the mucosal closure to be buried beneath the surface (Figs 15.28 and 15.29). After placing both lateral purse string sutures, the intervening seromuscularis can be closed with interrupted sutures like a partial-thickness bowel resection, working from each angle toward midline (Figs 15.30 and 15.31).

Integrity of the repair can be checked with underwater air pressure exam (Fig. 15.32) using a large irrigation syringe filled with air inserted into the rectum. Alternatively, the same large irrigation

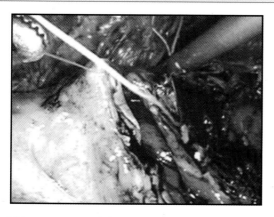

Fig. 15.25: The graspers at left are pulling on the mucosal suture to hold the tissue in position for easy suturing. The mucosal stitches can pass through muscularis without concern

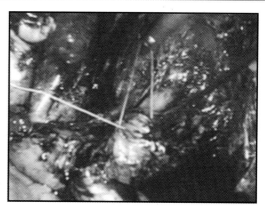

Fig. 15.26: The final mucosal stitch at the right angle. After the knot is tied, the suture will be cut long enough to cause the location of the angle to be obvious. The silk traction suture at the angle leads out of the abdomen alongside the accessory sheath and is optional for bowel repair. Some surgeons may find such traction sutures useful, others may not

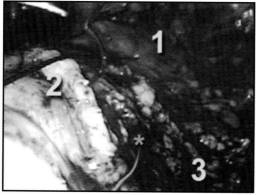

Fig. 15.27: The right edge of the mucosal closure is marked by the green asterisk and the end of the 3-0 vicryl suture which closed the mucosa can be seen. The seromuscular purse string suture of 2-0 silk is being placed around the mucosal angle to bury it. At least three separate bites of silk suture, indicated by the numbers, are needed to bury the mucosal angle

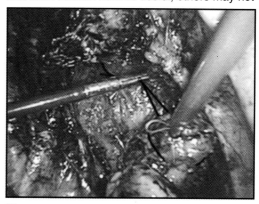

Fig. 15.28: The silk purse string suture has been placed and the free ends are held by the grasper on the left. The end of the vicryl mucosal suture is held by the needle driver and will be pushed down inside the purse string suture

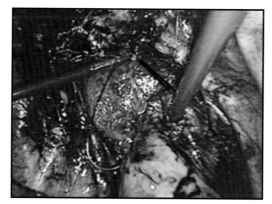

Fig. 15.29: As the grasper pulls on the ends of the purse string suture, the needle driver pushes the mucosal angle down, resulting in burial of the mucosal angle beneath the seromuscularis

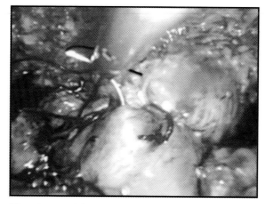

Fig. 15.30: After placement of a purse string suture on the opposite angle of the repair, the intervening seromuscularis is closed with interrupted 2-0 silk suture

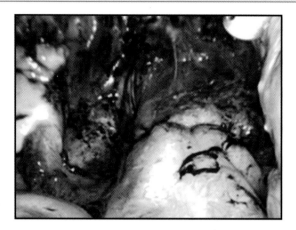

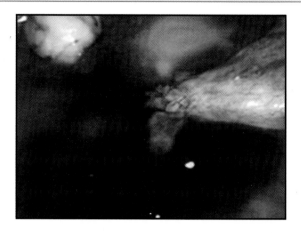

Fig. 15.31: The completed repair is shown, representing a dramatic improvement when compared to the original pathology

Fig. 15.32: An underwater air pressure examination proves that the bowel is air tight and that the closure is adequate

syringe may be used to administer an enema with an antiseptic solution. A leak will be signaled by escape of air bubbles or liquid solution. More stitches must be placed and the bowel wall integrity test repeated until the bowel wall no longer leaks.

CONCLUSION

The bowel is only one of many things that may require intracorporeal suturing during laparoscopy. If a surgeon makes an effort to become proficient in a simple protocol of suturing and knot-tying, suturing can also be used to control large bleeders, repair ureters, close myomectomy beds, and suspend ovaries for prophylaxis against adhesions.

REFERENCES

1. Redwine DB, Wright J. Laparoscopic treatment of obliteration of the cul-de-sac in endometriosis: Long term follow-up. Fertil Steril 2001;76:358-65.
2. Tsaltas J, Healy DL, Lloyd D. Complications of laparoscopy: a tautological audit. Gynaelogical Endoscopy 2001;10:17-1 9.
3. Harkki-Siren P, Sjoberg J, Kurki T. Major complications of laparoscopy: a follow-up Finnish study. Obstet Gynecol 1999;94:94-98.
4. Tu FF, Lamvu GM, Hartmann KE, Steege JF. Preoperative ultrasound to predict infraumbilical adhesions: a study of diagnostic accuracy. Am J Obstet Gynecol 2005;192:74 - 79.
5. Redwine DB. Complications of sharp and blunt adhesiolysis. In Corfman R, Diamond M, DeCherney A (Eds): Complications of Endoscopy. Boston: Blackwell (2nd edn), 1997;78-81.
6. Redwine DB, Wright J. Laparoscopic treatment of obliteration of the cul-de-sac in endometriosis: long-term follow-up. Fertil Steril 2001;76:358-65.
7. Redwine DB. Laparoscopic en bloc resection for treatment of the obliterated cul-de-sac in endometriosis. J Reprod Med 1992;37:695-98.
8. Redwine DB. Ovarian endometriosis: a marker for more severe pelvic and intestinal disease. Fertil Steril 1999;73:310-5.
9. Redwine DB. Intestinal endometriosis. In Redwine DB (Ed): Surgical Treatment of Endometriosis. London: Dunitz, 2003;157-73.

Ureteric and Bladder Injury and Repair

FARR NEZHAT, BAHAREH FAZILAT
CEANA NEZHAT, CAMRAN NEZHAT

Chapter Sixteen

URETERAL INJURY AND REPAIR

Introduction

Ureteral injuries occur at the rate of 1 to 2 percent during pelvic surgeries, with the majority in the field of gynecologic procedures, where the reported iatrogenic injuries range from 0.05 to 30 percent. Simple hysterectomy has the highest incidence of ureteral injury, accounting for an incidence rate up to 2.5 percent. The ureteral injury occurs about ten times more often during abdominal procedures than during vaginal surgery. In advanced laparoscopic procedures involving the pelvic sidewall such as oophorectomy, laparoscopic-assisted vaginal hysterectomy, endometriosis resection or ablation and lymph node dissection ureteral injuries occur more frequently. The ureter can be injured in its abdominal segment during certain procedures such as para-aortic lymphadenectomy or colon surgery.

Application: How and When They Occur

Common sites of injury of the ureter are:
1. At or below the infundibulopelvic ligament.
2. Along the course of the broad ligament.
3. At and below the cardinal ligament when the ureter passes beneath the uterine vessels.
4. Beyond the uterine artery where the ureter lies adjacent to the anterior vaginal wall and enters the base of the bladder.

Most common site of the injury is the lowest 3 cm. The varieties of injuries include: crushes, ligation, transection, angulation, and devascularization. Laparoscopic injuries could be thermal damage mostly caused by electrosurgery and occasionally by laser; sharp injury or it could also be due to stapling devices. Endoscopic stapling devices have been implicated in a large number of ureteral injuries during oophorectomy or hysterectomy.

Ureteral injuries are categorized into the following types:
1. Devascularization due to extensive dissection or thermal injury.
2. Partial ureteral transaction; such as a small laceration occurring during pelvic side wall dissection or resection of fibrotic endometriosis tissue or metastatic lesion.
3. Complete transaction.
4. Obstruction caused by suture or a stapler.

Intraoperative Diagnosis

Thirty percent of injuries are recognized at the time of surgery. The majority of the cases require additional procedures after the original surgery due to late recognition. If an injury is suspected, cystoscopy with intravenous indigo carmine injection should be performed. Give 5 to 10 ml intravenous indigo carmine and 200 ml sterile saline if bladder is empty and then observe for the flow of indigo carmine from ureteral orifices within 3 to 5 minutes. If non-spillage occurs, a stent or ureteral catheter can be placed by cystotomy/cystoscopy.

Remember the presence of peristalsis does not mean that the ureter has not been injured or damaged.

Management

Management of Thermal Injury/devascularization

When a significant periurethral devascularization has occurred especially when patient has a prior history of radiation, ureteral stents for few weeks postoperatively can decrease the chance of ureteral fistula formation or stenosis due to scarring and fibrosis formation.

It takes less than 2 weeks for re-epithelialization to occur. The placement of ureteral stent serves two purposes. It drains the urine and maintains the caliber of the ureter. If there is the possibility of an intra-abdominal leakage then a Jackson Pratt drain can be placed adjacent to the injury and brought out from the lower quadrant incision for a few days.

Management of Partial Resection

A small ureterostomy can be repaired as long as no significant devascularization has occurred. Transcystoscopic ureteral stent is placed first and ureteral defect is repaired using delayed absorbable 4.0 suture. An intraperitoneal drain should be placed as mentioned above.

Management of Complete Resection

Repair of the ureter depends upon the type and the level of the injury. The selection of the type of repair depends upon the distance from the ureteral defect to the bladder, and the condition of the vasculature to the ureter at the site of planned repair. Either a ureteroureterostomy or ureteroneocystomy can be performed. The principles of different techniques will be discussed briefly in the following section.

URETEROURETERAL ANASTOMOSIS. This is an appropriate procedure for the injuries of the ureter near the pelvic brim; for an intentional or an unintentional transaction of the ureter due to obstruction caused by fibrosis, endometriosis or malignancy (Figs 16.1A and B). The ureter is mobilized on both sides of the defect (Figs 16.2 and 16.3). This should be accomplished by being able to bring the two segments together without tension. The ends of the ureter are trimmed until good vasculature has been identified and spatulated (Fig. 16.4). One layer repair is performed using delayed absorbable 4.0 sutures

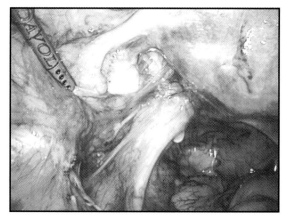

Fig. 16.1A: Left distal ureter obstruction due to infiltrative endometriosis

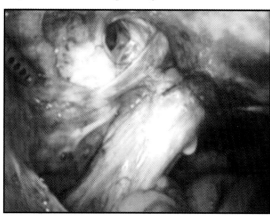

Fig. 16.1B: Magnified view of left distal ureter obstruction due to infiltrative endometriosis

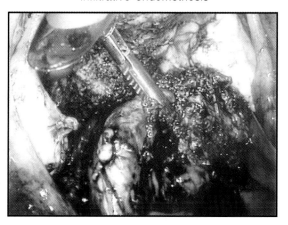

Fig. 16.2: Severe infiltrative endometriosis of the distal left ureter being mobilized and excised

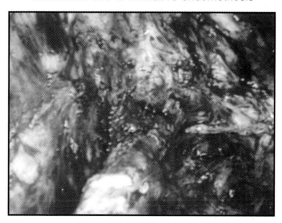

Fig. 16.3: Left distal ureter obstruction

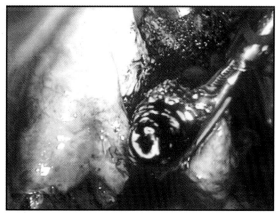

Fig. 16.4: Left distal ureter is being transected and a fish mouth incision is made in the ureter in the preparation for reimplantation to the bladder

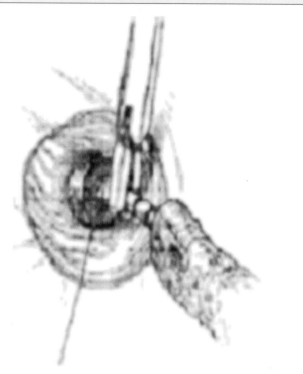

Fig. 16.5: Catheter being advanced through new ureteral opening. Under cystoscopic guidance, a 7 French ureteral catheter is passed through the ureterovesicle junction

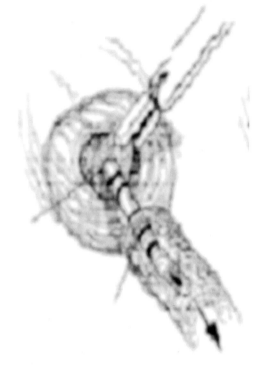

Fig. 16.6: New ureteral opening and patent ureter is identified. The catheter is advanced through the proximal part of the ureter to the renal pelvis

placing at 6, 12, 9 and 3 o'clock. Intracorporeal suturing and intacorporeal or extracorporeal knot tying is utilized. The anastomosis is done over a double-J stent (placed cystoscopically) which is kept in place for 4 to 6 weeks postoperatively (Figs 16.5 to 16.7).

URETERONEOCYSTOTOMY. This is a preferred procedure for most injuries within 4 to 5 cm of ureterovesical junction and maybe used for some injuries at the level of the pelvic brim. The proximal portion of the ureter is mobilized using sharp, electrosurgical scissors, laser or harmonic scalpel. Sharp scissors are used for removing any fibrotic, metastatic tumor, endometriotic nodules or devascularized tissue. If the ureter can be reached to the posterior aspect of the bladder, a 1 cm transverse incision is made in the posterior wall of the bladder and the incision is extended to the mucosa. The free end of the ureter is brought to the posterior incision and under cystoscopic guidance; a ureteral stent is passed through the ureterovesical junction (Fig. 16.8). Four interrupted 4.0 polydioxanone sutures are placed at 6, 12, 9, and 3 o'clock to approximate the ureter to the bladder using intracorporeal suturing and knot tying (Figs 16.9 and 10).

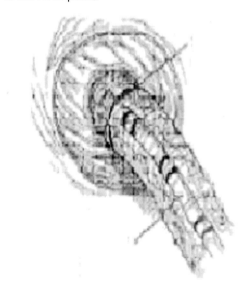

Fig. 16.7: Sutures in the ureter noted. Catheter is advanced to the left renal pelvis. The edges of the ureter are approximated

Psoas Hitch procedure. If the injury is more than 5 cm above the ureterovesicle junction or the ureter cannot be reached to the bladder without tension, the psoas hitch technique is used. The bladder peritoneum is incised from the involved lateral pelvic wall and the bladder is mobilized and anchored to

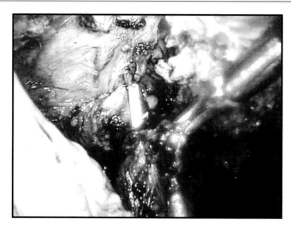

Fig. 16.8: First suture is applied at 6 o'clock and a transvesicle ureteral stent is passed through the ureter prior to the application of remaining reanastomosis sutures

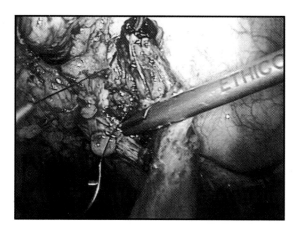

Fig. 16.9: Performing ureteroneocystotomy using a 4.0 polyglycolic and applying the suture at 9 o'clock

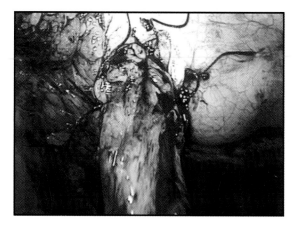

Fig. 16.10: Left ureteroneocystotomy after reimplantation of the ureter to the back of the bladder. Four sutures are applied at 6, 9, 12 and 3 o'clock using 4.0 polyglycolic sutures

the psoas muscle using 0 polydioxanone suture. Ureteroneocystotomy will be performed as described above.

Bori Flap procedure. This procedure is useful if a large segment of the ureter has to be removed. Additional length is obtained by constructing a flap from the tissue of the bladder dome. In combination with the psoas hitch procedure, this technique provides adequate length between the ureter and the bladder. After distending the bladder with saline solution, a U-shaped flap of bladder is marked out. The flap must be long enough to overlap the ureter without tension. A double-J-stent is placed cystoscopically in the proximal ureter. Then an oblique tunnel is made between the mucosa and the muscle of the Bori flap. The ureter is drawn through, spatulated, and sutured to the mucosa with 4.0 delayed absorbable suture. The bladder is closed with 0 polydioxanone suture.

Instruments and Suture Material Required

Standard laparoscopic instruments such as high resolution video camera, laparoscope, automatic fast insufflators, fine grasping forceps and laparoscopic needle holders are all required for the repair of any injuries to the bladder, ureter or the bowel. Number 6 or 7 double J ureteral stent and Jackson Pratt drain is also required during this procedure.

The 4.0 delayed absorbable polydioxanone sutures are preferred. Careful approximation not strangulating the tissue without tension should be accomplished.

Technique

Use noncrushing instruments, avoid unnecessary dissection, and avoid tension on the suture line. Place ureteral stents and leave them in place for a few weeks postoperatively. Consider placing a Jackson Pratt drain intraperitoneally at the time of the repair. This is done for prevention of the accumulation of urine which could interfere with the healing of the repair or anastomosis. The drain should not provide strong suction at the anastomosis site; encouraging a fistula formation by continuous flow of urine from the anastomosis site to the drain.

General principles for the repair of the injured ureter involve the following: The anastomosis has to be tension free, the anastomosed tissues must be well vascularized, the created anastomosis needs to be water tight, the connection must be widely patent to prevent stricture after post-surgical swelling and the ureter must not be kinked or twisted. In addition to the use of appropriate stents and drains, it is important that the ureteral adventitia and its blood supply are left intact to preserve the integrity of the ureter. Wrapping the anastomosis with an omental pedicle may reduce the risk for anastomotic leakage.

Pit Falls

Several steps can be taken to prevent ureteral injuries. The most important aspect is familiarity with the anatomy, the pathophysiology and contributing factors such as extensive endometriosis, adhesions, neoplasm and inflammation which could increase the risk of injury. Preoperative intravenous pyelogram, ultrasound, CT scan or MRI can be helpful in the detection of ureteral abnormalities such as obstruction or congenital anomalies. The placement of ureteral catheters preoperatively can be useful in patients with extensive retroperitoneal fibrosis due to severe pelvic endometriosis or malignancy or adhesions.

Prophylactic placement of the ureteral catheters may not assure the prevention of transmural ureteral injury, although they can assist in their immediate recognition. The reported incidence of ureteral injury as a direct result of catheter insertion accounts for 1.1 percent. Adequate exposure and visualization intraoperatively is an essential part of performing any surgery. Avoiding excessive dissection of the ureter and its blood supply is also essential. Intraperitoneal identification of the ureter or pelvic wall dissection and identification of the ureter retroperitoneally should always be done prior to securing the infundibulopelvic ligament, uterine vessels or resection of retroperitoneal mass or fibrosis.

If due to intraperitoneal adhesions, endometriosis or obesity, identification of the ureter is difficult, retroperitoneal dissection can be utilized for the identification of the ureter. The hydrodissection, which is done by injecting several ml of lactated Ringer or normal saline retroperitoneally, can be very helpful. The peritoneum is elevated and an incision is made over the peritoneum therefore the ureter can be identified. However, excessive dissection of the ureter can be associated with bleeding and control of this bleeding itself could cause damage to the

ureter. Should the blood vessels around the ureter be traumatized, thrombosed or ligated in dissecting the ureter from its tunnel, a segment of the ureter may become avascular resulting in fistula or stenosis with obstruction.

Studies have suggested that glomerular filtration is best preserved by rapid reversal of obstruction of the ureter, and function is best restored by immediate repair if possible.

Contraindications to immediate repair of ureteral injuries are: Extensive devascularization or injury, retroperitoneal cellulitis. It is important to note that limited blood supply leads to an increased risk of healing, stenosis and obstruction.

In any given clinical situation requiring ureteral reanastomosis or reimplantation, compliance with the following principles will improve successful outcome:
1. Gentle handling of the tissue.
2. Preventing tension on the anastomosis.
3. Meticulous hemostasis.
4. Proper drainage.
5. Use of sutures placed along the ureteric length.
6. Preservation of vascular supply by avoiding unnecessary dissection.
7. Careful mucosa to mucosa approximation avoiding urine leakage and tension will allow the ureteral defect to be bridged by new growth of transitional epithelium and the growth of new smooth muscle across the gap in a few weeks.

Most urologists and gynecologists prefer to insert a ureteral catheter for a few weeks post ureteral repair. The double end J-catheter is the most popular, although this catheter usually requires insertion over a guide by cystoscopy. The soft silastic #8 tube can be inserted through the ureteral defect.

Postoperative Management of Ureteral Injury

It maybe necessary to drain the anastomotic site retroperitoneally with a JP drain for a few days. This drain can be removed on the second or third postoperative day.

Patient has to be followed carefully for a possible peritonitis. Postoperatively the patient should be given prophylactic antibiotics for as long as the ureteral stents are in place. The foley catheter is discontinued on the second or third day; however if a ureteroneocystotomy is performed we recommend to catheterize the bladder for 5 to 7 days and obtain a cystogram prior to the discontinuation.

The internal ureteral stent is removed 4 to 6 weeks later after a laparoscopic ureterouretostomy or ureoneocystotomy operation. The time of removal of the stents are based on the degree of the injury. Reassessment of the integrity of the ureter maybe evaluated 7 to 14 days after the removal of the stents. The same radiography should be repeated at intervals after the catheter has been removed to assure continued function without the presence of hydroureter or hydronephrosis.

BLADDER INJURY AND REPAIR

Introduction

There are a wide range of bladder injuries during laparoscopic procedures. The incidence of bladder injury during laparoscopic procedures ranges from 0.02 to 8.3 percent of cases. An intraoperative diagnosis of bladder injury is made in about half of all bladder injury cases. The bladder dome is the most common site of injury. Less than half of the bladder injuries are corrected laparoscopically. Under magnification provided by video laparoscope, a skilled laparoscopist should be able to repair even a large intentional or unintentional cystotomy laparoscopically.

How and When They Occur

There are many predisposing factors that increase the chance of bladder injury during laparoscopic procedures. Any bladder pathology or any contiguous pelvic process (such as inflammation, endometriosis, malignant infiltration, previous surgery, adhesions, previous radiation, and bladder wall diverticula) may put the patient at increased risk for bladder injuries (Fig. 16.11). An overly distended bladder, as well as thin (less than 3 mm) bladder wall, may also predispose the bladder to injury during surgery. Erosions created by vaginal pessary, which may cause thinning of the bladder wall, as well as erosions around permanent sutures also pose as risk factors.

Most frequently bladder injuries occur during either total or laparoscopic-assisted vaginal hysterectomy. Sharp electrosurgical and blunt dissections are the leading cause of bladder injury. Bladder drainage prior to laparoscopy and gentle dissection of bladder are helpful measure, but do not prevent thermal injury from electrosurgery or during trocar place-ment. It is extremely critical to recognize the injury intraoperatively and not delay the immediate repair.

Intraoperative Diagnosis

Both abdominal distention due to CO_2 pneumoperitoneum and magnification by video laparoscope can assist in easily diagnosis of most intraoperative bladder injuries.

The surgeon should suspect bladder injury during laparoscopic surgery whenever air is noted in the Foley drainage bag, with hematuria, or when urine is seen within the operative field. When there is a doubt, distention of the bladder with normal saline and performing cyctoscopy is the best method to diagnose the bladder injury.

Management

In many cases, bladder perforation from a laparoscopic needle or a 5 mm trocar will heal spontaneously with the aid of an indwelling catheter for 1 to 2 weeks. However larger defects should be repaired. Applying the already established techniques of bladder injury repair by laparotomy to laparoscopic procedures is acceptable in most endoscopic settings.

Instruments and Suture Material Required

Instrumentations used for the bladder repair is similar to the instrumentations as described for the ureter repair.

2.0 or 0 absorbable polydioxanone or catgut (chromic) sutures are preferred.

Technique

Although two-layer repair and occasionally application of one or two endoloop for small injuries have been reported, our preferred method is one layer interrupted or continuous closure using 0 polydioxanone suture (Fig. 16.12). Identification of the ureteral orifices and insertion of ureteral stents are recommended when the injuries are close to the ureteral orifices. Cystoscopy and bladder distention is recommended for evaluation of the repair (Figs 16.13 and 16.14).

Pit Falls

Fistula formation is a sequel of bladder injury if it is not repaired appropriately or if the Foley catheter is

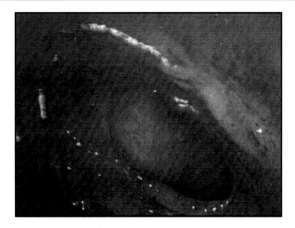

Fig. 16.11: Intentional cystotomy at the time of the removal of an infiltrating endometriosis of the bladder wall

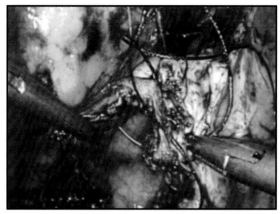

Fig. 16.12: An interrupted one layer repair using No.0 Polyglycolic suture to close the cystotomy

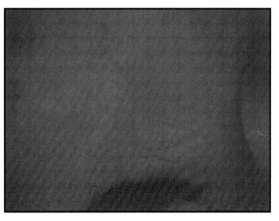

Fig. 16.13: Identification of the left ureteral orifice after injection of indigo carmine intravenously. The blue dye can be seen in the bladder

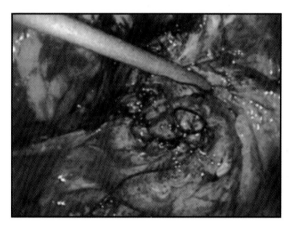

Fig. 16.14: Bladder has been distended with normal saline and it is water tight

removed prior to the completion of the bladder healing process. Adequate drainage and evaluation of the cystotomy repair by cystogram prior to the discontinuation of the Foley catheter is essential.

Postoperative Management of Bladder Injury

Oliguria is one of the postoperative symptoms of undetected bladder injury. Therefore adequate hydration and fluid intake-output monitoring during and after the surgery is essential to detect any potential problems.

- Transurethral or suprapubic bladder drainage is used for 7 to 14 days. Prior to the discontinuation a cystogram may be considered.
- Patients should receive antibiotics as prophylaxis.

BIBLIOGRAPHY

1. Nezhat C, Nezhat F. Laparoscopic repair of ureter resected during operative laparoscopy. Obstet Gynecol 1992; 80:543.
2. Nezhat C, Nezhat F. Laparoscopic segmental bladder resection for endometriosis: a report of two cases. Obstet Gynecol 1993; 81:882-4.
3. Nezhat C, Nezhat F, Nezhat CH, et al. Urinary tract endometriosis treated by laparoscopy. Fertil Steril 1996;66:920.
4. Carmel Jonathan Cohen, Farr Nezhat. Techniques of ureteral implantation. Nogyogyaszati Onkologia 1998;2:165-70.
5. Nezhat CH, Shazia Malik, Nezhat F, Nezhat C. Laparoscopic ureteroneocystotomy and vesicopsoas hitch for infiltrative endometriosis. JSLS 2004;8:3-7.
6. Rodney J Poffenberger. Laparoscopic repair of intraperitoneal bladder injury: a simple new technique. Urology 1996; 47:248-9.

Endoscopic Suturing in Gastrointestinal and General Surgery

PRADEEP CHOWBEY

Chapter Seventeen

INTRODUCTION

The practice patterns of general surgery have changed significantly with the advent of laparoscopic surgery. These changes have occurred over a short period of time and continue rapidly with the increasing use of advanced laparoscopic surgery. Accurate tissue approximation is essential for operative surgical repair of defects and execution of safe anastomosis. Apart from gentle handling of tissues and careful dissection, the approximation must be achieved without compromise of the integrity of blood supply essential to the healing process. Endoscopic approximation of tissues, by interrupted or continuous suturing, is an acquired craft based on established surgical principles. It involves the appropriate selection of suture materials and the deployment of correct technique with optimal spacing of atraumatic sutures which approximate the tissue edges without undue tension.

Compared to open surgery, the situation is different in endoscopic surgery. Manipulations are conducted viewing an indirect and magnified image of the operative field. Due to significant cerebral, perceptual and translational processing necessary, endoscopic tissue approximation, can never be conducted with the same ease and fluency as open surgery. The structured stepwise choreography of intracorporeal suturing lies at the heart of efficient and safe endoscopic tissue approximation. Special considerations apply to suturing techniques in the endoscopic surgery. These are restrictions of ergonomic maneuverability and visual perspective display problems. Neither of them is encountered in conventional open surgery.

PRINCIPLES OF ENDOSUTURING

The *position of the surgeon* in relation to instruments and intended suture line determines the challenge and the result. The visual path, coaxial alignment and triangulation of camera and operating ports are crucial aspects of the set up. The camera is positioned midway between two instrument ports; this set up mimics the normal relationship between the eyes and two hands. The port positioning, relative to the proposed suture line, provides the proper angle of access and a fulcrum for the instrument. Optical viewing angle is related to optical axis of telescope. Probably the best exposure for endosuturing is 30° forward oblique telescope.

To improve *visual perception* a three-chip camera and high-resolution 19 inch monitor, viewed from a distance of 5 feet, are utilized. The visualization in endoscopic surgery is affected by the type of laparoscope (the optical instrument) used, the flat two-dimensional image on the video monitor and the ability of the surgeon to adjust to the new viewing perspective.

Hand-eye Coordination

The surgeon must readjust eye-hand coordination and adapt to the speed of instrument movement. Visual memory and a trained eye are ideal cognitive instruments. The movement of instruments are magnified on screen. This shows how quickly instruments are perceived to move even when the surgeon is operating at his normal pace. The movements in endosurgery should be slower than in open surgery. Eliminating unnecessary movements and tightly choreographing the procedure help to make the most efficient use of time. It also increases precision. A proper formal training on a simulator and supervised practice help in overall success.

Motor Skill

The balance and coordination of perception, and sensory-motor coordination orchestrate the ideal procedure. Magnification and the use of long instrumentation create an imbalance. This is compensated by a special approach that is commonly referred to as principles of microsurgery. Familiarity with open microsurgery eases transition to endosuturing, as one is used to operate under a microscope, which is also a virtual image.

Ambidexterity

Ambidexterity is a very desirable attribute for laparoscopic surgery especially for endosuturing. The surgeon should make a conscious effort to enhance his level of coordinated ambidexterity, so that both hands supplement each other's activity.

EQUIPMENT

Needle Holders/Drivers

There are various types of needle drivers. They require either to be self-loading or to incorporate a click on and off mechanism to engage the needle. These should have ergonomic handles which are set in line with the long axis of the instrument and not at an angle to it.

Coaxial Handles

Instrument rotation is seriously limited with the traditional angled handles. A coaxial item to handle relationship allows for greater maneuverability and rotation necessary for laparoscopic suturing. Coaxial handles provide 360° rotation of the instrument.

Grips

It allows delicate, minute movements to be transmitted using a combination of the fingers, wrist and forearm for guidance. It facilitates rotation of instrument and allows the precision and control necessary for sophisticated maneuver and complex suturing.

Tips

The tips of needle driver and assisting grasper must be of multifunction design due to the limited accessibility and maneuverability within the laparoscopic field. The needle driver must be able to handle the tissues gently, firmly grasp and drive the needle, and handle the tissue and thread atraumatically. Another important feature, which facilitates internal knotting, in areas of difficult access, is for the end of one of the needle drivers to be coaxilly curved, which facilitates grasping the short tail and forming a loop over the assisting grasper.

A surgeon should choose one pair of needle holders/drivers and become thoroughly familiar with its use and avoid changing from one type to another. Needle holders must always be deployed in pairs. Atraumatic sutures must be introduced and withdrawn through access ports which incorporate sealing valves, i.e. sleeve reducers as otherwise the suture and needle tip might get engaged and damage the flap valve. The access port for the suture holder must be well ahead of the operative field and opposite to the converging axes of the two needle drivers. The needle driver in the non-dominant hand is called the assisting grasper. Every surgeon has a preference for these instruments. Special modulated needle holders/drivers are also available which ease out endosuturing.

Scissors

In endoscopic surgery, scissors are used for dissection, sharp division of tissues and for cutting the suture material during knotting. It is important that dissecting and cutting scissors are used exclusively for this purpose to preserve sharpness of the cutting blades. For endoscopic suturing, the instrument set should include 'suture scissors' reserved specifically for this purpose. Preferably the suture scissors should be of the hook variety.

Clips and Staples

Titanium clips are used for securing small blood vessels during endoscopic surgery. Provided the principles of application are observed and the clip is of right size, these appear to be relatively safe, but double clipping is recommended to ensure secure hemostasis. Clips are unsafe if the vessel is surrounded by fatty tissue or if the vessel is > 4 mm wide. In these cases, vascular cartridge stapler or intracorporeal suturing is preferred.

SUTURE AND LIGATURE MATERIAL

Surgical needles are penetrating devices, which are designed to pass sutures through tissues with minimal trauma. The function of needle are three-fold:

  i. to provide secure grip for the needle driver
 ii. to penetrate the object to be sewn and create a channel for the thread to enter
iii. to provide a mean by which thread can be trailed.

The especially designed endoski needle, which can be introduced through a 5 mm port greatly facilitates endoscopic suturing but entails a minor modification of the suturing technique. When the tip of the needle is driven through the entry point, it is not possible to determine the direction of the tip of the needle should any deflection take place since the straight shaft gives no clue as to the needle tip direction. The needles are introduced with the help of sleeve reducers. The needle should be held in the holder at 2/3-1/3 junction.

Many components related to suturing that have been developed for open and microsurgical operations can be applied with modifications to endosurgery.

Needle cross-sections can be round, oval, flattered hexagonal, rhomboid, triangular and the diamond shaped. The cross-section of the body influences the security of hold of the needle by the needle driver.

Needle Visibility

It has special significance in endosuturing. The needle should be hydrophobic and have light fluorescent surface color, contrasting sharply with the deeper hues of the surrounding tissues.

Prevention of Needle Loss

The critical points where chances of loosing the needle are high are, during introduction and retrieval through access port. An adequate length of thread should always be left attached to the needle, which should be trailed rather than picked during any translocation. The tip grasps the thread close to the needle, or otherwise, needle can easily catch tissues as it is not noticed and surgeon continues to pull.

Secure Grasping

Ensure the right match between the needle body configuration and the interface of the jaws of the needle driver. Application of ergonomic gentle suturing techniques, minimizes the force necessary to counter needle deflection during needle passage.

Needle Loading

The needle should be placed on adjacent smooth surfaces such as stomach and liver surface. The correct pick up is achieved by advancing the open jaws of the active needle driver across the shaft of this needle. It is important that the needle is picked up by the tip of the grasper's jaws.

There is a large element of personal preference with regards to suture materials used by individual surgeons. On the basis of safety and ease of use in endoscopic surgery the following suture ligatures are recommended. Commonly used suture ligatures in surgery are:

Absorbable

- Dry chromic catgut used in endoloops, e.g. for appendicectomy, sac ligation in TEP for hernia repairs.
- Vicryl for endoscopic suturing/ligation of cystic duct, for primary closure of CBD after exploration, enterotomy closure, bladder repair, etc. which may be interrupted or continuous, etc.

Nonabsorbable

Silk, ePTFE, Ethibond for interrupted suturing involved in fundoplication, rectopexy, securing large vascular pedicle for splenectomy, mesenteric pedicles during small bowel or colonic surgery, etc. Nonabsorbable sutures may act as nidus for infection and stone formation. So, these sutures should never be used for cystic dust ligation, closure of CBD, urinary bladder.

TECHNIQUES OF KNOT-TYING

Basic Stages

There are three steps of knotting which are taking the knot, drawing the knot and locking the knot. These are also known as configuration, shaping and securing. One should remember Clifford Ashley's classical saying, *A knot is never nearly right, it is either exactly right or hopelessly wrong.* The underlying rule for all knots is the over and underwriting sequence, which must never be violated. The length of ligature material used for knot tying can be considered as consisting of three sections, the end or the short tail, the bight, which refers to the short part of the knot and the standing part, the long tail. The C-loop is referred to as the bight.

Both intracorporeal and extracorporeal knot-tying techniques have an important role in laparoscopic surgery.

Intracorporeal

Intracorporeal knots replace a process that virtually duplicates the methods used during open surgical procedure. Intracorporeal tying is faster and uses less suture material.

Extracorporeal

Extracorporeal tying uses a special knot that is designed to slip one way but not the other with the help of a knot pusher with the surgeons knot being tied externally, e.g. Roeder's Knot.

Steps

Intracorporeal Suturing

Create a C-loop as the right instrument reaches over the left side of the field, grabs the long tail and brings it back to the right below the short tail. This loop must be in a horizontal plane, or else it will be difficult to wrap the thread. The right instrument can rotate the thread counterclockwise until it lies flat against the tissue. The right instrument holds the long tail and the left instrument is placed over the loop. One can tie a square knot as well as a surgeon's knot intracorporeally (Figs 17.1 to 17.26).

The right instrument holds the long tail and the left instrument is placed over the loop. The short tail should be long enough so that it cannot be pulled out accidentally, but not so long that its end is hidden. Use a large loop to allow ample space for both the instruments, moving slowly, when returning the short tail. Use the right instrument to wrap the long tail around the stationary tip of the left instrument forward to create an arch in the suture, assisting the wrapping motion. Rotate the right instrument. Keep the jaws of the instruments retrieving the short tail closed until ready to grasp the tail. Care should be taken not to handle the thread frequently and cause trauma to the thread.

By and large the situations which necessitate intracorporeal tissue approximation.

- Bypass procedures without excision, e.g. bilio-enteric bypass or entero-enteric bypass
- Repair of injuries to solid organs, e.g. liver and spleen
- Excisional procedures where the ends cannot be exteriorized, e.g. reconstruction after partial gastrectomy, esophageal transaction, esophago-gastrostomy
- Repair of defects, e.g. anti-reflux surgery and hiatal repair, repair of inguinal hernia rectopexy, bladder suspension, etc.

The good habits, which facilitate efficient intra-corporeal knotting, are:

- Always operate under good magnification

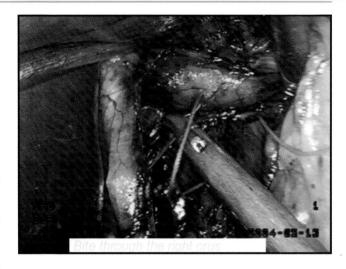

Fig. 17.1: Bite through the right crus

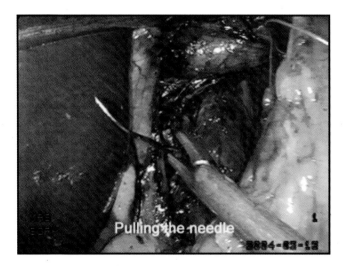

Fig. 17.2: Pulling the needle

- Precise and economic movements
- Ergonomic port placement
- Avoid instrument crossing
- Achieve expertise in knot tying choreography
- Knots should be executed close to the tissue surface
- Jaws of instruments should remain closed except during grasping
- Awareness of dominant versus assisting instruments during the knotting process.
- Wrapping technique should be good
- Knot should be configured and tied close to the tail

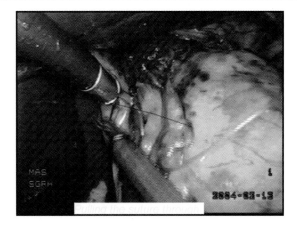

Fig. 17.3: Pulling the suture through the tissue

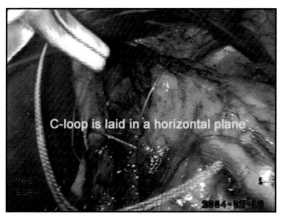

Fig. 17.4: C-loop is laid in a horizontal plane

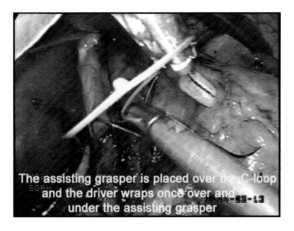

Fig. 17.5: The assisting grasper is placed over the C-loop and the driver wraps once over and under the assisting grasper

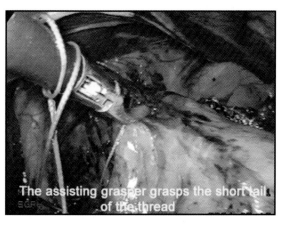

Fig. 17.6: The assisting grasper graps the short tail of the thread

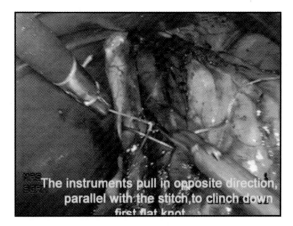

Fig. 17.7: The instruments pull in opposite direction, parallel with the stitch, to clinch down the first flat knot

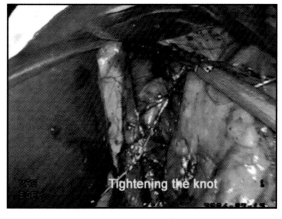

Fig. 17.8: Tightening the knot

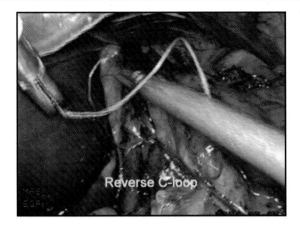

Fig. 17.9: Reverse C-loop

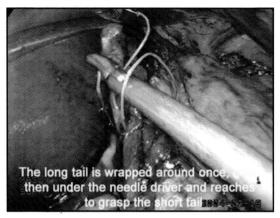

Fig. 17.10: The long tail is wrapped around once, over then under the needle driver and reaches to grasp the short tail

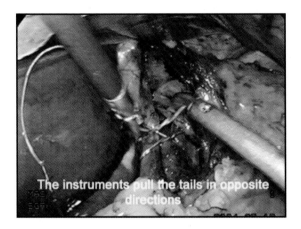

Fig. 17.11: The instruments pull the tail in opposite directions

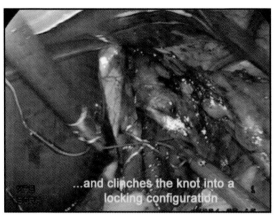

Fig. 17.12: Then clinches the knot into a locking configuration

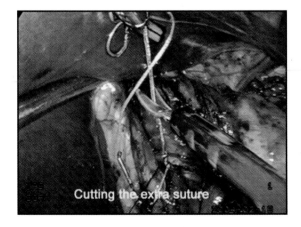

Fig. 17.13: Cutting the extra suture

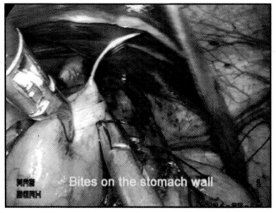

Fig. 17.14: Bites on the stomach wall

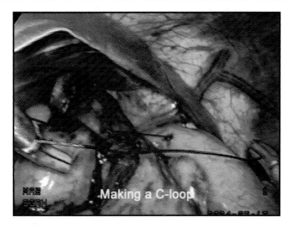

Fig. 17.15: Making a C-loop

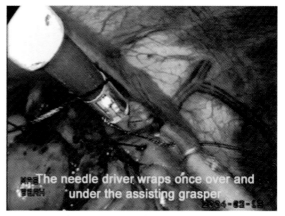

Fig. 17.16: The needle driver wraps once over and under the assisting grasper

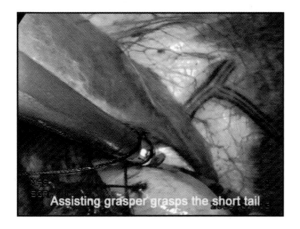

Fig. 17.17: Assisting grasper grasps the short tail

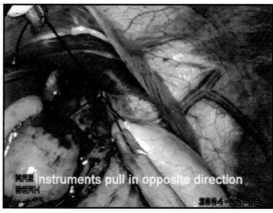

Fig. 17.18: Instruments pull in opposite direction

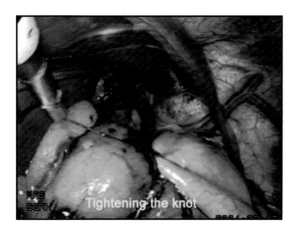

Fig. 17.19: Tightening the knot

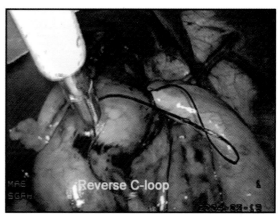

Fig. 17.20: Reverse C-loop

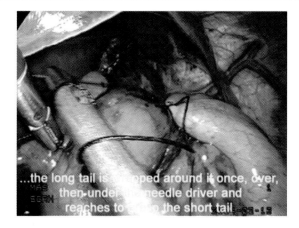

Fig. 17.21: The long tail is wrapped around it once, over, then under the needle driver and reaches to grasps the short tail

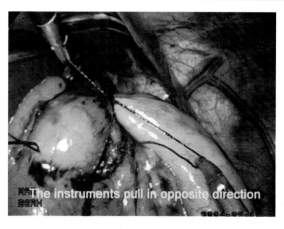

Fig. 17.22: The instruments pull in opposite direction

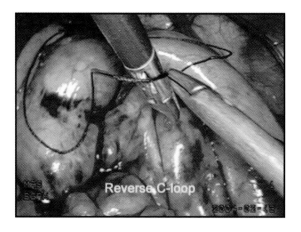

Fig. 17.23: Reverse C-loop

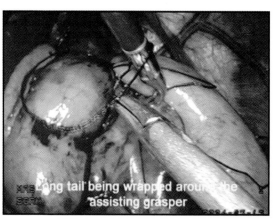

Fig. 17.24: Long tail being wrapped around the assisting grasper

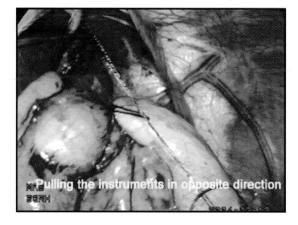

Fig. 17.25: Pulling the instruments in opposite direction

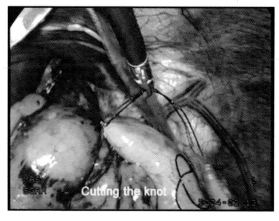

Fig. 17.26: Cutting the knot

Extracorporeal Knot

An extracorporeal knot is tied externally and slid down to the tissue with the aid of knot pusher. This method requires long threads and while extra-corporeal knotting appears to be a simpler approach, it requires a systematic and careful application to avoid trauma to the tissues and contaminating or damaging the suture. The Roeder's knot is widely used in endosuturing. It was developed around the term of the century and introduced to laparoscopic practice before intracorporeal suturing and knotting was developed. This is the knot used in commercially available pre-tied suture ligatures. There are other types of extracorporeal knoting techniques. Modified Tayside's is an example of such a technique knot.

THE APPLICATION OF ENDOSUTURING IN GENERAL AND GI SURGERY

Common usage of continuous suturing in laparos-copic surgery.

- Oversewing of seromyotomies
- Gastrojejunostomy
- Closure of stapler access enterotomies
- Cholecystojejunostomy
- Choledochojejunostomy
- Entero-enteric anastomosis
- Ilieo-transverse anastomosis
- Resection of Meckel's diverticulum
- Repair of small bowel injuries
- Closure of peritoneal defects during TEP for groin hernia.

Common usage of interrupted suturing in laparoscopic surgery:

- Pyloroplasty
- Stricturoplasty
- Cystojejunostomy
- Closure of choledochostomy
- Choledochojejunostomy
- Closure of mesenteric and other defects
- Repair of hiatal canal in anti-reflex surgery
- Rectopexy.

BIBLIOGRAPHY

1. Bowyer DW, Moran ME, Szabo Z. Laparoscopic surgery in urology: A model for vesicouretheral anastamosis following radical prostatectomy. Min Invas Ther 1993;4(2);165-70.
2. Crosthwaite G, Chung T, Dunkley P, Shimi S. Influence of imaging on surgical task efficiency in endoscopic surgery: comparison of direct vision and electronic display with 2-D and 3D system. Br J Surgery.
3. Cuscheiri A, Nathanson LK. Instruments and basic techniques. In Cuschieri A, Berci G (Ed): Laparoscopic biliary surgery (2nd edn). Oxford; Blackwell Scientific Publication 1992;62-63.
4. Cuschieri A, Shimi S, Banting S, Vander Velpen G Coaxial curved instrumentation for minimal access surgery. Endo Surgery 1993;1:30,3-5.
5. Cuschieri A, Szabo Z. Tissue approximation in endoscopic surgery. ISIS Medical Media.
6. Nelson MT, Nakashima M, Mulvihill SJ. How secure are laparoscopically placed clips? An in vitro and in vivo study. Arch Surgery 1992;127:718-20.
7. Szabo Z, Berci G. Extra and intracorporeal knotting and suturing technique. In Berci G ed. GI Endoscopy Clinics of North America.
8. Szabo Z, Hunter J, Berci G, Sachier K, Cusheiri A. Analysis of surgical movements during surgery in laparoscopy. End Surg 1994;2:55-61.

Laparoscopic Appendectomy for Gynecologists

MARK ERIAN, GLENDA MCLAREN

Chapter Eighteen

INTRODUCTION

The world's first laparoscopic appendectomy was performed by a German gynecologist, Professor Kurt Semm, Kiel University, and was published in 1983.[1] The laparoscopic approach is safe, efficacious, has many advantages over the traditional open appendectomy as the former offers the patient better cosmetic result, less postoperative pain and discomfort, less wound complications, shorter hospitalization, and quicker return to the workforce.[2-5] Despite initial skepticism,[6-8] laparoscopic appendectomy is the "gold standard" of management of appendicitis in many institutions, even in cases of complications, e.g. perforated, ruptured, abscess or gangrenous appendix.[9-16]

Training, knowledge, expertise of the performing surgeon, and availability of adequate facilities are important factors in determining whether or not the laparoscopic approach could be easily adopted.

THE ROLE OF LAPAROSCOPIC APPENDECTOMY

With the evolution of minimally invasive surgery, laparoscopic appendectomy was largely embraced by gynecologist and general surgeons alike.[17-19] With possible reservations, the procedure has rapidly gained ground in the management of both acute and chronic situations.[20]

In cases of acute right lower quadrant abdominal pain due to appendicitis, laparoscopic appendectomy may be performed in all cases of appendicitis with or without complications, and as an interval procedure following drainage of appendicular abscess. In chronic gynecological pelvic pain, laparoscopic appendectomy is advocated by many endoscopists especially in recurrent right iliac fossa pain of unknown origin.

Laparoscopic findings of injection of appendiceal peritoneum, peri-appendiceal adhesions, and induration of the appendix are particularly relevant factors influencing the decision of laparoscopic appendectomy.[21] In many cases, the pain would largely settle after laparoscopic appendectomy; complete or partial relief of abdominal pain in these circumstances happen in 74-93 percent of cases of right lower quadrant abdominal pain as the patient is asymptomatic in long-term.[22-25] In some cases of recurrent, persistent gynecological right lower abdominal pain, the resection of a "normal" appendix is beneficial by eliminating appendicitis in differential diagnosis.[26-29] In any case, there is no substitute for good clinical judgement.[30-32]

PROCEDURE OF LAPAROSCOPIC APPENDECTOMY

Instruments and Equipment

- A Verres needle (Ethicon)
- A 10 mm cannulae and sharp trocar (Ethicon)
- A Versaport trocar 12 mm (Auto-suture)
- Two reusable trocar and cannulae 5 mm (Apple Medical, Australia). These come in two lengths, with the long version used for obese patients, and the shorter for relatively slim patients.
- Two self-retaining atraumatic graspers, 5 mm length (Stortz), one/two self-retaining grasper, 5 mm (Stortz).
- Irrigation/suction, 5 mm cannular (Stryker)
- Three bags of 1 liter each of Ringer's solution
- "Suzie" (laparoscopic de-fogger) (Innovation Surgical Technology, USA)
- Three prettied Vicryl 0 endoloops (Ethicon)
- Laparoscopic endocatch (Ethicon)
- Bipolar diathermy generator (Valleylab, Australia)
- Bipolar diathermy grasper "basket" (Weck, USA)
- Long laparoscopy injection needle (Hoyland, Australia)
- Laparoscopic scissors (Hoyland, Australia)
- Laparoscopic "J" shaped needle (Hoyland, Australia) with 0 Vicryl (Ethicon) through the eye of the needle. The "J" shaped needle comes in three different sizes; large, medium, and small, to be used for obese, medium build and slim patients respectively.
- A 2/0 Vicryl stitch on small needle (Ethicon)
- Bellavac negative suction drainage (Hoyland, Australia)
- Sterile steri-strips ¼ inch (Johnson & Johnson)
- A Foley's catheter with a urine bag.

Telescope

- Stryker 30° 10 mm telescope
- Stryker camera three chip, 988 digital, high resolution Sony tele-monitor 21 inches.

- Stryker Digital Image Capture System, provided with CD and high quality printer to document the procedure. The video recording equipment has a medicolegal relevance to be able to fully counsel the patient postoperatively regarding the findings and the relevance of the procedure, the presence or otherwise of any complications and how these were managed.

Insufflator

Stryker high-flow carbon dioxide insufflator with fairly full carbon dioxide cylinder. The authors usually adjust the carbon dioxide to 2 liters per minute during the initial insufflator; then 12 liters per minute, for maintenance, with intraperitoneal pressure is automatically adjusted at 15 mmHg.

Chemicals and Drugs

- Povidone iodine 10 percent solution (Faulkner Pharmaceuticals, Australia).
- Bupivacaine (Marcaine) 0.5 percent/1: 200,000 adrenaline 20 ml.

SURGICAL TECHNIQUE

Anesthesia

Usually the procedure is performed under general anesthetic, unless if the attending anesthetist preferred regional analgesia, e.g. epidural or spinal.

Steps

- The anesthetist is requested to pass a nasogastric or orogastric tube to ensure complete emptying of the stomach contents to avoid the risk of stomach wall injury.[33]
- The abdomen is painted with an antiseptic solution, followed by the perineum, external urethra, vestibule, and the vagina. Draping is applied on the patient's lower limbs, pelvis and abdomen, but the operation area is well exposed. Foley's catheter is inserted into the urinary bladder, the balloon inflated and the catheter is attached to a urine bag.
- The anesthetist is requested to put the patient into exaggerated Trendelenburg position at 15-25°.

Ports Location (Fig. 18.1)

- A—10 mm wide and contains the telescope
- B—12 mm wide and contains the Versaport and is about midway between the pubic hairline and umbilicus.
- C and D—at the right and "left" McBurney's points. Both points C and D are 5 mm wide. The latter three points and insertion of trocar have to be done under laparoscopic guidance to avoid intraoperative injuries.
- S—Surgeon on left-hand side of patient
- OT—Operating Theater scrub sister next to surgeon
- E—Assistant

The advantage of this arrangement is that the location of ports C and D facilitates the parallel "chopstick" situation ideal for laparoscopic suturing if that was required at any stage during the operation. For that purpose, the authors employ Johnson and Johnson straight needle holder with monocryl (0) on a 36 mm needle (Ethicon) and a grasper via ports C and D to affect laparoscopic suturing.[34]

- Pneumoperitoneum is created via the well known open laparoscopy Hasson technique or Palmer's point (mid-clavicle line, about two fingers breadth below the lower left costal margin) and induced by the use of Verres needle. As with Hasson's technique, the use of Palmer's point approach is adequate for easy access and visualization of the

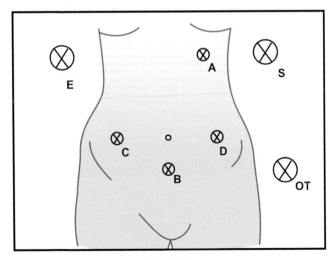

Fig. 18.1
(A = Palmer's Point, B = Suprapubic, C & D = Right and "left" McBurney's points, S = Surgeon, OT = Operating Theater scrub nurse, E = Assistant)

pelvic and abdominal organs. However, it is important to exclude splenomegaly clinically prior to using this point for induction of pneumo-peritoneum, if intraoperative splenic injury is to be avoided.

- Insertion of laparoscopy trocar cannula at the above mentioned point. The trocar is removed and cannula is connected to the carbon dioxide insufflation tube.
- Laparoscope, connected to the camera, is inserted with "Suzie" laparoscopic defogger applied between the eye piece and the light connection. White balance is done.
- Pelvi-abdominal cavity is inspected to exclude unsuspected injuries during introduction of Verres needle, or laparoscopic trocar.[35] However, these injuries are extremely rare in experienced hands.
- Initial thorough examination of pelvi-abdominal organs, to exclude any significant pathology is required.
- Two pairs of atraumatic graspers are introduced via ports C and D to retract the caecum upwards

towards the liver and expose the appendix. "Hand-under-hand" approach is followed.

- The appendix is identified and the tip is grasped with an atraumatic grasper. The whole length of the appendix must be visualized down to its caecal base. Adhesiolysis may be required to separate the appendix from adherent structures.
- The mesoappendix is identified and prophylactic bipolar diathermy followed by sharp dissection using laparoscopic scissors to skeletonize the appendix (Figs 18.1 to 18.4).
- Applying two successive Vicryl endoloops to the proximal part of the appendix flush with its caecal base, to eliminate the possibility of future "stump" appendicitis, and these are applied extremely tight (Figs 18.5 to 18.12). A third endoloop is applied about 0.5 cm above the previous endoloop. It has been suggested that one endoloop on either side is adequate.[36] However, it is the authors' technique to employ double endoloops at the base of the appendix to decrease the incidence of appendicolith.[37]

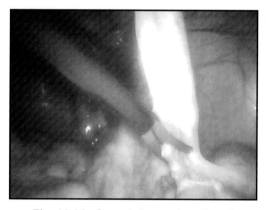

Fig. 18.2A: Coagulation and section of meso appendix

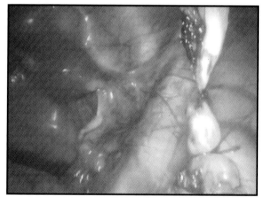

Fig. 18.2B: Two pretied endoloops

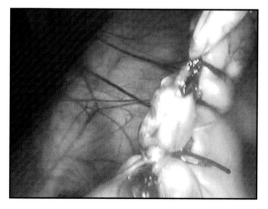

Fig. 18.3: One more endoloop passed

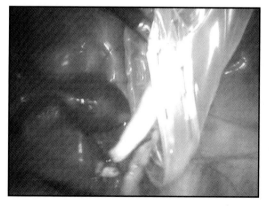

Fig. 18.4: Appendix put in the endo bag for retrieval

- The appendix is severed between the uppermost endoloop and the succeeding one using laparoscopic scissors; then it is carefully loaded inside a laparoscopic endocatch, passed into the peritoneal cavity via B port of entry, using a grasper, and the appendix is removed from the abdomen via incision B, and sent for histological examination.

- Appendectomy can be carried out by using free ties employing intracorporeal knot tying this can be done when endoloops are not available or surgeon more proficient with intracorporeal knot typing technique (Figs 18.5 to 16).

Appendectomy by Using Free-tie Sutures

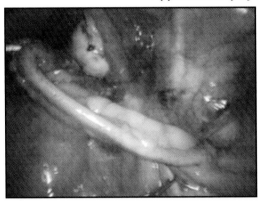

Fig. 18.5: Initial appearance of inflamed appendix

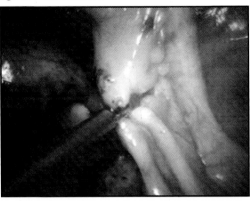

Fig. 18.6: Starting coagulation of the meso appendix

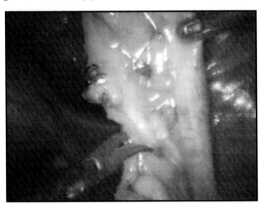

Fig. 18.7: Dividing the coagulated meso appendix

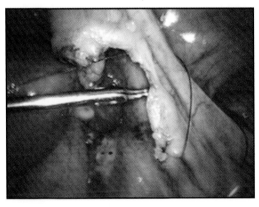

Fig. 18.8: After coagulation of meso appendix a free tie nonabsorbable suture is passed by needle holder

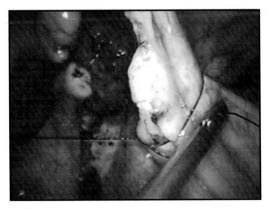

Fig. 18.9: Tightening the nonabsorbable free tie suture at the base of appendix

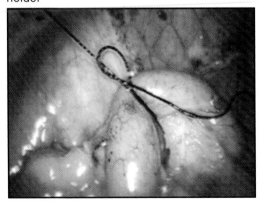

Fig. 18.10: This is secured by intracorporeal suturing by applying a standard square knot

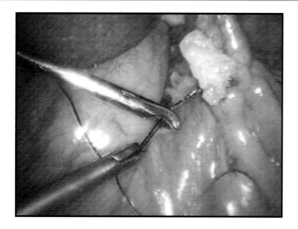

Fig. 18.11: First suture in situ

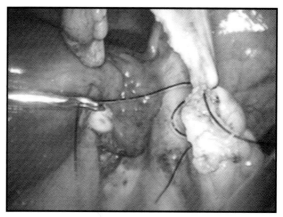

Fig. 18.12: Second suture placed 1cm proximal to the first suture applied by intracorporeal knot tying

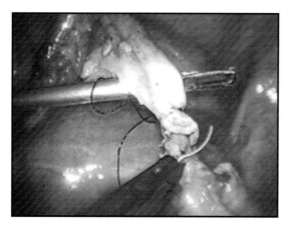

Fig. 18.13: Dividing the appendix between the two sutures

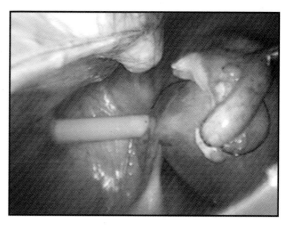

Fig. 18.14: Separated appendix with the proximal suture

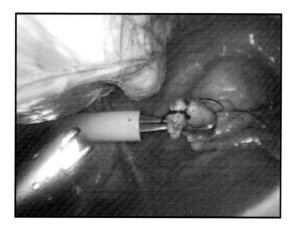

Fig. 18.15: Removal of appendix through 10mm port holding with claw forceps

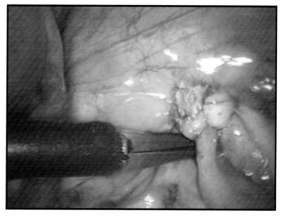

Fig. 18.16: Inspecting the base of appendix at end of procedure

- 10 ml of Povidone iodine 10 percent is applied on the appendicial stump, using a laparoscopic injection needle and a 10 ml syringe, to sterilize it; followed by irrigation/suction using Ringers solutions. In cases of perforated, ruptured, or gangrenous appendix, at least 3 liters of Ringer's solution have to be used for the process of irrigation/suction.[38]

- Recheck homeostasis and abdomen is examined to exclude a possible bowel injury.¼ inch Bellavac tube is located in the pouch of Douglas, under laparoscopic guidance. This removes the remains of blood, irrigation fluid and carbon dioxide from the peritoneal cavity and minimizes postoperative pelvic and shoulder tip pain. The Bellavac, with its negative pressure suction drainage tube and bag, is usually removed 4 hours postoperatively.

- A "J" shaped needle loaded with zero Vicryl suture, together with Foley's catheter, is used to suture the rectus in port B which contains the Bellavac tube, under laparoscopic guidance. Care must be exercised to avoid suturing the Bellavac tube itself. All instruments are removed from ports of entry under laparoscopic guidance to prevent a loop of bowel and/or omentum being sucked into an abdominal wound.

- The large (10-12 mm) abdominal wounds are closed using 2/0 vicryl suturing of the rectus of the port of entry and sterile steri-strips applied on the skin of all the ports of entry.

- A total of 10 ml of local anesthetic 0.5 percent marcaine/adrenaline 1:200,000, are injected under the skin of the 4 "ports of entry" (approximately 5 ml each) to relieve postoperative pain and discomfort.

- Patients are usually discharged home from the "Day Surgery" unit and advised to use "over the counter" oral analgesics for 24-72 hours as required.

COMPLICATIONS

Hemorrhage

Intraoperative Hemorrhage

a. *Parietal hemorrhage*—profuse bleeding may result from injury of an anterior abdominal wall blood vessel, e.g. inferior epigastric artery during inser-

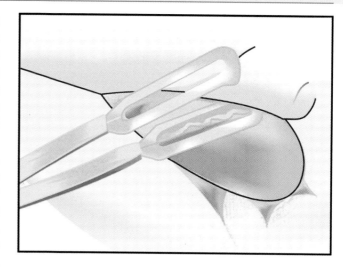

Fig. 18.17: Shows application of bipolar forceps to apply diathermy for hemostasis

tion of a trocar in a point of entry. The bleeding can be usually stopped by carefully applying bipolar diathermy at 50 watts under direct laparoscopic guidance (Fig. 18.17).

b. Bleeding from appendicular artery. Bipolar diathermy should be used to stop the bleeding. Irrigation/suction may be used to clearly identify the bleeding vessel. Care must be exercised to avoid contact of the prongs of the diathermy forceps with loops of intestines.

Accidental Bowel Injury

Rarely, caecal wall injury may happen with laparoscopic scissors during sharp dissection of tissues planes or severing of the appendix. The surgeon should be able to readily identify and manage such a complication.

Laparoscopic purse string suture using monocryl 0 is applied around the tear and firm extra- or intracorporeal knot applied (Fig. 18.18).

Usually the patient comes to no harm. However, admission to hospital for observation for at least 24 hours is warranted in these circumstances.

Laparotomy

Conversion to laparotomy may be required in some cases of perforated appendix or appendicular abscess, as the base of the appendix may acquire a "Swiss cheese" consistency and cannot hold sutures.[39]

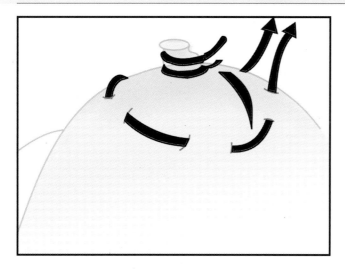

Fig. 18.18: Shows suturing to deal with an injury point in the intestine

However, the use of endoloops has largely solved this problem. 0 vicryl endoloops may be successfully directly applied under laparoscopic guidance; in effect creating a "mini partial caecotomy".

Conversion to open appendectomy carries a high risk of morbidity, slower recovery, and increased wound infection.[40-42] In general, the authors (Erian M, McLaren G) showed that conversion can be avoided if the endoscopist is experienced.[43]

Infection

Pelvic abscess may follow laparoscopic appendectomy especially in complicated cases of appendicitis.[44] Computerized tomography (CT) scan is a valuable diagnostic tool in these circumstances.[45]

The general rule of "pus means knife" applies. Drainage is necessary. CT scan guided drainage is recommended by some. However, the authors prefer to perform laparoscopy as this has advantage of inspecting pelvic abdominal organs, and ensuring that the endoloops applied on the stump of the appendix are still tight, and in situ. Copious irrigation/suction using 3-4 liters of Ringer's (or occasionally Hartmann's solution in case Ringer's solution is not available) is performed. ¼ inch Bellavac drain is normally left in the pouch of Douglas to ensure complete drainage. A broad spectrum antibiotic is used for a few days to avoid septicemia.

"Stump" Appendicitis

This complication occurs if the original appendectomy was not performed properly. During laparoscopic appendectomy, as in open appendectomy, the appendix must be ligated, and, then resected, flush with the caecum. "Stump" appendicitis is an easily preventable complication, and conforms clinical difficulty to diagnose appendicitis knowing that the patient had previously undergone appendectomy.[46–49]

SPECIAL CIRCUMSTANCES

In Pregnancy —Appendicitis in Pregnancy is a Serious Disorder that Carries

Considerable perinatal morbidity and mortality, and possible maternal mortality. Early diagnosis and prompt surgical intervention is vital.[50] Depending on the degree of the surgeon's expertise, manual dexterity, and knowledge, there is no contra-indication to the laparoscopic approach in pregnancy.[51-57] Clearly, the gravid uterus forms a pelvic/pelvi-abdominal swelling that may interfere with the smooth running of laparoscopic appendectomy. However, the laparoscopic "ports of entry" may have to be located different than the above description, to avoid the gravid uterus being in the way of the laparoscopic diagnosis, and surgical resection of the appendix in these circumstances.[58]

Obesity

In general, obese women are more difficult to operate upon, and tend to suffer from more intra- and postoperative complications. However, laparoscopic appendectomy may be a preferred option to open appendectomy with less post-operative analgesic requirements and wound complications.[59,60] The authors, as outlined above, use Palmer's point of entry to induce pneumoperitoneum. That provides an easy access and good view of the peritoneal cavity even in grossly obese patients, and those who underwent previous multiple laparotomies and have considerable pelvic and/or abdominal adhesions.

As in the case of pregnancy—especially past the first trimester, obese patients and those with expected adhesions as of multiple previous laparotomies should be operated upon by an experienced endoscopist.[61]

TRAINING

Laparoscopic appendectomy can be easily integrated within a well structured training program of residents and registrars of obstetrics and gynecology, and general surgery alike, without the need to resort to animal experimentation laboratories. Just like any other endoscopic procedure, there is a learning curve; the operating time decreases as one goes through the learning curve so that ultimately the surgeon would grasp knowledge and training to enable him/her to perform laparoscopic appendectomy competently, in both emergency and elective settings, to the benefit of the patient.[62–69]

QUALITY ASSURANCE

As in all surgical procedures, especially minimally invasive techniques, a well designed system of quality assurance is crucial.[70] We owe it to our patients to provide the best and highest possible standards of surgical care. An objective system, based on continuous constructive self-criticism, must be introduced to evaluate the efficacy, cost-effectiveness and the patient benefits from laparoscopic appendectomy in each center of excellence.

FUTURE DEVELOPMENT

Laparoscopic appendectomy, as many other laparoscopic procedures, can be successfully performed via robotic and tele-robotic surgery.[71-74] A program has been recently introduced by NASA (National Aeronautical and Space Administration), USA have shown that even non-surgeons may be able to perform these procedures successfully with good results. However, the financial costs at the moment may be prohibitive to some institutions. Most likely, with the passing of time these state-of-the-art techniques will be available, not only to private, but, indeed, public major teaching hospitals so that gynecologists working in provincial areas may be easily taught to perform laparoscopic appendectomy. This program may have a positive impact on teaching as well as recruitment and maintaining of gynecologists in provincial areas where staffing is often a problem in many parts of the world.

ACKNOWLEDGMENTS

The authors would like to thank Professor SK Khoo, Professor, and Director of Gynecology, Royal Brisbane and Women's Hospital, Queensland, Australia for critically reviewing this chapter, and Mrs Ann Hanson for typing the manuscript.

REFERENCES

1. Semm K. Endoscopic Appendectomy. Endoscopy 1983;15:59-64.
2. Hermans BP, Otte JB. Laparoscopic appendectomy: pros and cons—literature review of 4,190 cases. Acta Chir Belg 1997;97 (3):110-17.
3. Heinzelmann M, Simmen HP, Cummins AS, Largiader F. Is Laparoscopic appendectomy the new "gold standard"? Arch Surg 1995;130 (7):782-85.
4. Frazee RC, Roberts JW, Symmonds RE, Snyder SK, et al. A prospective randomized trial comparing open versus laparoscopic appendectomy. Ann Surg 1994;219 (6):725-28. Discussion 728-31.
5. Nowzaraden Y, Westmoreland J, McCarver CT, Harris RJ. Laparoscopic appendectomy for acute appendicitis: indications and current use. J Laparoendos Surg 1991;1(5):247-57.
6. Fingerhut A, Millat B, Bornie F. Laparoscopic versus open appendectomy time to decide. World J Surg 1999;23 (8):835-45.
7. Merhoff AM, Merhoff GC, Franklin ME. Laparoscopic versus open appendectomy. Am J Surg 2000;179(5):375-78.
8. Kald A, Kullman E, Anderberg B, Wiren M, et al. Cost-minimisation analysis of laparoscopic and open appendectomy. Eur J Surg 1999;165 (6): 579-82.
9. Khalili TM, Hiat JR, Saver A, Lau C, et al. Perforated appendicitis is not a contraindication to laparoscopy. Am Surg 1999;65 (10):965-67.
10. Johnson AB, Peetz ME. Laparoscopic appendectomy is an acceptable alternative for the treatment of perforated appendicitis. Surg Endosc 1998;12 (7):940-43.
11. Sosa JL, Sleeman D, McKenny MG, Deggert J, et al. A comparison of laparoscopic and traditional appendectomy. J Laparoendosc Surg (JSLS) 1993;3 (2):129-31.
12. Guller U, Jain N, Peterson ED, Muhlbaier L H, et al. Laparoscopic appendectomy in the elderly. Surgery 2004;135 (5): 479-88.
13. Ball CG, Kortbeck JB, Kirkpatrick AW, Mitchell P. Laparoscopic appendectomy for complicated appendicectomy—an evaluation of postoperative factors. Surg Endosc 2004;18(6):969-73.
14. Kang KJ, Lim TJ, Kim YS. Laparoscopic appendectomy is feasible for the complicated appendicitis. Surg Laparosc Endosc Percutan Tech 2000;10(6):364-67.

15. Yao CC, Lin CS, Yang CC. Laparoscopic appendectomy for ruptured appendicitis. Surg Laparosc Endosc Percutan Tech 1999; 9(4): 271-73.

16. Paya K, Rauhofer U, Rebhandle W, Deluggi S, et al. Performing appendicitis. An indication for laparoscopy. Surg Endosc 2000;14 (2):182-84.

17. Kumar R, Erian M, Kimble R, Sinnott S, et al. The role of laparoscopic appendectomy in modern gynaecology. J Am Ass Gyn Laparosc 2002;9(3):252-63.

18. Chiasson PM, Pace DE, Schlachte CM, Mamazza J, et al. Minimally invasive surgical practice: a survey of general surgeons in Ontario. Can J Surg 2004;47(1):15-19.

19. Nguyen DB, Silen W, Hodin RA. Appendectomy in the pre-and post-laparoscopic eras. J Gastrointest Surg 1999;3 (1):67-73.

20. Cervini P, Smith LC, Urbach DR. The surgeon on call is a strong factor in determining the use of a laparoscopic approach for appendectomy. Surg Endosc 2002;16(12):1774-77.

21. Greason KL, Rappold JF, Liberman MA. Incidental laparoscopic appendectomy for acute right lower quadrant abdominal pain. Its time has come. Surg Endosc 1998;5 (3): 275-81.

22. Popp L W. Gynaecologically indicated single-endoloop laparoscopic appendectomy. J Am Assoc Gynecol Laparosc 1998;5(3):275-81.

23. Protopepas A, Shushan A, Hart R, Chatzipapas I, et al. Is laparoscopic appendectomy a gynaecological procedure? Lancet 1998;14;351 (9101): 500.

24. Mattei P, Sola J E, Yeo C J. Chronic and recurrent appendicitis are uncommon entities or misdiagnosed. J Am Coll Surg 1994;178 (4): 385-89.

25. Mussack T, Schmidbaur S, Nerlich A, Schmidt W, et al. Chronic appendicitis as an independent clinical entity. Chirug 2002;73 (7):710-15.

26. Chiarugi M, Buccianti P, Decamini L, Balestri R, et al. "What you see is not what you get". A plea to remove a "normal" appendix during diagnostic laparoscopy. Acta Chir Belg 2001;101 (5):243-45.

27. Wang HT, Sax HC. Incidental appendectomy in the era of managed care and laparoscopy. J Am Coll Surg 2001;192 (2):182-88.

28. Popovic D, Kavjanic J, Milostic D, Kolar D, et al. Long-term benefits of laparoscopic appendectomy for chronic abdominal pain in fertile women. Croat Med Ju 2004;45(2):171-75.

29. Di Sebastiano P, Fink T, di Mola FF, Weihe E, et al. Neuroimmune appendicitis. Lancet 19997;354 (9177): 461-66.

30. Kraemer M, Ohmann C, Leppert R, Yang Q. Microscopic assessment of the appendix at diagnostic laparoscopy is reliable. Surg Endosc 2000;14 (7): 625-33.

31. Seidman JD, Andersen DK, Ulrich S, Hoy GR, et al. Recurrent abdominal pain due to chronic appendiceal disease. South Med J 1991;84 (7):913-16.

32. Chandler B, Beegle M, Elfrink RJ, Smith WJ. To leave or not to leave? A retrospective review of appendicectomy during diagnostic laparoscopy for chronic pelvic pain. Mo Med 2002;99(9):502-4.

33. Erian M, Goh J, Coglan M. Auditing the complications of laparoscopy in a major teaching hospital in Australia. Gynaecological Endoscop 2001;10:303-08.

34. Hasson HM. Open laparoscopy. Biomed Bull 1984;5 (1):1-6.

35. Schafer M, Lauper M, Krahenbuhl L. Trocar and Veress needle injuries during laparoscopy. Surg Endosc 2001;15 (3):275-80.

36. Beldi G, Muggli K, Helbling C, Schlumpf R. Laparoscopic appendectomy using endoloops: a prospective, randomized clinical trial. Surg Endosc 2004;18(5):749-50.

37. Guillem P, Mulliez E, Proye C, Pattou F. Retained appendicolith after laparoscopic appendectomy, the need for systematic double ligature of the appendiceal base. Surg Endosc 2004;18(4):717-18.

38. Stoltzing H, Thon K. Perforated appendicitis: is laparoscopic operation adviseable? Dig Surg 2000;17(6):610-16.

39. Krishner SL, Browne A, Dibbins A, Tkacz N, et al. Intra-abdominal abscess after laparoscopic appendectomy for perforated appendicitis. Arch Surg 2001;136 (4): 438-41.

40. Hellberg A, Rudberg C, Enochsson L, Gudbjarston T, et al. Conversion from laparoscopic to open appendectomy: a possible drawback of the laparoscopic technique? Eur J Surg 2001; 167(3): 209-13.

41. Piskan G, Kozik D, Rajpal S, Shaftan G, et al. Comparison of laparoscopic open and converted appendectomy for perforated appendicitis. Surg Endosc 2001;15 (7): 660-62.

42. Liu S I, Siewert B, Raptopoulos V, Hodin R A. Factors associated with conversion to laparotomy in patients undergoing laparoscopic appendectomy. J Am Coll Surg 2002;194(3):298-305

43. Erian M, McLaren G. Laparoscopic appendectomy—gynaecologist or general surgeon? Proceedings of the 11th International Congress, Society of Laparoendoscopic Surgeons, New Oreleans, USA, September 2002;231-32.

44. Katkhouda N, Friedlander M H, Grant S W, Achanta K K, et al. Intrabdominal abscess rate after laparoscopic appendectomy. Am J Surg 2000;180(6): 456-9; discussion 460-1.

45. Maniatis V, Chryssikopoulos H, Roussakis A, Kalamara C, et al. Perforation of the alimentary tract: evaluation with computer tomography. Abdom Imaging 2000;25 (4):373-79.

46. Demartines N, Largiader J. "Residual" appendicitis following incomplete laparoscopic appendectomy. Br J Surg 1996;83(10):1481.

47. Sommerville PG, Lavelle MA. Residual appendicitis following incomplete laparoscopic appendectomy. Br J Surg 1996;83(6):869.

48. Fillippi de la Palavesa MM, Vaxmann V, Campos M, Tuchmann C, et al. Appendiceal stump abscess. Abdom Imaging 1996;21 (1):65-66.

49. Mangi AA, Berger DL. Stump appendicitis. Am J Surg 2000;66.

50. Guttman R, Goldman R D, Koreri G. Appendicitis during pregnancy. Can Fam Physician 2004;50: 355-57

51. Andreoli M, Servakou M, Meyers P, Mann W J Jnr. Laparoscopic surgery during pregnancy. J Am Assoc Gynecol Laparosc 1999;6 (2):229-33.

52. Thomas S J, Brisson P. Laparoscopic appendectomy and cholecystectomy in pregnancy: six case reports. JSLS 1998;2(1):41-46.

53. Curet MJ, Allen D, Josloff R, Pitcher D E, et al. Laparoscopy during pregnancy. Arch Surg 1996;131 (5): 546-50; discussion 550-51.

54. Ueberrueck T, Koch A, Meyer L, Hinkel M, et al. Ninety-four appendectomies for suspected acute appendicitis during pregnancy. World J Surg 2004;28(5):508-11.

55. Schreiber J H. Laparoscopic appendectomy in pregnancy. Surg Endosc 1990;4(2):100-02.

56. Fatum M, Rojansky N. Laparoscopic surgery during pregnancy. Obstet Gynecol Surv 2001;56 (1):50-59.

57. Lachman E, Schierfeld A, Voss E, Gino G, et al. Pregnancy and laparoscopic surgery. J Am Assoc Gynecol Laparosc 1999;6 (3):347-51.

58. Barnes SL, Shane MD, Schoemann MB, Bernard AC, et al. Laparoscopic appendectomy after 30 weeks pregnancy—report of two cases and description of technique. Am Surg 2004;70 (8):733-36.

59. Scott-Conner CD, Hall TJ, Anglin BL, Muakkassa FF. Laparoscopic appendectomy. Initial experience in a teaching program. Ann Surg 1992;215(6): 660-7; discussion 667-68.

60. Enochsson L, Hellberg A, Rudberg C, Fenyo C, et al. Laparoscopic vs open appendectomy in overweight patients. Surg Endosc 2001;15 (4):387-92.

61. Curet M J. Special problems in laparoscopic surgery. Previous abdominal surgery, obesity and pregnancy. Surg Clin North Am 2000;80(4):1093-110 (8):739-41.

62. Meinke A K, Kossuth T. What is the learning curve for laparosopic appendectomy? Surg Endosc 1994;8(5):371-5; Discussion 376.

63. McCormick PH, Tanner WA, Keane FB, Tierney S. Minimally invasive techniques in common surgical procedures—implications for training. Ire J Med Sci 2003;172 (1):27-29.

64. Letterie GS, Hibbert ML, Morgenstern LL. A program of instruction in operative laparoscopy in a residency in obstetrics and gynaecology. J Gynecl Surg 1993 Winter;9 (4):187-90.

65. Carresco-Prats M, Soria Aledo V, Lujan-Mompean J A, Rios-zambu, et al. Role of appendectomy in training for laparoscopic surgery. Surg Endosc 2003;17(1):111-14.

66. Sackier J M. Laparoscopy in the emergency setting. World J Surg 1992;16(6):1083-88.

67. Duff S E, Dixon AR. Laparoscopic appendicectomy: safe and useful for training. Ann R Coll Surg Eng 2000;82 (6):388-91.

68. Adrales GL, Chu UB, Hoskins JD, Witzke DB, et al. Development of a cost effective laparoscopic training program. Am J Surg 2004;187 (2):157-63.

69. Adrales GL, Donnelly MB, Chu UB, Witzke DB, et al. Determinents of competency judgements by experienced laparoscopic surgeons. Surg Endosc 2004;18(2):323-27.

70. Erian M, McLaren G. Quality assurance of Gynaecological laparoscopic procedures in a major Teaching Hospital in Australia. Proceedings of the 12th International Congress of Society of Laparoendoscopic Surgeons, Las Vegas, USA, September 2003. Pages S10-11.

71. Gadiere GB, Hinpens J, Germeny O, Izizaw R, et al. Feasibility of robotic laparoscopic surgery: 146 cases. World J Surg 2001;25(11):1467-77.

72. Rosser JC Jr, Herman B, Giammaria LE. Telementoring. Semin Laparosc Surg 2003;10 (4): 209-17.

73. Moorthy K, Munz Y, Dosis A, Hernandex J, et al. Dexterity enhancement with robotic surgery. Surg Endosc 2004;18 (5):790-95.

74. Satava RM. Disruptive visions: a robot is not a machine. Systems integration for surgeons. Surg Endosc. 2004;18(4):617-20.

Endosuturing in Abdominal Wall Hernias

PRADEEP CHOWBEY

Chapter Nineteen

INTRODUCTION

Currently, both inguinal and ventral hernias are performed laparoscopically. Inguinal hernia repairs are commonly performed by two techniques:
1. Total extraperitoneal repair (TEP)
2. Transabdominal preperitoneal (TAPP) repair.

Ventral hernia repair is performed commonly by Intraperitoneal onlay mesh (IPOM) repair.

ENDOSCOPIC TEP GROIN REPAIR

Endoscopic TEP groin repair is an advanced laparoscopic procedure. The essential feature of TEP repair is the reinforcement of the transversalis fascia by a large prosthesis that extends well beyond the myopectineal orifice. All potential groin hernia defects / weakness (direct, indirect, femoral) are thus covered effectively with a prosthesis (usually a polypropelene mesh) that envelops the visceral sac. The mesh is held in place by intra-abdominal pressure and later by ingrowth of connective tissue. The repair conforms to the current standard practice of being both anatomical as well as "tension-free". This technique is the absolute weapon to eliminate all types of groin hernias, especially difficult and recurrent hernias.

TRANSABDOMINAL PREPERITONEAL REPAIR (TAPP)

As this name suggests, the preperitoneal space is reached through the abdominal cavity for repairing the defect, whereas TEP repair is carried out without breaching the peritoneum. The advantages of TAPP approach are—it is simpler to learn, provides more working space, familiar anatomic orientation, and therefore, is more frequently performed. Disadvantages of TAPP approach are necessitates violation of the peritoneal cavity during entry and subsequent performance of the surgical procedure, requires general anesthesia and is an indirect route to access to the preperitoneal space. TEP has several advantages over TAPP, such as fewer complications and lower recurrence rate. Once the mesh is placed inside the abdominal cavity or in the extraperitoneal space it is secured with the help of helical tacks (Autosuture, Tyco Healthcare, USA).

The role of endosuturing is very limited for hernia repair. It is done mainly for fixation of the mesh to the pubic bone, suturing of large peritoneal tears, ligation of sac, taking control of an incompletely dissected bleeding vessel and reperitonealization after a TAPP repair.

Endosuturing is being used for herniotomy in pediatric group of patients. A purse suture is tied to close the internal ring.

VENTRAL HERNIA REPAIR

Ventral abdominal wall hernias consist of primary abdominal wall hernias (e.g. umbilical, paraumbilical, epigastric, spigelian), traumatic hernias and incisional hernias. It is estimated that between 2 to 11 percent of coeliotomies eventually result in an incisional hernia. The recurrence rates of conventional primary repair of these hernias may range from 30 to 50 percent.

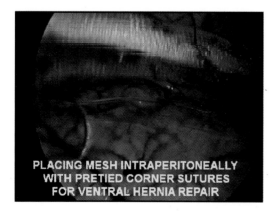

Fig. 19.1: Placing mesh intraperitoneally with pretied corner sutures for ventral hernia repair

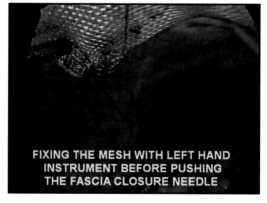

Fig. 19.2: Fixing the mesh with left hand instrument before pushing the fascia closure needle

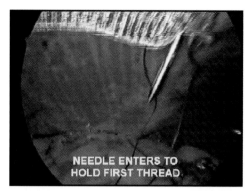

Fig. 19.3: Needle enters to hold first thread

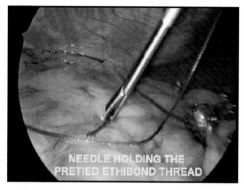

Fig. 19.4: Needle holding the pretied ethibond thread

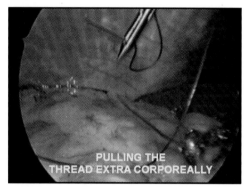

Fig. 19.5: Pulling the thread extracorporeally

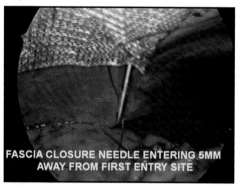

Fig. 19.6: Fascia closure needle entering 5 mm away from first entry site

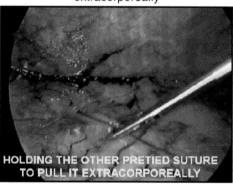

Fig. 19.7: Holding the other pretied suture to pull it extracorporeally

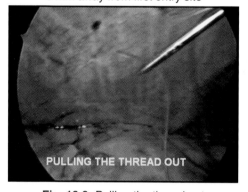

Fig. 19.8: Pulling the thread out

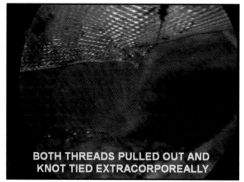

Fig. 19.9: Both threads pulled out and knot tied extracorporeally

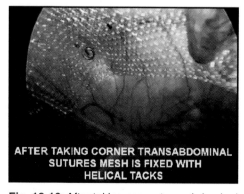

Fig. 19.10: After taking corner transabdominal sutures mesh is fixex with helical tacks

The basic principles underlying a sound laparoscopic hernia repair by intraperitoneal onlay mesh are the following:

- Tensionless closure of the defect
- Prosthetic reinforcement with the biocompatible material lending support to the attenuated tissues of the abdominal wall
- Eliminating the continuity between the access port used for introduction of the mesh and the site of mesh placement to reduce the chances of mesh contamination and infection.

The mechanical characteristics of a mesh are strength, fixation retention and durability. The biological characteristics are infectibility, adhesion formation and erosion/fistulization.

The suturing technique was devised to obtain strong fixation to the anterior abdominal wall. Stapling is very effective in laparoscopic hernioplasties. Use of a large mesh extending 3-5 cm beyond the edge of the defect on all sides utilizes Pascal's law, which states that pressure in a closed space, when increased is distributed in all directions equally. Thus, if the patch is larger than defect, the patch is implanted against the inner surface of the anterior abdominal wall and is stabilized in position by the very forces that tend to push the patch through the defect. However, fixing the mesh with transabdominal sutures is mandatory as meshes are known to contract over a period of time. We apply transabdominal retention sutures on the 4 corners of mesh using a fascia closure needle. The corner sutures are sutured to the mesh extracorporeally and once mesh is placed intraperitoneally these are withdrawn using a fascia closure needle. Knots are tied extracorporeally and lie in the subcutaneous tissue. All 10 mm ports are also closed using the same fascia closure needle to prevent future herniation through these defects.

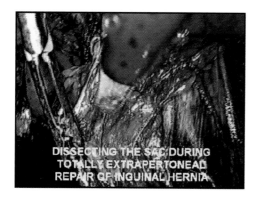

Fig. 19.11: Dissecting the sac during totally extrapertoneal repair of inguinal hernia

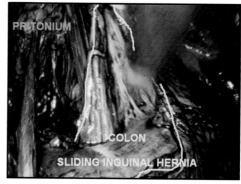

Fig. 19.12: Sliding inguinal hernia

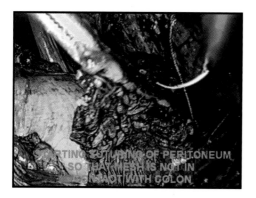

Fig. 19.13: Starting suturing of peritoneum so that mesh is not in contact with colon

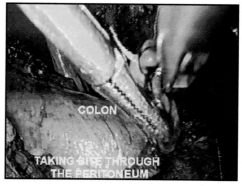

Fig. 19.14: Taking bite through the peritoneum

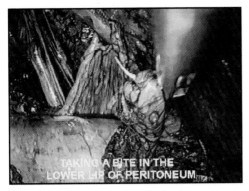

Fig. 19.15: Taking a bite in the lower lip of peritoneum

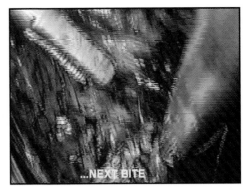

Fig. 19.16: Next bite

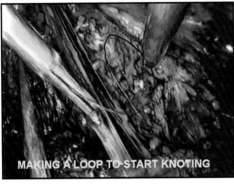

Fig. 19.17: Making a loop to start knoting

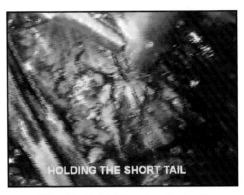

Fig. 19.18: Holding the short tail

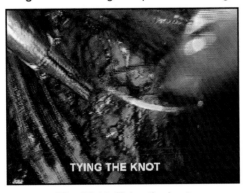

Fig. 19.19: Tying the knot

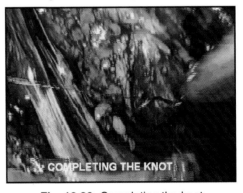

Fig. 19.20: Completing the knot

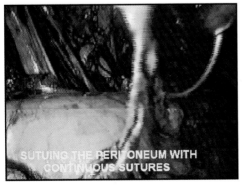

Fig. 19.21: Suturing the peritoneum with continuous sutures

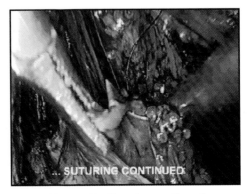

Fig. 19.22: Suturing continued

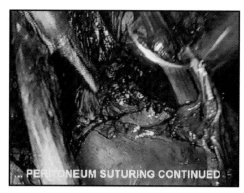

Fig. 19.23: Peritoneum suturing continued

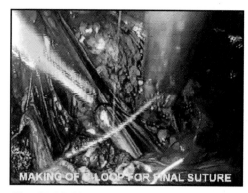

Fig. 19.24: Making of C-loop for final suture

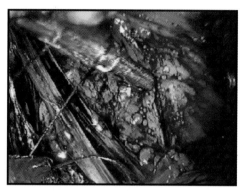

Fig. 19.25: Taking two throws

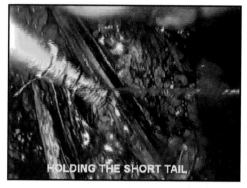

Fig. 19.26: Holding the short tail

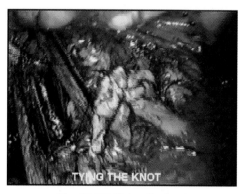

Fig. 19.27: Tying the knot

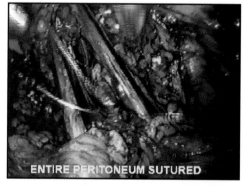

Fig. 19.28: Entire peritoneum sutured

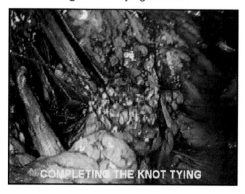

Fig. 19.29: Completing the knot tying

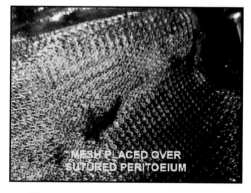

Fig. 19.30: Mesh placed over sutured peritoneum

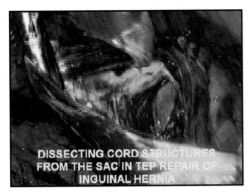

Fig. 19.31: Dissecting cord structures from the sac in tep repair of inguinal hernia

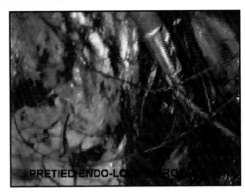

Fig. 19.32: Pretied endo-loop introduced

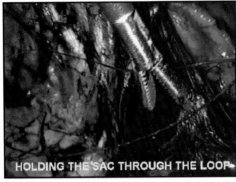

Fig. 19.33: Holding the sac through the loop

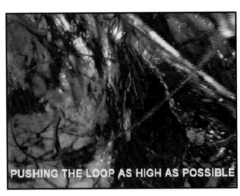

Fig. 19.34: Pushing the loop as high as possible

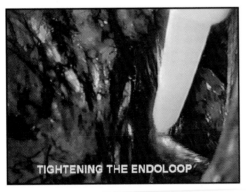

Fig. 19.35: Tightening the endoloop

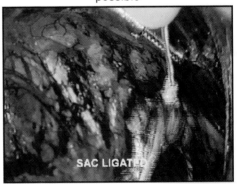

Fig. 19.36: Sac ligated

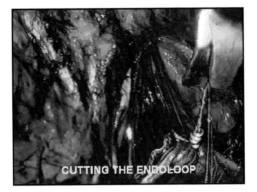

Fig. 19.37: Cutting the endoloop

REFERENCES

1. Voeller GR. Laparoscopic repair of ventral hernias. In Arregui ME, Eubanks S, Olsen DO, et al (Eds): Laparoscopic Surgery of the Abdomen. MacFadyen BV; Springer-Verlag, New York, Inc. 2004, pp327-334.
2. Chowbey PK. Endoscopic repair of abdominal wall hernias. First edition: 2004, New Delhi : Byword Viva Publishers Pvt. Ltd.

Laparoscopic Microsurgical Suturing

NUTAN JAIN

Chapter Twenty

Microsurgical suturing is quite a new concept, a transition of conventional microsurgery into laparoscopic arena. Laparoscopy is undergoing a sea change in clinical applications and indications and so are microsurgical applications. Medical fraternity the worldover has embraced microsurgical applications to give better surgical and reproductive outcomes. With advances in instrumentation and overall manual dexterity achieved in laparoscopic suturing laparoscopic microsurgical suturing has come a long way come into being accepted as a principal modality to carry out certain specialized procedures. The traditional operating microscope was the hallmark of successful outcome of open microsurgery (Fig. 20.1). Microsurgical applications using the operating microscope soon become widely acceptable and were the Gold standard. Early pioneers were Gomel[1] who gave the world initial series of highly convincing results. Main applications being tubotubal reanastomosis, adhesiolysis and eversion of fimbria in neosalpingostomy. The pioneers were keenly followed and within no time there was no dearth of open microsurgical[2] enthusiasts. It soon was established as the principal modality to carry out microsurgical procedures. Though difficult to learn and master it attracted a lot of workers in the field of infertility to embrace it. The era of open microsurgery flourished till the advent of in vitro fertilization with the birth of Louis Brown in 1978[3] it became evident that blocked fallopian tubes could be bypassed and conception possible even in absolutely damaged and blocked fallopian tubes. Though the results of IVF were not comparable to microsurgery but the option appeared. This was also the time Laparoscopy started making inroads into the gynecologist office. The beginning of laparoscopy was humble, restricted to diagnostic scopies in infertile patients. But since the first laparoscopic hysterectomy by Reich[4] it soon became evident that laparoscopy is only an access route and any application you imagine can be carried out laparoscopically. Good results of laparoscopy had started coming in for adhesiolysis, Salpingo-ovariolysis and the bright idea of Bruhat[5] of employing thermal energy for fimbrial eversion in neosalpingostomy. So a combination of above all was the catalytic point of early workers like Dr Charles H Koh and Dr Grace Janik in 1992[6] to try tubotubal reanastomosis employing microsurgery via the laparoscopic route.

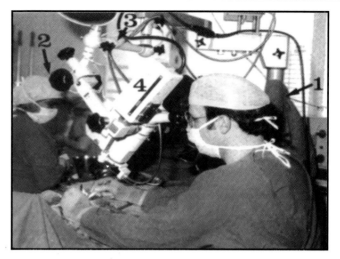

Fig. 20.1: Open microsurgical armamentarium

The medical world was taken by surprise when reports of laparoscopic microsurgery started coming in.

LAPAROSCOPIC MICROSURGERY

Laparoscopy by it is inherent qualities appear to be giving the most ideal environment to carry out microsurgery. The first and foremost requirement of microsurgery is to work under magnification without recourse to a bulky instrument like operating microscope just by bringing the telescope closer to the target organ does it all. Magnification is required to differentiate normal from abnormal tissue and to facilitate dissection and suturing by ultramicro instruments, needles and sutures. By laparoscopy, magnification of the entire viewing field, rather than of a fixed and limited field, is achieved very naturally. The magnification can be increased by up to 40 times by the movement of the laparoscope, by bringing the telescope closer to the organ of interest. Coupled with the three-chip camera which offers zoom facilities and digital enhancement, laparoscopy provides excellent view and magnification.

Laparoscopy offers a closed working environment hence avoids tissue drying, there is least chance of infection and above all thorough suction irrigation and lavage easily continues all through the procedure. The use of patient's positioning in steep Trendelenburg and CO_2 pneumoperitoneum offers the advantage of spontaneous retraction of bowel without recourse to bulky retractors and this offers unique, comfortable exposure of pelvic organs. Last but not the least, several trials have demonstrated reduced occurrence of postoperative adhesion following laparoscopy compared to laparotomy.[7] Using laparoscopic armamentarium one could perform this superior microsurgery today. This with a added ease of working with delicate micro instruments specially designed to carry out super specialized tasks render laparoscopic suturing a virtual reality. The ingredients of success appear to be passion for microsurgery, prior expertise with microsurgical techniques and readiness to dedicate long practising hours on bovine models, virtual simulator and pelvic trainers. Laparoscopic microsurgical suturing is no different from other intracorporeal suturing; it is only familiarity to use very small needles and fine suture materials to execute the surgical task.

CLINICAL APPLICATIONS OF MICROSUTURING

As discussed early all infertility procedure could give better results if carried out giving respect to microsurgical principles. Acquiring an operating microscope was unusual but now as laparoscopic armamentarium is present and easily available in all operating rooms of this century, all reproductive surgeries like adhesiolysis, management of ectopic pregnancy, management of hydrosalpinx, tubotubal reanastomosis or tubal cornual implantation can be done by laparoscopic route. Hence, the modern day laparoscopic microsurgical suturing is a "Concept" which can be applied to any visceral closure. Laparoscopic myomectomy could be carried out keeping microsurgical principles and give anatomically gratifying results. As indications for laparoscopy and surgical procedures are widening there would be more instance of visceral, vascular injures. Endometriosis is a growing Enigma, so is its surgical management. Radical excision of endometriosis poses a threat to ureter, rectum and at times bladder. The microsurgical closure of ureter[8] not only obviates need of laparotomy but also promises a better repair under laparoscopic guidance. My own case of ureteric transection during TLH for a very large uterus with multiple fibroids near the lower uterine segment and a posterior cervical fibroid resulted in a deft laparoscopic reanastomosis of the ureter employing 4-0 sutures. This was easily done in the background of surgical expertise acquired in carrying out laparoscopic tubotubal reanastomosis. In fact, it appeared simpler as the ureter is much more rigid than the soft pliable fallopian tube which is more mobile, difficult to stabilize during reanastomosis. So to say, acquiring the skill of microsuturing is not only to carry out selected few laparoscopic tubal reanastomosis but empowers one to tide over any surgical catastrophe in challenging situations.

Suture Materials

The principles of microsurgery require a suture material which is less adhesiogenic and as fine as possible. Earlier it was common place during the era of open microsurgery to use 6-0, 8-0 prolene but now with universal acceptance of polyglycolic acid (vicryl), extra fine vicryl sutures are highly acceptable and over the years have proved to be less adhesiogenic. They have less memory compared to prolene so lot more easier to handle laparoscopically. Most of the pioneers of laparoscopic microsuturing are using fine vicryl as the suture material of choice. For bowel and bladder 3-0 or 4-0 vicryl or PDS is good to give proper tissue approximation and tensile strength in postoperative healing phase. Vascular repair has been attempted as reported in literature by recourse to 7-0, 8-0, sutures. The last word is that finer the suture and smaller the needle with which the operator can work comfortably should be the material of choice.

Instrumentation

The laparoscopic gamut should be complete with a high-resolution three-chip camera, which provides facilities of zoom, light enhancement, auto iris and auto focus. I presently find the new HDF camera from Stryker Endoscopy (Fig. 20.2) favorite. It offers all the features highly favorable for laparoscopic microsuturing. It has a preset for microscope, which give distinct advantages over currently available laparoscopic cameras. A good light source is a bare minimum requirement. A high-resolution monitor to transfer the minute tissue details are a boon for laparoscopic microsurgical suturing. Software for documentation and image capturing render the learning process easier by reviewing them after the surgery.

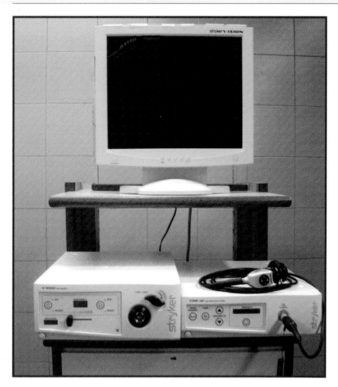

Fig. 20.2: High definition stryker camera with light source and 19 inches flat pannel monitor

Microsurgical Hand Instruments (Figs 20.3A to F)

There is a sea change in the instruments of bygone days and the most sophisticated laparoscopic instruments of today. Microsurgical needle holders and graspers pioneered by Dr Charles H Koh manufactured by Karl Storz, GmbH are delicate, yet very sturdy instrument giving lot of precision in tissue holding, dissecting and suturing. They are surgical masterpieces. They have unique sandblasted tip, which avoids glare and have a very firm, precise hold by ultra micrograspers and microneedle holders. We have made indigenously available micro probes, suction irrigation cannula and microunipolar needle and microbipolar forceps. All this completes the surgical instrumentation.

Delicate microsurgical laparoscopic hand instruments require very special care in cleaning and handling. So, the OR team should use them only in the intended manner, cleaning to be very good otherwise the jaws, tips and ratchet mechanism could suffer.

No instrument alone can transfer the skill of microsuturing hence a lot of practice outside the human body is required to handle these delicate instruments intraoperatively with ease by the prospective endoscopic microsurgeon.

Port Placement

The port placement for microsurgery is no different from a routine one. The difference comes from two aspects. Use of finer 3 mm instrument and ports for ipsilateral suturing style works better. The ports and port placement are shown in Figures 20.4A to C. Universal port placement is a 10 mm intraumbilical port, a 3 mm left paraumbilical port and 3 mm port on the side of assistant, i.e. lower right quadrant port. I prefer to use a 5 mm port with 3 mm reducer in lower left quadrant to be able to use, if needed, any of the 5 mm instruments. The suturing is done by ipsilateral technique so this is most beneficial when coapting delicate tissue like of tubal lumina, fimbria, bowel or ureter. In this technique both hands work on the same side as the surgeon stands rather than crossing over to the contralateral side. Contralateral suturing would be less precise more stressful and at worst could be damaging for such delicate surgical tissue. Pioneered by Dr Charles H Koh, it remains the cornerstone to achieve good anatomical, surgical outcome.

TUBOTUBAL REANASTOMOSIS

Patients are worked up in the preoperative phase by a transvaginal sonography and other investigations but there does not seem to be any need for a diagnostic laparoscopy or hysterosalpingography. Patients are taken up in immediate postmenstrual phase. Patient is in general anesthesia, modified lithotomy. Port placement is as shown earlier in the chapter, i.e. micro ports for ipsilateral suturing two on the left side and the right lateral lower quadrant port. General inspection of the pelvis is done and necessary adhesiolysis carried out. Then the tubes are looked for the site of filshie clip, fallope ring or diathermy coagulation. Dilute vasopressin, one ampoule in 100 ml saline is injected. A special micro needle is used to inject vasopressin in the mesosalpinx and on both the sides of the fallope ring. Once blanching occurs we prepare and fashion out the tubal stumps, proximal and distal. Koh and Janik use a special cutter the Guillotine, which cuts the tube precisely. If that is not available a curved mayo

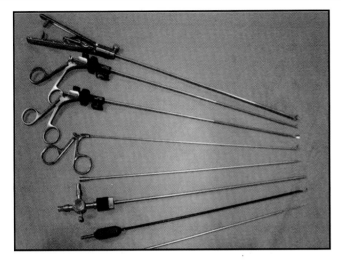

Fig. 20.3A: Instruments for laparoscopic microsurgery

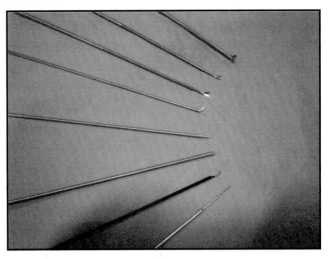

Fig. 20.3B: Tips of laparoscopic microsurgery instruments

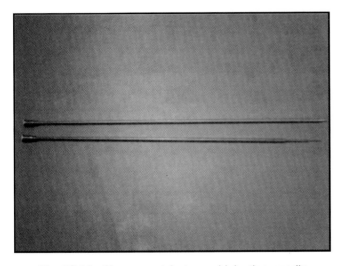

Fig. 20.3C: Chromopertubator and injection needle

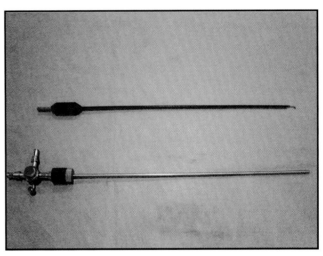

Fig. 20.3D: Suction irrigation cannula and curve monopolar hook

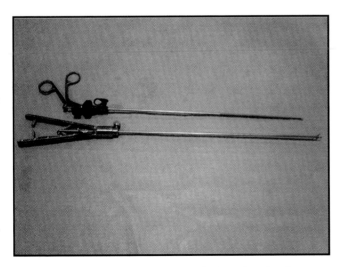

Fig. 20.3E: Microneedle holder and micrograsping forceps

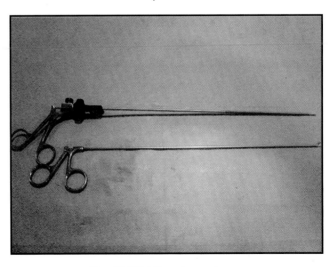

Fig. 20.3F: Ultramicro scissors

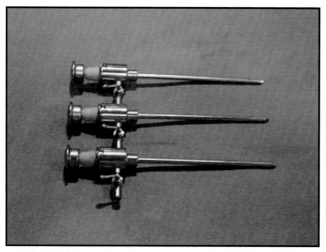

Fig. 20.4A: 3.5 mm microtrocars with automatic valve

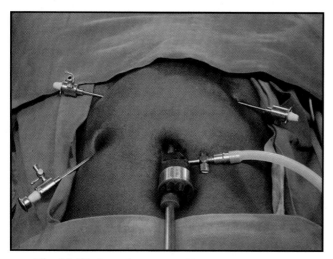

Fig. 20.4B: Port placement with 3 mm micro trocars

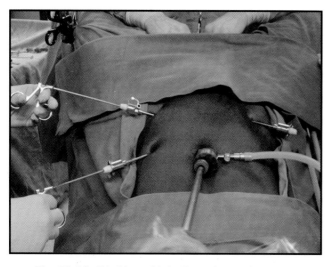

Fig. 20.4C: Working with ipsilateral port placement

scissors is used to transect the tube. The scissors approaches the fallopian tube exactly at right angle and tries to cut in just one go avoiding ragged edges and inaccurate cutting. Once the tube is cut on either side of the fallope ring, with very low setting monopolar needle we transect the portion of tube and mesosalpinx containing the fallope ring. There are usually no bleeders at the cutting of the fallopian tube and even if these is some bleeding excessive cautery is avoided. Now the proximal stump is tested for patency by injecting dilute methylene blue through the cervical canal and using a specialized chromopertubator, which is introduced from the fimbrial end, checks the distal stump patency. The egress of dye noted from both ends. If there is no free flow of dye from either side then further cuts are made either by scissors or by guillotine until free dye comes out from the proximal as well as the distal stump. The next step is to carry out the tubotubal reanastomosis. A study uterine elevator, like, RUMI is ideal for a good range of movement for suturing, grasping and cutting as the uterus actually participates in the surgery.

The first stitch is applied at the mesosalpinx. This stitch is crucial as it brings the two cut ends of the tube together and is important to avoid putting tension on the anastomosis. It gives a firm support of mesosalpinx over which the tubal anastomosis rests. The suture material used is 6-0 vicryl and the suture length is 8-10 cm. Two half knots are applied in opposite direction to give a secure knot. With such fine sutures usually a single throw is sufficient. The next suture to be applied is the 6'0 clock stitch. It is usually easy to pass distal to proximal for the right-handed surgeon. I do anastomosis of both the sides by standing on the left of the patient but many operators change sides and operate on the corresponding fallopian tube by standing on the right or left of the patient. In this particular application of suturing being ambidextrous helps by being more precise and faster. The next suture to be applied is at 12 o' clock position. The suture length is same 8-10 cm. The suture can be left little longer for holding to facilitate in applying the 3 o' clock and 9 o' clock sutures, which are applied after this. When all four sutures are tied (Figs 20.5A to F) then the long suture can also be cut. All the sutures are placed in the tubal muscularis, avoiding the serosa. If the suture enters

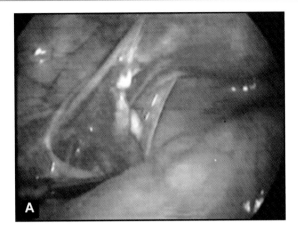

Fig. 20.5A: Initial view of the tube with a fallope ring

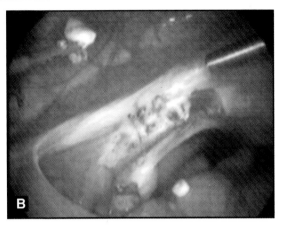

Fig. 20.5B: Fallope ring and midtubal segment removed

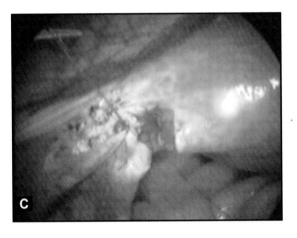

Fig. 20.5C: Tying the mesosalpingeal stitch

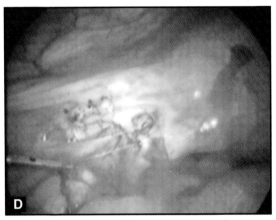

Fig. 20.5D: Tying the 6 o' clock stitch

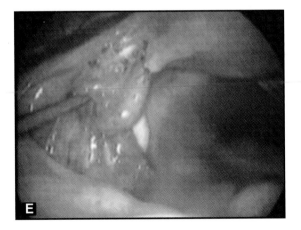

Fig. 20.5E: Final appearance of anastomosis

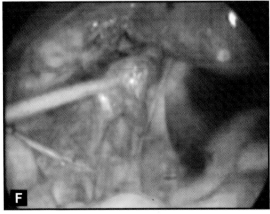

Fig. 20.5F: Chromopertubation to check patency postoperatively

the mucosa it does not make a difference in future reproductive outcome. Separately, one or two sutures with 6-0 vicryl are applied for serosal approximation, making the second layer of closure. Chromo-pertubation is carried out. There could be leakage from the anastomotic site. The contralateral tube is then repaired. No stents are applied as trying to put one at laparoscopy could be very difficult. A thorough suction irrigation lavage is carried out all through the procedure. There is usually no need of any cauterization around the anastomosis as bleeding is hardly there. Postoperative recovery is very quick. Pregnancy rates as cited in literature[9–12] are at 12 months completed follow-up the true pregnancy rates are 35.5 percent at 3 months, 54.8 percent at 6 months, 67.7 percent at 9 months and 71 percent at 12 months, with an ectopic pregnancy rates of 5 percent. In our series of tubotubal anastomosis we have achieved very good pregnancy rates almost up to 60 percent at one year. Most encouraging being three patients conceived from those done in workshops where the familiar operation room conditions and own operating team is not present. If working in an unfamiliar conditions with assistants not aware of microsurgical instruments and techniques can give equal results it shows that microsurgical suturing is not difficult to master, only a matter of patience and perseverance.

Tubocornual Anastomosis

Tubocornual anastomosis is reserved for the patients with proximal tubal obstruction. It may be due to salpingitis isthmica nodosa, fibrosis, or endometriosis. First patients are offered hysteroscopic guided tube cannulation. After a period of waiting if patient does not conceive, then tubocornual implantation is performed. Patient is counseled about the prospects of conception after surgery. Preparation of distal stump is the most important factor for determining the success. All the steps are similar to tubotubal anastomosis. A linear slit is made at the 12 o' clock position in the cornual muscularis using the microneedle electrode after pitressin injection. This allows some mobility of the interstitial portion of the tube so that it can be aligned to the needle and the needle holder to effect suturing.

Following this, preparation of the distal stump is done. A mesosalpingial stitch is taken to approximate

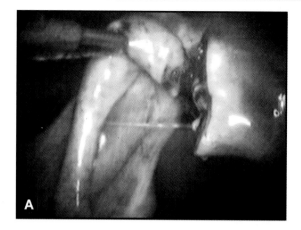

Fig. 20.6A: Checking the patency of the proximal tubal segment

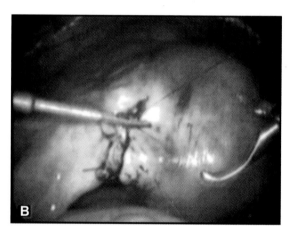

Fig. 20.6B: Completed picture of tubocornual implantation

the proximal and distal stumps by using 6-0 vicryl suture. Four interrupted stitches are taken by using 6-0 vicryl for tubocornual anastomosis (Figs 20.6A and B). Every suture includes the muscularis and mucosa. Then one or two interrupted serosal sutures are taken. Suction irrigation and lavage done and dye test is done at the end of procedure.

Neosalpingostomy is the operation, which attempts to recreate a new ostia when the tube has a hydrosalpinx. So, as to say that when there is complete obstruction and original fimbria have completely disappeared or buried beneath adhesions then, neosalpingostomy is carried out. First of all adhesiolysis is carried out and when the end of the tube is free, then methylene blue is injected under high pressure to distend the hydrosalpinx The most important point is to determine the opening point on the former ostium. It is sometimes easy to find, and is situated at the tubal puncture point of the methylene blue (Fig. 20.7A) or at the convergence of several fibrous folds separating the underlying mucosa. Otherwise, the point of the first incision will be chosen at the center of the hydrosalpinx. Atraumatic forceps are used to hold the preampullary portion of the tube and present it to the laparoscopic scissors or CO_2 laser.[21,22] A pinhole incision is then made, enlarged with the scissors or CO_2 laser (25 watt focused shots) in a star pattern towards the four quadrants of the hydrosalpinx (Figs 20.7B and C). The scissors must then be removed and 2 pairs of atraumatic forceps with long jaws are used to widen the opening by pulling the peritoneum gently in opposite directions. The avascular zones must be left intact. In the case of bleeding, microbipolar coagulation is performed with continuous irrigation. It is useful to make one of the incisions at the 12 o' clock position down to the mesosalpinx in order to recreate a Richard "neofimbria".

The condition of the terminal portion of the intra-ampullary tubal mucosa is then assessed directly or by means of the salpingoscope. The latter is inserted under continuous irrigation with warm saline to improve the view and try to collapse the intratubal intermucosal adhesions. Finally, this evaluation can lead to the decision of a salpingectomy in the case of advanced grade four adhesions.

Eversion of Fimbria

After sufficient experience in suturing in other conventional situations microsurgical suturing for fimbrial eversion can be attempted. Most of the time in laparoscopic neosalpingostomy fimbrial eversion is done by Bruhat maneuver, i.e. tissue heating effect but there is a case control data suggestive of a higher fertility rate by open microsurgery. This could be explained by the fact that only difference in laparotomic approach and laparoscopic is in fimbrial eversion.[23] In laparotomy it is more precise with help of four or five sutures,[24] taken from fimbrial rim.

The exact technique is replicated in laparoscopy. Very fine 4-0 or 5-0 vicryl (PGA) sutures are taken on an atraumatic needle (Figs 20.7D to H). The needle first picks up the peritoneum just beneath the exposed fimbria and then the corresponding bite of peritoneum at a distance of 1 to 1.5 cm from the edge. As

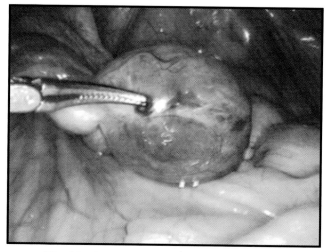

Fig. 20.7A: Initial appearance of hydrosalpinx

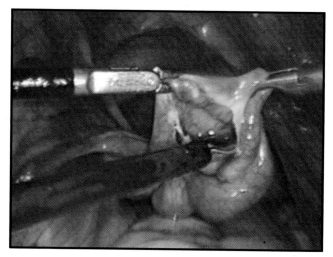

Fig. 20.7B: Cruciate incision over the hydrosalpinx

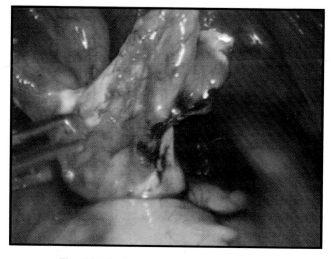

Fig. 20.7C: Appearance of normal fimbria after cruciate incision

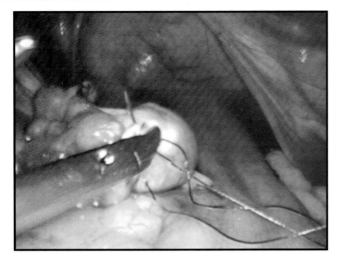

Fig. 20.7D: Passing the suture through 12'0 clock position

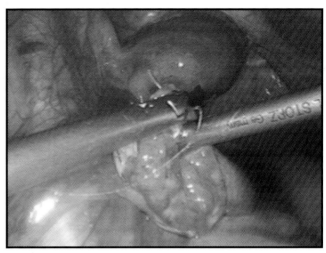

Fig. 20.7E: Passing the suture through fimbria

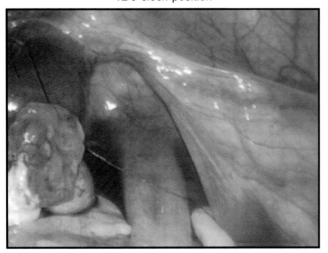

Fig. 20.7F: Tying the suture

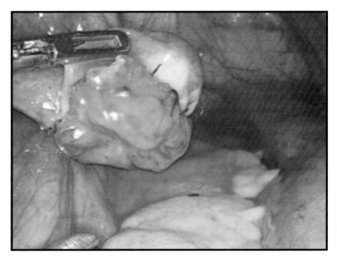

Fig. 20.7G: Final appearance after tubal reconstruction with four sutures

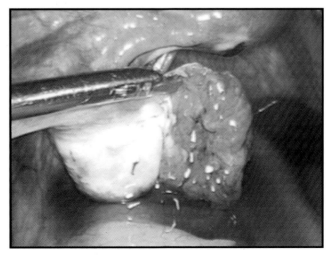

Fig. 20.7H: Chromopertubation at the end of procedure

the suture is tied fimbrial edge is everted and the ostium is opened up. Four stitches are placed at equal distance keeping all atraumatic precautions. Thorough suction irrigation lavage is continuously done. There is hardly any bleeding, but if at all there is, then the same is secured by a wolf microbipolar forceps kept at a low wattage. The end result is very gratifying with use of fine sutures. Laparoscopy offers all the benefits of traditional microsurgery like minimal tissue handling, less tissue trauma, no tissue drying and the capability to use microsutures. So laparoscopic neosalpingostomy with fine sutures promises to give better result than open laparotomy in surgical hands adept with laparoscopic suturing.

Microsurgical Adhesiolysis

By adherence to principles of microsurgery viz minimal tissue handling, avoidance of tissue drying by thorough suction irrigation and lavage and proper dissection in correct tissue planes thus avoiding bleeding and if any, achieving proper hemostasis by microbipolar, adhesiolysis in infertility patient becomes very precise and less adhesiogenic in postoperative phase. By using micrograsper and microscissors (Figs 20.8A to F) and an underwater examination, adhesions are visualized better; more so by utilizing the magnifications offered the camera. By precisely locating adhesions and by atraumatically but firmly grasping delicate tissue by ultra-micrograsper (Koh instruments) and then dissection by small jaws of ultra-microscissors adhesiolysis proceeds atraumatically. Delicate handling assures less adhesiogenic potential in the healing phase. This microsurgical adhesiolysis is most suited for infertility evaluations or second look procedures. A little more patience on the part of the operator and the results are much more rewarding. In the case depicted here the patient had been infertile with dysmenorrhea, dyspareunia. Microsurgical instrumentation, i.e. ultramicrograsper, ultramicroscissors, microsuction irrigation cannula and a microbipolar has been used. The initial appearance is only of fimbrial end stuck to the ovary, uterosacral ligament and rectosigmoid. By delicate grasping of the tube dissection carried out and during mobilization a small extra ovarian endometrioma drained. The tube was freed by sharp dissection with ultra microscissors. Then the ovary lifted up exposing implants in ovarian fossa. By micrograsper the retroperitoneal dissection continued and all implants fulgurated and excised. Ureter was also enmeshed in fibrotic adhesions. All adhesions removed by ultra-microscissors and microbipolar coagulation. Ureter traced till the lower end. Complete clearance of endometriotic implants in ovarian fossa achieved. Rectosigmoid lysed away again only by microbioplar scissors and grasper. Thorough suction irrigation and lavage done. At end a very normal tubo-ovarian relationship restored by being minimally invasive. Thus, microsurgical adhesiolysis proves to offer better surgical and reproductive outcome.

Difficulties in Microsuturing

The only drawback or difficulty, which could arise, could be lack of precision in handling and suturing with delicate materials and fine needles. The only substitute to learning microsuturing in, today's scenario is, robotic surgery. Short of that only option is to master the technique of microsurgical suturing on pelvic trainers and other tissues like placenta. No instrument or equipment can carry out good microsuturing unless the operator is deft with suturing skills. So to overcome these difficulties the prospective endoscopic microsurgeon will have to recourse to long training session with a lot of dedication and motivation, which will make him, succeed on table. Gradually attempting more complex procedure in a logical manner would be other suggestion. Tubotubal reanastmosis could be the most complex surgical feat, so, this to be accomplished in the end, starting from passing sutures in neosalpingo-stomy or ovarian reconstruction or at times suturing the salpingectomy site in an ectopic pregnancy. Microsurgically carrying out salpingo-ovariolysis would obviously be the first, surgical drill. Closure of serosal layer of myoma with 4-0 PDS would still be simple. So, it is suggested to the readers to venture into microsurgical suturing in a more gradual logical manner.[17]

Remedial Step

The only problem comes from taking long suture lengths which keep getting entangled. Dictum is not to exceed 10 cm of suture length, so that when trying to tie the knot the tail end is just close by and easy to grasp. The temptation of taking long suture length to take all sutures by one suture should be resisted

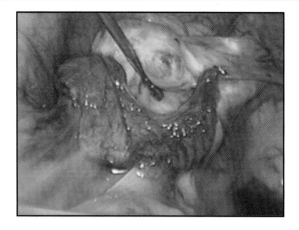

Fig. 20.8A: Left ovary fimbrial end, and rectosigmoid all adherent due to endometriotic implants in the ovarian fossa

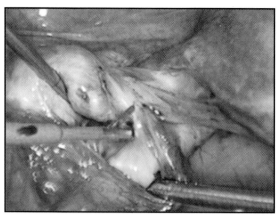

Fig. 20.8B: Salpingo-ovariolysis started

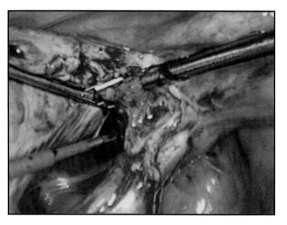

Fig. 20.8C: Salpingo-ovariolysis in progress by microscissor and grasper

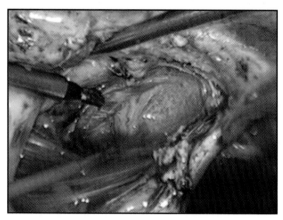

Fig. 20.8D: Ovary lifted up from the ovarian fossa and deep endometriotic implants fulgurated by bipolar coagulation

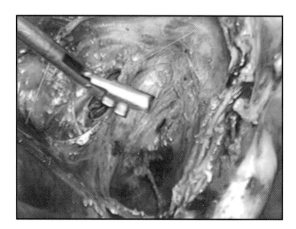

Fig. 20.8E: Completed dissection and fulguration of endometriotic implants in left ovarian fossa, ureter is seen under the micrograsper

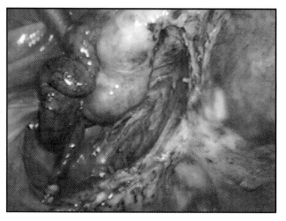

Fig. 20.8F: Final appearance of fallopian tube, ovary, ovarian fossa and uterosacral ligament after adhesiolysis

and for each microsurgical suture, a separate suture length around 10 cm should be taken.

Complications

There really appears to be no complication of micro-surgery except operator dependant so adjudge your skills before undertaking a certain procedure rather than facing failure or doom.

Postoperative Management

Patients are discharged within 12 hours of the surgery since the incisions are just 3 mm. Postoperative recovery is excellent due to adherence to strict microsurgical principles.

CONCLUSION

Laparoscopic microsurgery offers all the benefits of traditional microsurgery coupled with the inherent advantages of laparoscopy. The two together are a unique surgical tool, which appear to be patient friendly, capable of carrying out complex yet delicate tissue repair. Endoscopist endowed with such suturing skills would definitely pass on the benefits to the patient by giving good reproductive outcome. Hence in the times to come laparoscopic microsurgery will see more and more applications in the ever-expanding field of endoscopic surgery.

REFERENCES

1. Gomel V. Tubal reconstruction by microsurgery. Fertil Steril 1977; 28:59-65.
2. David H. Lees, Albert Singer, Robert M.L. Winston in Microsurgery for Infertility. A Colour Atlas of Gynaecological surgery. Infertility Surgery 1981;5(10):131.
3. Steptoe PC, Edwards RC. Birth after re-implantation of a human embryo. Lancet 1978;2:366.
4. Reich H, DeCaprio J, McGlynn F. Laparoscopic hysterectomy. J Gynecol Surg 1989;5:213-16.
5. Bruhat MA, Mage G, Manhes H, Soualhat C, Report JF, Pouly JL. Laparoscopy Procedures to Promote fertility ovariolysis and salpingolysis. Results of 93 selected Cases. Acta Eur Fertil 1983;14(2):113-15.
6. KOH CH, Janik GM. Laparoscopic Microsurgical Tubal Anastomosis. Video presented at the Third International Congress of Endocrinology and Metabolism, April 1-3, 1992, Royal London Hospital; London.
7. Lundorff P, Thorburn J, Lindblom B. Fertility outcome after conservative surgical treatment of ectopic pregnancy evaluated in a randomized trial. Fertil Steril 1992;57(5): 998-1002.
8. Janik GM, KOH CH. Surgical Treatment of Endometriosis of the Urinary Tract. Operative Technique in Gynecologic Surgery 1997;2(2):115-21.
9. Koh CH, Janik GM. Laparoscopic microsurgical tubal anastomosis. Obstet Gynecol Clin North Am 1999;26(1):189-200.
10. Koh CH, Janik GM. Laparoscopic microsurgical tubal anastomosis. In Adamson GD, Martin DC (Eds): Endoscopic Management of Gynecologic Disease. Philadelphia: Lippincott-Raven, 1996;119-45.
11. Koh CH, Janik GM. Laparoscopic microsurgical tubal anastomosis. Results of 40 consecutive cases (abstract). Presented at the American Society of Reproductive Medicine, 52nd Annual Meeting, November 2-7, 1996, Boston, Ma.
12. Koh CH, Janik GM. Laparoscopic microsurgery: current opinion in Obstetrics and Gynecology 1999;11:401-07.
13. Bruhat MA, Mage G, Manhes H, Pouly JL. Utilization dulaser CO2 par coelioscopie. Rev Fr Gynecol Obstet 1981;76:397-99.
14. Daniell J, Herbert CM. Laparoscopic neosalpingostomy using CO_2 laser. Fertil Steril 1984;16:139-45.
15. Canis M, Manhes H, Mage G, Pouly JL, Wattiez A, Bruhat MA. Laparoscopic distal tuboplasty: report of 87 cases and a 4-year experience. Fertile Steril 1991;56:616-21.
16. Gomel V. Salpingostomy by microsurgery. Fertility and Sterility 1978;29-380-87.
17. KOH CH, Janik GM. Laparoscopic microsurgical tubal anastomosis: Difficulties and pitfalls. In Corfman, Dia-mond, DeCherney (Eds): Complications of Laparoscopy and Hysteroscopy, (2nd edn) 1997;107-13.

Robotic Suturing in Advanced Gynecologic Surgery

ARNOLD P ADVINCULA

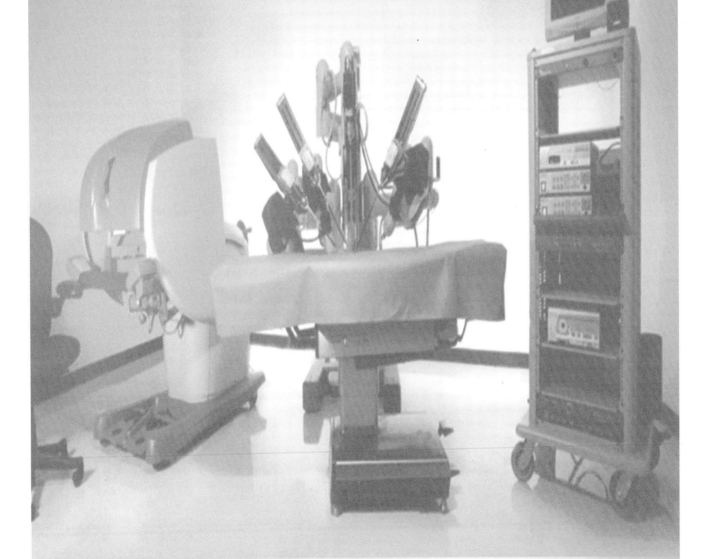

Chapter Twenty One

INTRODUCTION

The first known report of a rudimentary endoscopic procedure dates back to 1807 when a physician by the name of Bozzini visualized the urethra with a candle and simple tubelike device. Over a century later, laparoscopy found its way into gynecology and by the early 1970s revolutionized the field. Since then minimally invasive surgery has become increasingly popular and demanded by both surgeons and patients in the field of gynecologic surgery.

As technical advancements have brought about improvements to modern day laparoscopy, studies have clearly shown that laparoscopic surgery allows faster recovery with less postoperative pain. Despite these technological advancements and benefits, more complex procedures such as the management of advanced endometriosis, and procedures that require extensive suturing such as myomectomy, pelvic reconstructive surgery, and tubal reanastomosis are typically still managed by laparotomy.

One major obstacle to the more widespread acceptance and application of minimally invasive surgical techniques to gynecologic surgery has been the difficulty encountered with laparoscopic suturing. In an attempt to facilitate this process, pioneers such as Clarke and Semm developed techniques for both extracorporeal and intracorporeal suturing.[1-2] Although many devices have been developed through the years to facilitate laparoscopic suturing, limitations still exists. These limitations include counter-intuitive hand movement, two-dimensional visualization, and limited degrees of instrument motion within the body. Additional challenges have centered on the training and acquisition of these advanced skills. In order to overcome these obstacles, modern day gynecologic surgeons have begun to apply robot-assisted surgery to their endoscopic armamentarium. The following chapter will review the evolution and current state of robot-assisted laparoscopy in gynecology as it pertains to suturing.

HISTORY

One of the early predecessors and first applications of robotic technology to the field of gynecologic endoscopy was with a voice-activated robotic arm known as Aesop® (Computer Motion Inc.®, Goleta, CA). Although a study by Mettler et al found that the time required to perform surgery was faster with the robotic device, the primary role of Aesop® was to operate the camera during laparoscopic surgery.[3] The authors concluded that efficiency was improved because the robotic device allowed two surgeons to use both hands for operating. Suturing was still limited by the skill level of the surgeon and the design of the instruments.

Another predecessor to the current platform of surgical robots was Zeus® (Computer Motion Inc.®, Goleta, CA). This system was comprised of three remotely controlled robotic arms that were attached to the surgical table and a workstation called a robotic console. This console possessed the instrument controls while three-dimensional vision was obtained with the aide of special glasses. The robotic arms operated the camera and provided the surgeon with two operating arms that possessed interchangeable "microwrist" instruments. Although these instruments more closely mimicked the movements of the human wrist when compared to conventional laparoscopic instruments, their movements were not totally instinctive.

Early studies reported on its successful application to tubal reanastomosis, a procedure in which the ability to suture laparoscopically is of utmost importance. In one prospective study, pregnancy rates were evaluated in ten patients with previous tubal ligations who underwent laparoscopic tubal reanastomosis using the identical technique used at laparotomy.[4] A postoperative tubal patency rate of 89 percent was demonstrated in 17 of the 19 tubes anastomosed with a pregnancy rate of 50 percent at one year. There were no complications or ectopic pregnancies. Overall, this study clearly demonstrated the ability of a robotic device to facilitate replication of open surgical techniques during laparoscopy.

The daVinci® surgical system (Intuitive Surgical®, Sunnyvale, CA), represents that latest platform in surgical robotics. This system is comprised of three components (Fig. 21.1). The first component is the surgeon console where the surgeon controls the robotic system remotely through hand and foot controls while using a stereoscopic viewer. The second component of the daVinci® surgical system is the InSite® vision system which provides the three dimensional imaging through a 12 mm endoscope containing stereoscopic cameras and dual optical lenses. The third component of the daVinci® surgical system is the patient-side cart with telerobotic arms

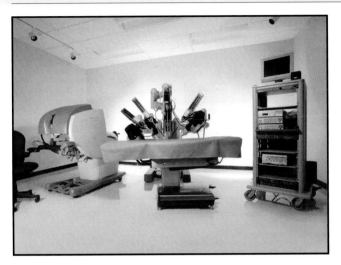

Fig. 21.1: Photograph of the da Vinci® Robotic System. From left to right: surgeon's console, patient-side surgical cart, and InSite® vision tower. Photo courtesy of Intuitive Surgical®, Inc.

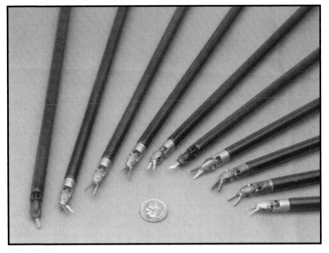

Fig. 21.2: Endowrist® instruments (8 millimeters). Photo courtesy of Intuitive Surgical®, Inc.

and Endowrist® instruments. This component is available with either three or four robotic arms. One of the arms holds the laparoscope while the other two to three arms hold the various laparoscopic surgical instruments known as Endowrist® instruments (Fig. 21.2).

The Endowrist® instruments are unique in that they possess seven degrees of freedom which replicates the full range of motion of the surgeon's hand thereby eliminating the fulcrum effect seen with conventional laparoscopy (Fig. 21.3). These seven degrees of freedom are (i) in and out movement, (ii) axial rotation, (iii) opening and closing of instrument, (iv) lateral movement at the articulation, (v) vertical movement at the articulation, (vi) right movement at each articulation, and (vii) left movement at each articulation. A significant improvement over earlier prototypes is that these movements allow instrument manipulation to be instinctive.

For years, only open and vaginal surgery provided the surgeon with a variety of angles of approach to the target tissue during suturing. The only real limitation was the degree of exposure provided by the surgical assistant. Laparoscopic surgery provided better exposure but at the expense of limited angles of approach to the target tissue. This approach was determined and limited by the location and orientation of the tissue with respect to the ports through which suturing was performed. The development of wrist-like instrumentation has over-

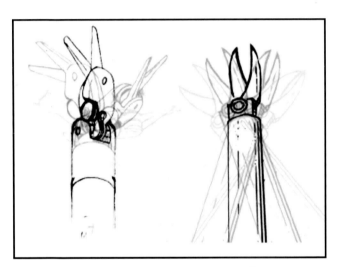

Fig. 21.3: Schematic comparison of Endowrist® instrument on left with conventional laparoscopic instrument demonstrating fulcrum effect on right

come these technical limitations while maintaining the improved visualization gained with laparoscopy.

Since its clearance for laparoscopic use by the FDA in July 2000 and most recently for gynecologic applications in April 2005, the use of the daVinci® surgical system to facilitate laparoscopic procedures in gynecology has rapidly increased. In numerous studies across various disciplines, it has been shown to be a safe and effective alternative to conventional laparoscopic surgery, particularly when dealing with advanced pathology that requires the ability to perform complex tasks. In the area of gynecology, there are reports of robot-assisted laparoscopy with the daVinci® surgical system for tubal reanastomosis, hysterectomy, myomectomy, and the repair of vaginal vault prolapse.[5-8]

The focus of this chapter will be on laparoscopic suturing techniques with the daVinci® surgical system, the only robotic surgical system currently in production. These techniques will be discussed in the context of both laparoscopic myomectomy and total laparoscopic hysterectomy. Emphases will be placed on uterine repair after enucleation of a leiomyoma and ligation of major vascular pedicles with closure of the vaginal cuff.

ROBOTIC MYOMECTOMY

The primary surgical management of symptomatic leiomyomata for women desiring future fertility or uterine conservation is myomectomy. Although many cases of intramural and subserous leiomyomata are managed with laparoscopic myomectomy as a result of the advent of modern day minimally invasive surgery techniques, the vast majority are still performed through laparotomy.[9] The management of leiomyomata endoscopically is one of the more challenging procedures in minimally invasive surgery and requires a skilled surgeon. Critical to the success of a laparoscopic myomectomy is the ability to repair the uterus with a multilayer sutured closure. For many surgeons, this technically challenging aspect of a laparoscopic myomectomy has been thought to affect conversion rates to laparotomy and possibly play a role in cases of uterine rupture. This ability to adequately suture a uterine defect laparoscopically has always been a subject of debate. In fact, laparoscopically-assisted myomectomy has been suggested in the past with enucleation of myomas performed laparoscopically and uterine closure done through a mini-laparotomy incision.[10]

Advincula et al described a technique that was successfully applied to 32/35 attempted robotic myomectomies.[7] Interestingly in their series, there were no conversions to laparotomy as a result of suturing difficulty. This was attributed primarily to the Endowrist® instruments that replicated the complex motions of the surgeon's hands. The majority of myomas removed were preoperatively assessed to have diameters greater than 5 cm and regardless of the location of the myoma in the uterus,

all defects were able to be closed with a multilayered technique.

The low conversion rate noted by Advincula et al was also significant given the fact that the daVinci® surgical system provided no tactile or haptic feedback. Although this limitation played a role in two of the conversions as a result of an inability to enucleate leiomyomata, this did not affect the surgeon's ability to suture once enucleation was accomplished. One limitation of the current state of the art in robot-assisted laparoscopy is the absence of tactile feedback to the surgeon operating the Endowrist® instruments remotely at the surgeon's console. The ability to allow tactile feedback to be relayed to the surgeon in robot-assisted laparoscopy has not yet occurred due to the expense of the technology however the improved visualization gained with the tree-dimensional imaging seems to overcome this deficit.

TECHNIQUE

The following technique represents a practical approach to successful robotic suturing during a myomectomy. All patients are placed in low dorsal lithotomy position with arms padded and tucked at their sides after general endotracheal anesthesia is administered (Fig. 21.4). The bladder is drained with a Foley catheter and a uterine manipulator is placed. Four trocars are typically utilized after pneumo-peritoneum is obtained. A 12 mm trocar is placed either at or above the umbilicus depending on the size of the uterus (Fig. 21.5). This trocar accommodates the endoscope. Occasionally a left upper quadrant entry with a 3 mm microlaparoscope is performed in order to help guide operative trocar placement in patients with a markedly enlarged uterus or who were at risk for pelvic adhesions such as prior abdominal surgery. Two-8 mm trocars which mount directly to the surgical carts two operating arms are placed in the left and right lower quadrants respectively. A fourth trocar which serves as an accessory port is placed between the camera port and the right lower quadrant port. This is typically 12 mm in order to facilitate introduction of a tissue morcellator, suction/irrigation instruments and suture along with any needle type such as the straight, ski tipped, or curved variety. Once all four trocars are in place, the patient is placed in steep

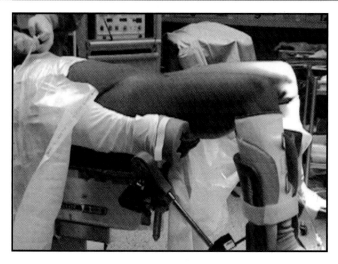

Fig. 21.4: Proper positioning for robotic cases with patient in dorsal lithotomy and arms padded and tucked at sides

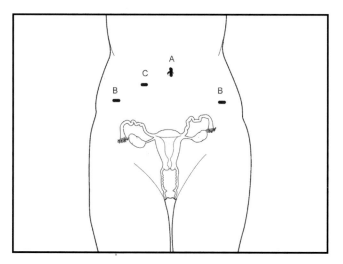

Fig. 21.5: Port Placement. The camera port (A) - 12 mm either at the umbilicus or above depending on the size of the uterus. The lateral ports (B) - 8 mm da Vinci® ports in the right and left lower quadrants of the abdomen. (C) The assist port (12 -15 mm) placed between the camera port and the right lower quadrant port

Trendelenburg and the surgical cart with three robotic arms is brought between the patients legs and docked, meaning that each trocar is attached to the assigned robotic arm with the exception of the accessory port.

A survey of the operative field is performed, after which a dilution of vasopressin is administered via a spinal needle transabdominally into the myometrium as an adjunct for hemostasis. The serosal incision and enucleation of leiomyomata are completed robotically

(Figs 21.6A and B). Countertraction is provided by the bedside surgeon assistant through the accessory port with a myoma grasper or cork screw. Once the myoma(s) are enucleated, attention is directed towards closure of the myomectomy resection bed(s) which is where the daVinci® surgical system significantly enhanced the procedure. Endowrist® instruments are changed to a Debakey forcep and needle driver. A three layer closure modeled after traditional open surgical technique is utilized (Figs 21.7 to 21.10). Interrupted six inch sutures of 0-Vicryl™ on CT-2 needles are used to close the first two layers with interrupted figure-of-eight stitches followed by a running baseball stitch of 3-0-Vicryl™ on a SH needle for the serosa. This suture is cut to eleven inches. All knots are tied intracorporeally via instrument tying. The gamut of surgical knots ranging from half-hitches to surgeon's knots can be thrown. Once the uterine defect(s) are repaired, a tissue morcellator is used to extract the specimen(s).

ROBOTIC HYSTERECTOMY

Approximately 600,000 hysterectomies are performed annually in the United States with the majority due to benign conditions.[11-12] Hysterectomies are traditionally approached by either a vaginal or abdominal route. In the late 1980s, Reich introduced laparoscopic-assisted vaginal hysterectomy.[13] Since the 1990s, a definite trend toward laparoscopic hysterectomy has been seen. Despite the increasing acceptance of laparoscopy, laparotomy remains the most common approach for hysterectomy. One explanation for this slow acceptance is the learning curve with conventional laparoscopy and its associated complications.[14] A significant impediment to this learning curve has been the ability to adequately control major vascular pedicles and close the vaginal cuff or cervical stump. Accomplishing these tasks by laparoscopic means can be daunting to many surgeons during total or subtotal hysterectomy. Given these concerns, robotics with its ability to facilitate suturing, may provide a way to overcome these difficulties.

TECHNIQUE

Two studies by Advincula and Reynolds demonstrate the ability to successfully apply robotic suturing techniques to hysterectomies that involve patients

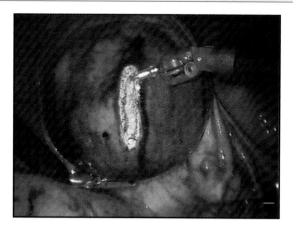

Fig. 21.6A: Serosal incision over leiomyoma with Endowrist® permanent cautery hook

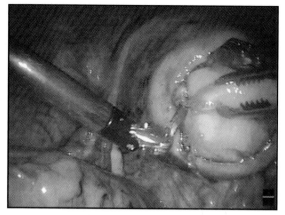

Fig. 21.6B: Enucleation of intramural leiomyoma

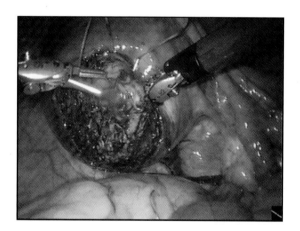

Fig. 21.7: Start of multilayer-sutured closure of uterine defect with interrupted 0-Vicryl™ sutures on CT-2 needles

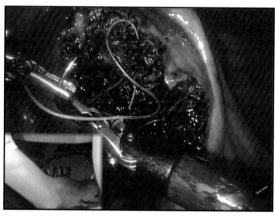

Fig. 21.8: Finger controls at surgeon console manipulate Endowrist® instruments (Debakey forceps and needle driver)

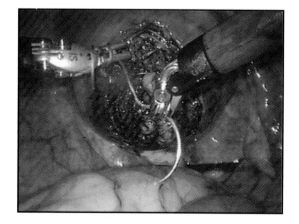

Fig. 21.9: Instrument tying with Endowrist® instruments (Debakey forceps and needle driver)

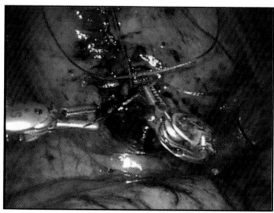

Fig. 21.10: Closure of serosal layer with running baseball stitch. Suture is 3-0-Vicryl™ on a SH needle cut to 11 inches

with either benign or malignant conditions.[15–16] The authors' technique is a practical approach to suture ligation of vascular pedicles and closure of the vaginal cuff or cervical stump.

The overall approach to robotic suturing during either a subtotal or total laparoscopic hysterectomy is identical to that seen with a robotic myomectomy, particularly as it relates to patient positioning and port placement. An attempt to replicate open surgical techniques is made throughout the hysterectomy. All of the procedures are consistent with either AAGL type IVE or LSH III laparoscopic hysterectomies.[17] A RUMI® uterine manipulator with a Koh® colpotomy ring and vaginal pneumo-occluder balloon (all Cooper Surgical®, Trumbull, CT) is used to facilitate completion of either a subtotal or total laparoscopic hysterectomy (Fig. 21.11). All vascular pedicles including the infundibulopelvic ligament and the uterine artery pedicles are skeletonized and subsequently suture ligated with either 0-Vicryl™ on CT-2 needles or free ties of 0-Vicryl™ prior to transection (Figs 21.12A and B). In cases where a total laparoscopic hysterectomy is intended, once the uterus and cervix are completely detached, the specimen with or without adnexa is delivered into the vagina. The uterine fundus is used to maintain pneumoperitoneum during the closure of the vaginal cuff which is closed with interrupted six inch sutures of 0-Vicryl™ on CT-2 needles. All knots are instrument tied (Figs 21.13A and B). Once the vaginal cuff is closed, the specimen is removed from the vagina.

In cases where laparoscopic subtotal hysterectomy is intended, the uterine corpus is robotically amputated below the internal os followed by extraction

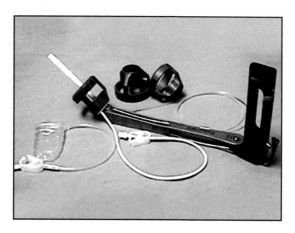

Fig. 21.11: RUMI® uterine manipulator in conjunction with Koh® colpotomy cups and a vaginal pneumo-occluder balloon (all Cooper Surgical®, Trumbull, CT)

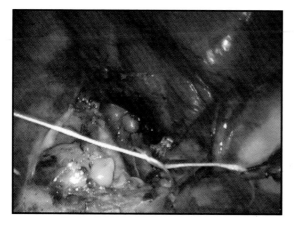 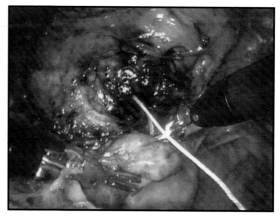

Figs 21.12A and B: (A) Placement of 0-Vicryl™ free tie around isolated left infundibulopelvic ligament. (B) Suture ligation of right uterine vascular pedicle

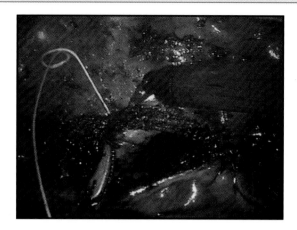 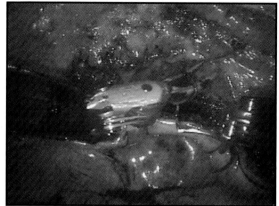

Figs 21.13A and B: Closure of vaginal cuff with interrupted sutures of 0-Vicryl™ on CT-2 needles

of the specimen through the accessory port with a tissue morcellator. The cervical stump is closed with interrupted six inch sutures of 0-Vicryl™ on CT-2 needles.

CONCLUSION

As technology evolves, the current platform of robotics holds the promise of continuing to overcome many of the limitations seen with conventional laparoscopy, particularly as it relates to suturing. Several advantages are obtained with the daVinci® surgical system when applied to suture-based procedures such as pelvic floor reconstruction, myomectomy, hysterectomy, and tubal reanastomosis. The first is the ability to repair any defect during a myomectomy regardless of location thereby bypassing the triangulation issues inherent to conventional laparoscopy. The second is the ease with which any needle type can be manipulated or knot thrown while instrument movement remains intuitive for the surgeon seated at the console. Finally, the systems improved dexterity and precision coupled with advanced imaging allows for the completion of complex suturing procedures in a fashion analogous to open surgical technique despite the absence of tactile feedback. These advantages should facilitate the acquisition of laparoscopic suturing skills for the surgeon-in-training.

REFERENCES

1. Clarke HC. Laparoscopy—new instruments for suturing and ligation. Fertil Steril 1972; 23:274-77.

2. Semm K. Tissue puncher and loop ligation—new ideas for surgical therapeutic pelviscopy (laparoscopy) and endoscopic intra-abdominal surgery. Endoscopy 1978;10:119-24.

3. Mettler L, Ibrahim M, Jonat W. One year of experience working with the aid of a robotic assistant (the voice-controlled optic holder AESOP) in gynecologic endoscopic surgery. Hum Reprod 1998;13:2748-50.

4. Falcone T, Goldberg JM, Margossian H, Stevens L. Robotically assisted laparoscopic microsurgical anastomosis: a human pilot study. Fertil Steril 2000; 73:1040-42.

5. Degueldre M, Vandromme J, Huong PT, Cadiere GB. Robotically-assisted laparoscopic microsurgical tubal reanastomosis: a feasibility study. Fertil Steril 2000;74:1020-23.

6. Diaz-Arrastia C, Jurnalov C, Gomez G, Townsend C. Laparoscopic hysterectomy using a computer-enhanced surgical robot. Surg Endosc 2002; 16:1271-73.

7. Advincula AP, Song A, Burke W, Reynolds RK. Preliminary experience with robot-assisted laparoscopic myomectomy. J Am Assoc Gynecol Laparosc 2004; 11(4):511-18.

8. Dimarco DS, Chow GK, Gettman MT, Elliott DS. Robotic-assisted laparoscopic sacrocolpopexy for treatment of vaginal vault prolapse. Urology 2004;63:373-76.

9. Falcone T, Bedaiwy MA. Minimally invasive management of uterine fibroids. Cur Opin Obstet Gynecol 2002; 14:401-407.

10. Nezhat C, Nezhat F, Bess O, et al. Laparoscopically assisted myomectomy: a report of a new technique in 57 cases. Int J Fertil Menopausal Stud 1994; 39:39-44.

11. Farquhar CM, Steiner CA. Hysterectomy rates in the United States, 1990-1997. Obstet Gynecol 2002; 99:229-34.

12. Wilcox LS, Koonin LM, Pokras R, et al. Hysterectomy in the United States, 1988-1990. Obstet Gynecol 1994;83:549-55.

13. Reich H, Decaprio J, McGlynn F. Laparoscopic hysterectomy. L Gynecol Surg 1989;5:213-16.

14. Wattiez A, Cohen SB, Selvaggi L. Laparoscopic hysterectomy. Cur Opin Obstet Gynecol 2002;14:417-22.

15. Advincula AP, Reynolds RK. The Use of robot-assisted laparoscopic hysterectomy in the patient with a scarred or obliterated anterior cul de sac. JSLS 2005;9:287-91.

16. Reynolds RK, Burke WM, Advincula AP. Preliminary experience with robot-assisted laparoscopic staging of gynecologic malignancies. JSLS 2005;9:149-58.

17. Olive DL, Parker WH, Cooper JM, Levine RL. The AAGL classification system for laparoscopic hysterectomy. J Am Assoc Gynecol Laparosc 2000;7:9-15.

Index